AF531532

PHARMACOGENOMICS

PHARMACOGENOMICS

By
Dr. G.P. Garg
&
Dr. M. Prakash

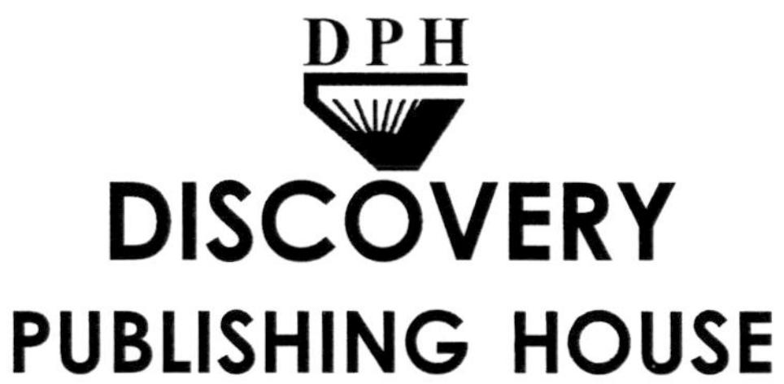

Published by:

DISCOVERY PUBLISHING HOUSE

4383/4B, Ansari Road, Darya Ganj
New Delhi-110 002 (India)
Phone : +91-11-23279245; 23253475; 43596065
E-mail : discoverybooksindia@gmail.com
discoverypublishinghouse@gmail.com
namitwasan9@gmail.com
web : www.discoverypublishinggroup.com

***First Edition:* 2011**
***Reprinted:* 2026**

ISBN: 978-81-8356-740-4

Pharmacogenomics

Printed at:
Infinity Imaging Systems
Delhi

Preface

The present title "Pharmacogenomics" has been written for those in the pharmaceutical research and those responsible for the education and training in pharmaceutical science and technology of graduate and undergraduate students. Medicine is an ever changing science. As new research and clinical experience broaden our knowledge, changes in treatment and drug therapy are required. This branch of life science has progressed enormously in recent years and the significant advances in therapeutics and an understanding of the need to optimize during delivery in the body have brought about an increased awareness of the valuable role played by the dosage forms. This statement is as true as it was back in ninteenth century and perhaps more so, given the increasing emphasis being placed on discovery, development, and use of large molecular entities as therapeutic and diagnostic agents. Development of these abilities requires an integration of knowledge, skills, attitudes, and values that can be acquired only through structured learning process including independent study, hands on practice and the availability of advanced literature. This tittle has designed to meet such needs of learners in the health professions.

In the last two decades, the pharmaceutical industry has experimented and successfully adopted several integrated and multidisciplinary approaches in the research areas of dring compound screening, toxicological evaluation, and pharmaceutical product development. The book is written in a concise style that facilitates an in-depth level of understanding of the essential concepts. The objectives of the present title are three folds: (i) to serve as a useful tool to help guide scientists in research and development by out-lining the theory and successful practice of in vitro - in vivo correlation, (ii) to help formulators apply the tool in designing and developing prototypes that enable selection of clinical formulations, and (iii) to help formulate strategy(ies) for product life-cycle management.

To make the work more comprehensive and informative, the author has consulted many authoritative books, research journals, abstracts, monographs etc., so there can be no claim to originality except in the manner of treatment.

The author expresses his thanks to his friends and colleagues whose continue inspirations have initiated him to bring out this book.

The author expresses his gratitude to Mr. Wasan and staff of M/s Discovery Publishing House Pvt. Ltd. for their whole hearted co-operation in the publication of this book.

Author

CONTENTS

1

Introduction

Pharmacogenomics is an extension of pharmacogenetics, a science described here in terms of five stages of development: (1) some clinical observations predicted genetic alterations of drug response; (2) additional case discoveries led to the term "*pharmacogenetics*," a concept broadened by (3) many systemic case studies, and the realization of its wide applicability; (4) came the recognition of systematic pharmacogenetic differences between human populations. Then it became clear that (5) most human drug-repsonse differences were multifactorial, caused by many genetic alterations plus environmental factors. The recognition of these complexities, and the advance of genetics into genomics led to the broader science of pharmacogenomics. This led to plans to create "*personalized medicine*," that is, making drug use more effective and safer by giving drugs that fit a person's genes.

Much of the science of genetics, dealing with gene structure, was changed by the realization that gene expression and thereby gene function was variable; this leads to systematic studies of drug action on genes, reversing the traditional studies of genes affecting drug action. Finally, the realization that gene-protein variations contribute to most common diseases leads to efforts of creating new drugs that act on these variants.

Pharmacogenomics is a recent offspring of pharmacogenetics. Both sciences deal with hereditary impacts upon the action of drugs, and their goals are overlapping. Any proper account of the history of pharmacogenomic must include a look at the development of pharmacogenetics. Thus, in this chapter pharmacogenetic history will be outlined first, concentrating on its development in terms of succeeding stages.

Pharmacogenetics: Its Stages of Development

Visions and Some Predictive Observations

Some visionaries and some keen observers predated pharmacogenetics as a science. Garrod' s 1902 studies of alcaptonuria and of phenylketonuria indicated to him that there was such a thing as human biochemical individuality. Haldane summarized his views in 1949 by stating, "It is an advantage to a species to be biochemically diverse. For the biochemically diverse species will contain at least some members capable of resisting any particular pestilence."

There were also some observational forerunners. In 1932, Snyder described a heritable disability of some people to taste phenylthiocarbamide. In 1943, Savin and Glick noticed a genetic lack of atropine esterase in some rabbits; these animals died while eating belladonna leaves, whereas most rabbits were not affected. These cases were perceived as isolated observations; they preceded the definition of pharmacogenetics but they helped later investigators to establish pharmacogenetics as a science.

Pharmacogenetics Lives: Systematic Case Studies

Several separate observations in the 1950s indicated clearly the dependence of drug effects on the genetic constitution of the recipient. The data were convincing because they were based on combinations of biochemical, clinical, and genetic observations. The cases included genetic variation of isoniazid acetylation, failing cholinesterase activity affecting succinylcholine action, and primaquine-caused hemolysis owing to deficiency of glucoses-6-phosphate dehydrogenase. All these cases became subjects of subsequent studies that showed that each of the enzymes could vary in many ways because of different mutations.

These clear-cut cases raised in several people the opinion that pharmacological heritability was a clinically important subject. Thus, the American Medical Association (AMA) invited the geneticist Arno Motulsky to consider the problem; he summarized it in a 1957 paper entitled "Drug Reactions, Enzymes, and Biochemical Genetics." Vogel in Germany was aware of the same problem and coined the term "Pharmacogenetics." Kalow began to summarize all available knowledge in a book that appeared in 1962, indicating that the concept of pharmacogenetics had been fundamentally accepted.

Broadening of Pharmacogenetic Knowledge

In the following years, many centers contributed new data, but all the data represented monogenic variations, i.e., differences between individuals caused by mutations of single genes. Weber's 1997 book listed 15 variable drug-metabolizing enzymes, 11 variable drug receptors, and 14 other variable proteins in humans that affected drug actions. In 2001, Kalow counted 42 variable drug-metabolizing enzymes. In short, the knowledge of different kinds of protein variants that may affect drug responses was growing.

Drug-metabolizing enzymes represent the category with the largest number of known variants, which probably has historical and methodological reasons. To measure a change of drug metabolism, all one needs are chemical methods, many of which are dated. To find a drug receptor variation, one has to identify the receptor protein and its gene, processes that require sophisticated procedures of more recent date. Thus, measurements of drug metabolism are older than some other procedures.

In the history of drug metabolism, prominent were the discoveries of genetic variability of the metabolism of debrisoquine and of sparteine. Subsequent studies indicated that both drugs are metabolized by the same enzyme, which turned out to be the P450 cytochrome CYP2D6. The enzyme's variations were found to be complex: enzyme activity could be absent because of frameshift mutations, splicing defects, gene deletion, or the presence of a stop codon. The enzyme may function slowly because of various kinds of mutation, whereby some mutations affected only the interaction with specific substrates. Enzyme duplication or multiplication could lead to very fast action.

Many clinical case studies and observations could be mentioned. For example, as summarized by Meyer, patients with deficient CYP2D6 activity experienced exaggerated or prolonged responses to metoprolol, encainide, perhexiline, or thioridazine; however, codeine had no analgesic effect in such cases because it must be activated to morphine by CYP2D6.

More than 60 alleles of CYP2D6 are known today, characterized by different combinations of some 45 mutations. Approximately 60 different drugs are metabolized by CYP2D6. A Pubmed search indicated that there are more than 2300 publications dealing with CYP2D6. The studies of CYP2D6 helped to give pharmacogenetics the deserved clinical attention.

Genetic failure of drug-metabolizing enzymes can lead to a patient's death. For instance, mercaptopurine or thioguanine have been fatal in cases of failing activity of thiopurine methyltransferase. Regulatory agencies are considering recommendations and official acceptance of pharmacogenetic testing before the administration of dangerous drugs.

Pharmacogenetic Differences Between Populations

Pharmacogenetics began with the observation of interindividual differences of some drug responses or of drug metabolism that started pharmacogenetics. This recognition, that there are pharmacogenetic differences between populations, truly widened and altered the science. Various older observations that led to the recognition of a pharmacogenetic difference between human populations were first considered to be odd cases. In 1921, Paskind injected atropine sulfate into 20 Caucasian and 20 African-American men in Chicago. He found that the drug caused an initial slowing of the heart rate in the white but not the African-American subjects. In 1929, Chen and Poth measured the pupillary size after applying various mydriatic eye drops into the eyes of a number of people. The increase in size was largest in Caucasians, intermediate in Asians, and smallest in African-Americans; the authors thought that the color of the iris affected its movability.

During World War II, American soldiers stationed in tropical countries received primaquine as antimalarial prophylaxis; it turned out that only soldiers of African descent developed hemolysis from the administration of primaquine. The explanation came later: The affected soldiers had a genetic deficiency of glucose-6-phosphate dehydrogenase; this deficiency was frequent in Africans because it protected the carrier from malaria, but it was rare in countries without malaria. After discovery of the genetic deficiency of isoniazid acetylation, other investigators found substantial interethnic differences in the frequency of this deficiency. The deficiency was rare in Eskimos (Inuit), relatively frequent in Europeans and Africans, and intermediate in East Asians.

In the early 1970s, my laboratory studied the metabolism of amobarbital (an at that time widely used drug) in a class of students. When we did not observe its normal metabolite in 7 of the 140 students, we assumed a laboratory error. When calling the students back for reinvestigation, it turned out that all 7 were of Asian origin and that our first measurements had been correct. At the same time, our laboratory ran tests with debrisoquine because a genetic variation of its metabolism had just been discovered. Again, we saw a substantial difference of its metabolic destruction between students of Asian and non-Asian origin (the difference was later defined in terms of DNA variation by Swedish investigators. These unexpected observations with amobarbital and debrisoquine caused us to search the literature and to publish in 1982 the first article on interethnic differences in drug metabolism.

In the mean time, studies of interethnic differences in drug response or metabolism have become frequent research projects. Computerized Pubmed lists more than 2000 articles dealing with the combined entries "drug" and "race." It is now quite clear that the interethnic differences may be divided into two kinds: first, a given mutation of a particular gene may occur with different frequencies in different populations. Second, there are mutations that appear to be specific for a particular population. Some of the differences may be there because they provide a population with a biological advantage; however, some mutations may simply differ because they have arisen in a population after it separated from others.

This difference is suggested by some overview data. The occurrence of 11 mutations that affect the function of the P450 cytochrome CYP2D6 was tested by various investigators in populations from Europe, China, Japan, and Africa. Of these 11 mutations, Europeans carried 7, Chinese 4, Japanese 3, and Africans 2. Only one mutation (G4268C) was found in all countries, suggesting that it arose before humanity separated into different ethnicities.

Inter-ethnic differences occur frequently. As stated previously, 42 drug- metabolizing enzymes have shown pharmacogenetic variability within one or other population. When checking the literature for the occurrence of interethnic differences between these variants, researchers discovered that 28 (66%) showed such differences. This percentage is considered high, particularly when noting the fact that interethnic comparisons had never been made for many drugs. In short, if we view a pharmacogenetic variation between people, it is likely absent in other populations or occurring with a different frequency. Is this a rule that holds for all mutations in any gene?

Rise of Multifactorial Pharmacogenetics

Differences between people in their response to drugs are regular occurrences. This observation was formalized in 1927 by introduction of the term and the concept of ED50; it indicates the dose of a drug sufficient to produce a given effect in 50% of the members of a population. In other words, all drug effects are variable. This result is not surprising because there are numerous factors that can affect a drug response.

As a simple example, let us consider the rate of metabolism of any particular drug. The metabolism may fail because of a genetic change of the enzyme structure. Perhaps the metabolism failed because not enough enzyme was formed, perhaps because of low gene expression or because of a failure of transcription or translation. Was there the absence of an inducing or regulating hormone, or was the enzyme degraded too quickly? Perhaps a genetic abnormality of the promoting region prevented the normal response to the inducer. Perhaps the drug could not reach the enzyme because it was bound somewhere else or a transporter was missing. Thus, even a single step in the drug's fate may be complex and affected by many genes; the genes may interact, and environmental factors also may contribute to the variation.

The causes of most differences generally remain uninvestigated, but the presence of both genetic and environmental causes is common. It is of considerable interest to know the relative contribution of the two causes. The classical method of investigation, used prominently, for example, by Vesell, consisted of twin studies: that is, the magnitude of differences between the two members of a pair of identical and a pair of fraternal was measured. Repeating such studies in many twins and averaging and comparing the differences allowed a calculation of heritability. Unfortunately, the recruiting of a sufficient number of twins often is difficult.

However, a simpler method is now available that is based on the fact that one can give a drug repeatedly to a person and measure each response and the difference between the responses. When giving a drug at an appropriate interval two or more times to a group of people, one can measure two magnitudes: first, one can calculate the average and standard deviation of the response differences between the first and subsequent applications in the same people; second, one can equally calculate and record the difference between subjects. Let us designate the standard deviations of the within-subject variations as SD_w, of the between-subjects as SD_b, and the genetic component of the between-subject variation as r_{GC}. Squaring the standard deviations, the genetic component is then calculated by the following equation:

$$r_{GC} = (SD_b^2 - SD_w^2)/SDb^2$$

A value close to 1.0 indicates overwhelming heredity, close to 0 indicates mostly environmental influence. A recent example of the use of this method has been the assessment of genetic and environmental determinants of cytochrome CYP3A4 activity.

Often forgotten is the fact that there may be a clinically significant drug response difference between two populations even if the average response differences are small, perhaps not even statistically significant. If population data are represented by a normal distribution (Gauss) curve, the persons with abnormal responses may be represented by one of the edges of the curve.

For example, let us consider a normally distributed metabolic destruction rates of drug X. Assume that 2% of the persons have a destruction rate low enough to suffer toxicity from the drug. In another group of people, destruction of the same drug may have a somewhat lower average rate, a fact that is immaterial for most subjects; however, if the distribution curves have equal spread in the two populations, many more people in the second population will have the critically low drug destruction rate and will be intoxicated than in the first population. In short, the difference between the edges of the distribution curves may be of clinical and statistical significance even if the averages are similar.

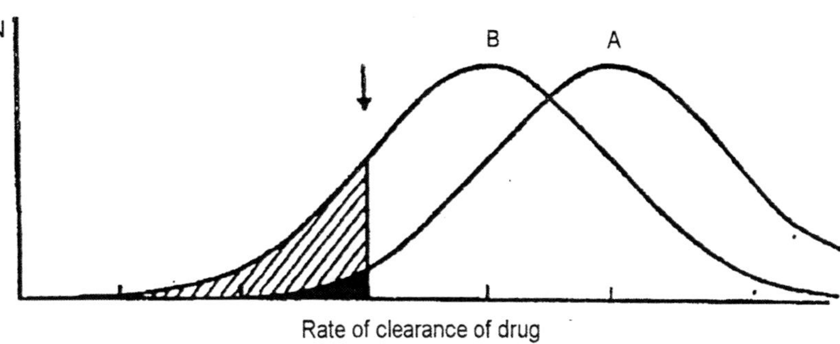

Fig. 1.1. Variation of drug clearance in two populations.

PHARMACOGENOMICS

Pharmacogenetics began with the study of single gene differences between individuals but developed into a broad science. Methodological advances expanded the science further into pharmacogenomics; one may say that pharmacologists followed the geneticist's adoption of genomic techniques. The consequence should be a better understanding of the multiplicities and complexities of drug–gene interactions; not only may genes affect drug action, but drugs may affect gene function. Pharmacogenomics represents attempts by researchers to medically use these new understandings together with the old ones. The hope is to optimize the efficacy of drugs, to minimize adverse drug reactions, and to facilitate drug discovery, development, and approval.

AIMS OF PHARMACOGENOMICS

Creation of a Basis for Personalized Medicine

Current medicine is based on statistical likelihood and often fails the individual. The incidence of serious or fatal drug reactions depends in many or most cases on genetic variation. Studies from U.S. hospitals suggested that 6.7% of patients had serious adverse and 0.32% had fatal, drug reactions. The latter caused approx 100,000 deaths per year in the United States. Many researchers hope that adverse reactions or therapeutic failures will be eliminated by the introduction of personalized medicine, meaning that the drug to be given to a patient will be determined by the patient's genes.

To reach this aim, we must learn much more about the genetic variants that may affect drug action. The most frequently occurring genetic variants are single-nucleotide polymorphisms (SNPs). The human genome contains approx 3 billion basepairs, and SNPs occur on the average in approx 1 per 1000 bases; thus, they cause genetic variation of many human proteins. These variants are important objects of study because human individuals usually differ from each other by less than 1% of their genes; thus, SNPs are important. Besides being most common, SNPs are the most technically accessible class of genetic variants. Using genomic methods, high-density maps of SNPs can be created and hopefully used as distinguishing markers of xenobiotic response, even if the drug target is not specifically identified.

By correlating SNPs and drug response data, one will have gained an ability to predict drug efficacy or toxicity within reasonable limits for any individual. Although variants other than SNPs are able to affect drug responses, this detection will happen less frequently than the SNP-related ones. Nevertheless, screening of the genome for all known and for unknown pharmacogenomics-related variations will be tasks for years to come.

Personalized medicine can also be said to be based on the identification of biomarkers. They extend to a broad variety of indirect manifestations of underlying, but often unrecognized, sequence variations. Because of their variety, their study or discovery may require various kinds of investigations.

Many published examples concern cancers. To name a few, prostate cancer is subject to transcriptional regulation, and there are prostate-specific antigens.

Cervical neoplasia may depend on the human papilloma virus. Many other examples apply to cardiovascular diseases. For example, high levels of C-reactive protein or interleukin 6 affect ischemic heart disease and its mortality risk. Low-density lipoprotein cholesterol is used to profile cardiac risks. A strange example in a different field is the fact that excessive alcohol consumption can be assessed by the serum level of carbohydrate-deficient transferrin. Thus, the complexity of biomarkers is frightening; even if we have reached personalized medicine, it will not be without problems.

Drugs Affecting Gene Expression

For a gene to form a protein, its DNA has to be converted into RNA, which acts within a ribosome. Various studies have shown that the amount of RNA can vary, indicating functional variation of the gene, quantified in terms of gene expression. Microarray experiments represent a genomic technique that has yielded expression information of thousands of genes.

The understanding that gene expression is variable has changed genetics, which was for a long time concerned only with structural differences between genes. We now know that gene interaction may mean that one gene affects expression and function of other genes.

Furthermore, gene expression may be changed by hormones, by disease, by food, or by drugs. In pharmacology, a good example of variable gene expression is drug-increased drug metabolism, a newer one is drug addiction caused by drugs that act on genes in brain. We sometimes do not know whether a drug action is the result of the drug affecting a protein or a gene.

This question may be answered by using gene expression changes. Using repeat studies, one can measure expressions obtained before and after exposure to a drug. Any difference of expression tells which, if any, genes are affected by the drug. One can test gene expression in specific cells, be it leukocytes or liver cells. If tested in brain cells, one may learn whether the drug affects a gene of interest in brain.

Identification of New Targets for Future Drugs

Common diseases are usually caused by a combined action of several or of many genes, in addition to environmental influences. Genomic methods that allow an investigation of numerous genes may help to identify a gene that contributes importantly to a disease. If so, one may look for a chemical that targets that gene or its protein product; this chemical may then become a drug that helps to combat the disease. This kind of effort has been called a search for "*drugable targets*," that is, for targets that can be approached by small molecules of the size of drugs. Thus, genomic studies may lead to new medical therapies.

Because the set of genes responsible for a given disease may differ somewhat between people, the targets able to be drugged may not be exactly the same in different subjects. This hypothesis is not classical pharmacogenetics, but it explains why a given drug may cure the disease only in some people. Genomic studies that tell ahead of time which person may benefit from the drug are a part of personalized medicine.

The search for disease-causing genes may also be helped by gene expression studies. By comparing genes in the presence and in the absence of a disease, one may get some indication of which genes are affected by the disease, or which genes cause the disease. In exceptional cases, one may be able to compare gene expression in a person before and after onset of the disease. Usually, it is necessary to compare groups of healthy and diseased subjects because there will be differences of gene expression that are unrelated to the disease.

Another set of target studies is the attempt to create new antibiotics or infection-fighting drugs by investigating the genetic structure of bacteria or other infectious agents. Thereby, one may identify potential targets for new drugs. Even if the targets are known, finding such new drugs may require intensive systematic searches.

Genetics and pharmacology are two sciences that interact in many different ways. The study of such interactions was aroused by some simple observations that indicated that monogenic differences could cause persons to respond differently to a drug. Unfortunately, both the effects of drugs and the effects of genes can vary a great deal, and the interactions of these two turned out to be often so complex that they are frequently hard to understand. Nevertheless, pharmacogenomics is the science that studies these interactions. Its purpose is to unlock some of the difficulties, to use as many facts as possible to improve medicine, and thereby to help all human beings.

2

GENOME-WIDE ANALYSIS

Human variation is largely caused by deoxyribonucleic acid polymorphism and difference in gene expression. Common disease/common variant hypotheses suggest that quantitative differences among different alleles may be the basis for complex diseases. Quantitative difference in gene expression between alleles may affect most complex diseases. We have developed a gene chip-based method to quantitatively examine allele- specific gene expression of 1063 transcribed single-nucleotide polymorphisms using Affymetrix HuSNP oligo arrays. Among the 602 genes that were heterozygous and expressed in kidney or liver tissues from seven individuals, 326 (54%) showed preferential expression of one allele in at least one individual. The genes that showed allele-specific expression are distributed throughout the genome. We showed that variation of gene expression between alleles is common and that this variation may contribute to human variation. Our studies demonstrate the feasibility to perform genome-wide analysis of allele-specific gene expression.

Polymorphism and variation in gene expression provide the genetic basis for human variation. Mendelian diseases are caused by mutations in a single gene or a few genes. To date, mutations in more than 2000 genes have been identified. Most of these mutations change the protein structure and function. Increasing efforts have been made toward understanding the genetic basis of common complex diseases. It is commonly believed that the complex diseases are caused by combination of common single-nucleotide polymorphisms (SNPs), each of which contributes quantitatively to the diseases. Most of the efforts so far have been focused on nonsynonymous SNPs. However, most of the SNPs in the genome are not nonsynonymous SNPs. They instead are synonymous SNPs, SNPs in untranslated region, intronic SNPs, or intergenic SNPs. These SNPs can affect complex diseases through their effects on gene expression.

Currently, there are more than 2 million SNPs deposited in GenBank. It is daunting task to perform association studies for all those SNPs. Several initiatives have been taken to prioritize a subset of those SNPs for association study of various types of diseases. Those include Haplotype Map Project and candidate SNP approaches. A SNP outside coding region may affect gene product quantitatively by altering gene expression. This type of SNP should show difference in gene expression between the two alleles of an individual. Identifying this class of SNPs could have significant impact in our efforts to identify genes that are associated with complex diseases. Several recent studies have shown that allelic variation in gene expression is common in the human genome. Also, variation in allelic gene expression was shown to be transmitted by Mendelian inheritance. To address the feasibility to analyze allele-specific gene expression at genome-wide level, we modified an existing genotyping technology, the Affymetrix HuSNP chip system, to analyze allele-specific gene expression.

The HuSNP chip was designed for simultaneous typing of 1494 SNPs of the human genome. It has been applied successfully to study loss of heterozygosity in human cancer. The HuSNP chip contains 16 probes for each SNP locus, with four matching perfectly to allele A and the other four matching perfectly to allele B. The other eight probes differ from the first eight probes by having one mismatched base in the center of the probe. In this report, we summarize the method that we used to perform both genotyping and allele-specific gene expression using HuSNP chips. Our studies demonstrate that the HuSNP chip system is a reliable way to simultaneously measure allele-specific gene expression for hundreds of genes.

Materials

Fetal Tissues

Fetal tissues were obtained from the Birth Defects Research Laboratory, University of Washington. The tissues were snap-frozen after surgery and were stored in liquid nitrogen. Kidney and liver tissues from seven individuals, five male and two female, were used in this study. The ages of the fetuses ranged from 78 to 103 d.

DNA Isolation

Genomic DNA was isolated using the QIAamp DNA mini kit.

1. Tissues of 25 mg were cut into small pieces and were placed in a 1.5-mL tube.
2. The tissues were mixed with 180 μL of Buffer ATL and 20 μL of proteinase K and incubated at 56°C until tissue was completely lysed, using shaking water bath to ensure mixing of sample.
3. The tissues were mixed with 200 μL of Buffer AL by vortexing for 15 s and then incubated at 70°C for 10 min, followed by addition of 200 μL of ethanol.
4. Tissue mixture was applied to QIAmp spin column without wetting the rim and was spun at 6000*g* for 1 min.
5. The samples were washed with 500 μL of Buffer AW1 (with ETOH added) and then 500 μL of Buffer AW2.
6. Genomic DNAs were eluted with 200 μL of Buffer AE or distilled H_2O.

RNA Isolation

1. RNAs were isolated from fetal tissues using RNAzol^B according to the manufacturer's protocol.
2. Tissues of 50 mg were homogenized in 4 mL of RNAzol^B and were mixed thoroughly with 0.8 mL of $CHCl_3$ and incubated on ice for 5 min.
3. The samples were spun at 9300*g* for 10 min at 4°C.
4. Aqueous phase (2 mL) were collected and mixed with 2 mL of isopropanol and incubated at room temperature for 5 min.
5. The samples were spun at 13,400*g* for 10 min at 4°C and washed with 4 mL of cold 75% EtOH.
6. RNAs were suspended in 50 μL of DEPC-treated H2O containing 1 μL of 40 U/ μL RNase inhibitor and were stored at -70°C.
7. Poly-A RNAs were isolated using the Micro-Fast Track kit. We mixed 20 μL of RNA with 1 mL of lysis buffer.
8. The mixture was incubated at 65°C for 5 min and chilled on ice for 1 min.
9. The samples were transferred back to room temperature and mixed with 63 μL of 5 *M* NaCl.
10. The samples were mixed with oligo (dT) cellulose for 20 min at room temperature and spun at 133*g* for 5 min at room temperature. The pellet was suspended in 1.3 mL of binding buffer. The above step was repeated until OD_{260} in the supernatant is less than 0.05.

11. The pellet was washed with 500 μL of Low Salt Wash buffer twice and eluted with 100 μL of elution buffer.
12. Poly A RNA was precipitated with NaAc and EtOH and resuspended in 20 μL of DEPC-treated H_2O, containing 1 μL of 40 U/μL RNase inhibitor and was stored at −70°C.

cDNA Synthesis

1. Complimentary deoxyribonucleic acid (cDNA) synthesis was conducted in 50-μL reaction. Poly-A RNA (60 ng) was mixed with 1 μg of oligo dT, 3 μg of random hexamer, and DEPC-treated water to a final volume of 34 μL.
2. The sample was incubated at 70°C for 10 min and put back on ice.
3. We added 10 μL of 5X buffer, 4 μL of dNTP (each at 2.5 m*M*), 1 μL of 20 U/μL RNase inhibitor, and 1.5 μL of 2.5 U/μL AMV reverse transcriptase to RNA/primer mixture.
4. The mixture was incubated at 42°C for 1 h and stored cDNA at −70°C.

METHODS

HuSNP Experiments

1. The HuSNP experiments were conducted according to the GeneChip HuSNP Mapping Assay Manual. Genomic DNA (120 ng) or cDNA (6 ng) was used for each set of 24 multiplex polymerase chain reactions (PCRs).
2. We prepared PCR I mixture by adding 35 μL of 10X buffer, 70 μL of 25 m*M* $MgCl_2$, 70 μL of 2.5 m*M* dNTP, and 7 μL of 5 U/μL AmpliTaq gold DNA polymerase (Applied Biosystems, Foster City, CA).
3. We took 223 μL of PCR I mixture and added 34 μL of 4 ng/μL DNA (or 34 μL of 0.2 ng/μL cDNA).
4. We dispensed 9.5 μL of the mixture into each well of a 96-well plate.
5. We added 3 μL of multiplex primers (24 primer sets for each DNA) to 96-well plate, sealed the plate with a film, did a quick spin, and put the plate on a thermal cycler.
6. The PCR condition had one cycle of 95°C for 5 min, 30 cycles of 95°C for 30 s, 52°C approx 57.8°C for 55 s (starting from 52°C and increasing the temperature by 0.2°C per cycle), 72°C for 30 s, and followed by five cycles 95°C for 30 s, 58°C for 55 s, 72°C for 30 s, and extension at 72°C at 7 min.
7. PCR II mixture contained 187.5 μL of H_2O, 62.5 μL of 10X buffer, 100 μL of 25 m*M* $MgCl_2$, 100 μL of 2.5 m*M* dNTP, 50 μL of 10 μ*M* biotin-T7 primer, 50 μL of 10 μ*M* biotin-T3 primer, and 12.5 μL of U/μL AmpliTaq gold DNA polymerase.
8. We aliquoted 22.5 μL of PCR II mixture into the 96-well plate, added 2.5 μL of 1:1000 dilution of PCR I product (from serial dilution of 3X 1:10), sealed the plate with a film, did a quick spin, and put on the thermal cycler.
9. PCR condition II contained one cycle of 95°C for 8 min, 40 cycles of 95°C for 30 s, 55°C for 90 s, 72°C for 30 s, and extension at 72°C for 7 min.
10. We used 1 μL of the PCR II product to check PCR reaction by gel electrophoresis.
11. We took 23 μL of PCR II products and combined those (12 wells per tube), put the PCR products into a Microcon-10 concentrator, and spun at 13,000*g* for 10 min.
12. We then inverted the concentrator into a fresh tube to collect samples and spun at 3000*g* for 3 min. You should get about 30 μL from each tube.
13. The samples were stored at −20°C.

14. Hybridization solution: mix 4 μL of H_2O, 81 μL of 5 *M* TMAC, 1.4 μL of control oligo B1, 1.4 μL of 1 *M* Tris-HCl, pH 7.8, 1.4 μL of 1% Tween-20, 1.4 μL of 0.5 *M* EDTA, 1.4 μL of 10 mg/mL sonicated Salmon Sperm DNA, 13.5 μL of 50X Denhardt's solution, and 30 μL of concentrated PCR II products.
15. The hybridization mixture was denatured at 95°C for 5 min and was added to a HuSNP chip.
16. The hybridization was carried out at 44°C for 16 h.
17. Washing buffer A: 140 mL of H_2O, 60 mL of 20X SSPE, and 0.2 mL of 10% Triton X-100.
18. Washing buffer B: 160 mL of H_2O, 40 mL of 20X SSPE, and 0.2 mL of 10% Triton X-100.
19. Staining solution: 305 μL of H_2O, 150 μL of 20X SSPE, 10 μL of 50X Denhardt's solution, 5 μL of 1% Tween-20, 12.5 μL of 1 mg/mL SAPE, and 5 μL of 0.5 mg/mL Biotinylated anti-streptavidin.
20. The HuSNP chip was washed and stained with the following Fluidics Protocol.

Washing A1 temperature (°C)	25
Number of wash A1 cycles	2
Mixes per wash A1 cycle	2
Washing B temperature (°C)	35
Number of wash B cycles	6
Mixes per wash B cycle	5
Staining time (s)	1800
Staining temperature (°C)	25
Washing A2 temperature (°C)	25
Number of wash A2 cycles	6
Mixes per wash A2 cycle	4
Holding temperature (°C)	25

21. The chip was then scanned in a HP GeneArray Scanner. Genotyping calls were made using the Affymetrix MicroArray Suite (MAS) software version 4.0. Allele-specific gene expression was analyzed by the method described below.

Computational Analysis of HuSNP Data

We mapped SNPs in the transcribed region using the annotation in dbSNP and Blast search. The criteria for Blast search were: (1) at least two EST hits; (2) E-value $< 10^{-10}$; and (3) alignment > 40 bp. We were able to map 1063 SNPs to the transcribed regions of genes.

We extracted the intensity values for each probe from the .CEL files generated by Affymetrix MAS 4.0. The .CEL files contain the fluorescent intensity values for each of the probes. HuSNP chip contains minimally 16 probes for each SNP locus. Four of the 16 probes match perfectly to allele A, four to allele B, four have one mismatch to allele A, and the other four have one mismatch to allele B. Allele A and allele B represent the two alleles of the SNP. Each probe contains 20 nucleotides. Affymetrix defines a mini-block as a group of four probes that include a perfect match probe for allele A (PMA), a mismatch probe for allele A (MMA), a perfect match probe for allele B (PMB), and a mismatch probe for allele B (MMB).

The mismatch probe has one mismatch base in the center of the probe. There are four miniblocks for each SNP, with the center nucleotide of the probe corresponds the base at –4, –1, 0, and 1 of the original SNP sequence. Ninety-five SNPs have an additional probe with the center base at +4 position of the SNP. The value for each probe pair was computed by subtracting the mismatch intensity from the perfect match intensity. A *t*-test was used to calculate a *p* value for the presence of signal (intensity greater than 0) for each allele of each SNP. We considered a signal to be present if at least one allele had signal ($p < 0.01$, t-test). For those SNP with signal, we set (PMA – MMA) = 50 if (PMA – MMA) is less than 50 for each miniblock. Similarly, baseline for allele B was set at 50. Fraction of the A allele, defined as f = (PMA-MMA)/(PMA-MMA + PMB-MMB), was computed for each mini-block, and the mean of the fractions among the four mini-blocks was computed for each SNP. The ratio of allele A/allele B can be computed from f/(1 – f). Two scans, scan A and scan B, are taken for each chip. Generally, we used the intensity values from scan A. We used the intensity values from scan B if scan A doesn't have a signal defined by t-test. The ratio of two alleles in cDNA was further normalized by the ratio of genomic DNAs for the SNP. Among the 602 SNPs analyzed in our studies, 39 had at least five heterozygous fetuses. We computed the 95% confidence interval for the allelic ratio of genomic DNA for each of these 39 SNPs, and the average confidence interval was between 0.5 and 2.0. This value was used to select those genes that show significant difference in the expression between the two alleles.

Notes

1. It is essential to start with high molecular weight genomic DNA. The quality of the genomic DNA was analyzed by 1% agarose gel electrophoresis with and without a restriction enzyme digestion. There should be only high molecular weight DNA before restriction enzyme digestion and generation of a mixture of variable sizes of DNA fragments after digestion.

Table 2.1. A Report From HuSNP Array

Pool	*%Pass*	*%A*	*%AB*	*%B*	*%AB_A*	*%AB_B*	*%No signal*
A01	79.8	17	36.2	24.5	2.1	0	20.2
A02	72.9	25.9	28.2	14.1	4.7	0	27.1
A03	86.7	32.5	20.5	30.1	2.4	1.2	13.3
A04	65.8	27.6	10.5	25	1.3	1.3	34.2
A05	91.7	27.8	13.9	47.2	2.8	0	8.3
A06	63.4	26.8	15.5	19.7	1.4	0	36.6
A07	60	16	21.3	18.7	2.7	1.3	40
A08	76.3	23.8	26.3	25	0	1.3	23.8
A09	79.3	23.2	31.7	24.4	0	0	20.7
A10	72.9	21.2	15.3	32.9	0	3.5	27.1
A11	77.9	25.6	18.6	31.4	2.3	0	22.1
A12	87	35.1	27.3	24.7	0	0	13
A13	85.2	26.1	25	33	1.1	0	14.8
A14	80	30	22.9	24.3	1.4	1.4	20
A15	78.1	23.3	26	26	0	2.7	21.9
A16	71.1	22.4	26.3	21.1	0	1.3	28.9
A17	69.2	16.7	28.2	20.5	3.8	0	30.8
A18	62	6	18	34	4	0	38
A19	78.4	31.4	17.6	27.5	0	2	21.6
A20	59	15.4	20.5	23.1	0	0	41
A21	69.2	20.5	17.9	30.8	0	0	30.8
Total	75	23.8	23	25.9	1.5	0.8	25

2. The protocol used 120 ng genomic DNA. It is generally believed that 2 to 5% of genomic DNA contains transcribed sequences. Therefore we used 6 ng of cDNA made from poly-A RNA. It is also possible to do the allele-specific gene expression using cDNA made from total RNA. Contamination of genomic DNA will increase the call for bi-allelic expression. However, genes that displayed preferential expression of one allele are not owing to any trace amount of genomic DNA contamination.
3. We always check the PCR II by a 4% agarose gel before hybridization. The expected PCR products are around 90 to 100 bp in all 24 multiplex PCRs.
4. We used Affymetrix MAS 4.0 in this study. You should see a sharp image with HuSNP 2K label and signals evenly distributed across the chip. A1 to A21 correspond to 1 to 21 of the 24 multiplex PCRs, which contain 1494 SNPs. The calling rate varies among different multiplex PCR reactions. We have used MAS 5.0 in recent studies. MAS 5.0 outputs RAS values that are similar to the fraction generated by the method described in this chapter.
5. The reproducibility of the HuSNP system can be assessed by correlation between duplicated experiments. To evaluate concordance between two duplicate experiments, we computed the Pearson correlation coefficient between the two experiments using the mean intensity of the probe pairs from each allele of a SNP. Pearson correlation coefficient is 0.98 to 0.99 for genomic DNA and 0.88 to 0.96 for cDNA.
6. The method described here can also apply to the study using Affymetrix 10k chip and 100k chip. The new high-density oligo arrays use GCOS software, which outputs RAS values in addition to genotype call.

3

ASPECTS INFLUENCING GENOTYPE

The variety of genotyping methods currently available and the evolution of their capabilities have facilitated an expansion of the field of pharmacogenomics. Traditionally, limited genotyping capabilities have restricted the generation and application of genotyping data for pharmacogenomic studies. With the variety of platforms and chemistries available for flexible, high-throughput genotyping, it is important to keep in mind the limitations imposed by both the polymorphisms that are to be interrogated and the type of pharmacogenomics study for which the data are being generated.

The completion of the human genome draft sequence and the ongoing annotation of genes and genetic variants have provided the foundation for an expanding role of genotyping in pharmacogenomics. Detailed information on genomic variants of all types is being constantly compiled and should be considered an invaluable resource for the identification and screening of these polymorphisms and their association with clinical phenotypes. As this wealth of genomic information has grown, so have the number of methods available for genomic interrogation. The effective integration of genotyping data into a pharmacogenomics study requires an understanding of the factors influencing the efficiency of different genotyping methods and the priorities required of different study designs. A variety of genotyping chemistries are available for interrogating all types of deoxyribonucleic acid (DNA) sequence variants. The physical nature of the variants in question will render some techniques uninformative. Because of this, the selection of a genotyping chemistry requires an initial assessment of the types of variants that are going to be investigated.

The type of pharmacogenomics study for which the genotyping data are being generated also will limit the usefulness of some of the available methods. Different study designs have different priorities for the number of assays necessary, the stringency of their physical location, and their minimum call rate. Prioritizing these aspects of the investigation at the outset can greatly increase the effectiveness of the genotyping method selected and in turn efficiently generate more useful data. The first portion of this chapter is dedicated to a discussion of different types of genomic variants and their effects on selection of a genotyping technique. The later sections highlight the different types of pharmacogenomic studies and the unique constraints they apply to selection of a genotyping technique. The aspects influencing method selection covered in this chapter are considered independent of platform as the application of different methods are covered in-depth in the following chapters. It also should be mentioned that often the overriding influence on the application of a genotyping method is dictated by the platforms that are available rather than its suitability for a given genotyping project. In this instance it is still important to keep the following information in mind in order to maximize the application of the available technology to new investigations in Pharmacogenomics.

Types of Variation

Genome databases currently contain information on millions of genetic variants located throughout the genome. These variants can be classified both by their effect on nearby genes and by their physical attributes. It is these classifications that dictate the application of different genotyping chemistries. The investigation of single nucleotide polymorphisms (SNPs) often requires a different chemistry than more substantial DNA variations, such as tandem repeats. Careful consideration of these aspects in the experimental design process will aid in the generation of high quality genotyping data.

Functional Classification

Variants fall into two categories, functional and nonfunctional, based whether the change at the genomic sequence level has an effect on normal gene function. The magnitude of the variant at the sequence level can range from single base changes to the deletion of entire genes. The resulting functional effect can be equally as diverse and manifest as changes in the amino acid sequence, vary rates of transcription by modification of promoter sequence, vary the sequence of intron/exon boundaries resulting in alternatively spliced ribonucleic acid (RNA) products, or cause the deletion of entire genes. These functional changes represent the genetic portion of observed clinical phenotypes. Thus, the identification and characterization of the functional variants responsible for the clinical phenotypes involved in a pharmacogenomics study are the ultimate goal.

Although they do not directly influence the clinical phenotype, nonfunctional variants can be critical to the effective application of genotyping to a pharmacogenomics study. Nonfunctional variants are much more abundant genome wide as there is no genetic selection against their accumulation in the population. Although the individual alleles of a given nonfunctional variant may have no direct impact on normal function of a particular gene, its physical location may place it in linkage disequilibrium with a functional variant. This provides the opportunity to use the more common nonfunctional variants as markers to localize novel functional variants via linkage analysis and association studies. Additionally, their relative abundance can provide the opportunity to be used in place of directly screening the functional variants for which validating a high performance genotyping assay cannot be achieved.

Physical Classification

Single nucleotide polymorphisms

SNPs are the most common type of genetic variant. An estimated 10 million or more SNPs are dispersed throughout the human genome. Their abundance and consistent occurrence throughout the genome have made them an increasingly useful target for pharmacogenomic investigations. More recently their utility has been reinforced by the accumulation of evidence, that suggests much of the heritable portion of common disease is attributed to minor sequence variations as opposed to more substantial gene defects such as insertions or deletions. As a natural recourse to their abundance, there is a dispersal of SNPs of both nonfunctional and functional significance. From the perspective of their applicability to genotyping in pharmacogenomic studies, this provides a critical resource. Currently, there is information on more than 9 million SNPs deposited in public databases. Projects are underway that are compiling genotype, gene frequency and, in some cases, validated assays for a variety of SNPs throughout the genome. These data should be considered a primary resource for any project that will involve SNP genotyping.

Simple sequence repeats

Simple sequence repeats (SSR) are stretches of DNA that are composed of various numbers of repeated DNA segments in which the core repeat unit is 1 to 4 bp in length. These variants are dispersed throughout the genome, are shown to be both functional and nonfunctional in nature, and are highly variable, resulting in the accumulation of multiple alleles for each SSR locus. These factors make many of these loci very informative as markers for studies of association and linkage analysis. Commonly referred to as microsatellites, these markers have been used extensively for mapping, association, and human identification studies since their discovery. Studies of population stratification have suggested that on average the genotypic information available from a single microsatellite marker is equivalent to that provided by five to eight SNP markers.

The primary drawback of using micro-satellites for mapping is that they are not as common as SNPs; thus, there may not be the density of markers necessary to investigate a specific region of interest. Additionally, as more data are generated on the number, location, and functional significance of SNPs in the human genome, it has been shown that specific SNPs can be even more informative than some dinucleotide microsatellite markers. Combined with increasing efficiency of genotyping SNPs the advantage of microsatellites being more informative is being overcome.

Specific SSRs have been associated with variation in gene function and clinically observed phenotypes. As would be expected, the expansion or contraction of a region of DNA sequence can have functional consequences that are highly dependent on its proximity to coding or regulatory DNA sequence. Different alleles of a 2-bp SSR in the 5' promoter region of the gene UGT1A1 have been shown to be associated with changes in efficiency of irinotecan metabolism. A common method of genotyping of this polymorphism involves the measurement of polymerase chain reaction (PCR)-amplified fragments that contain the polymorphic sequence. Two base pair variations in length of the amplified fragment can be detected by capillary electrophoresis or some gel electrophoresis-based systems.

Variable number tandem repeats

Variable number tandem repeats (VNTRs) are the sequential and repeated insertion of DNA sequences whose basic repeat unit is larger than those represented by SSRs. These tandem repetitions of DNA sequence can be tens of bases long and their insertion can rapidly change the structure of a gene at the sequence level. Because of the more substantial alteration of gene sequence caused by the VNTR polymorphisms, genotyping methods generally have focused on the detection of size variation in PCR amplicons containing the repeats. Selection of a genotyping method for the screening of these types of polymorphisms must take into account not only the length of the repeat sequence, but also the number of repeats likely to be present in the study population. Because the number of repeat units increases so does the length of the PCR product. Careful consideration must be taken to keep the resulting amplicons within the detection capabilities of the genotyping platform.

The presence of a 28-bp VNTR in the promoter region of the thymidylate synthase (TYMS) gene has been shown to be associated with changes in in vitro expression levels of the gene. TYMS is an important target for several chemotherapy drugs. Genotyping for the TYMS promoter VNTR has commonly been performed by analysis of variation in PCR amplicon length to calculate the number of repeat units. This method is robust; however, special consideration must be taken to keep the length of the amplified fragments within the detectable range of the platform being used for analysis. Thus far, there have been up to nine repeats of the 28-bp repeat identified, which requires the detection of fragments varying throughout a range of 250 bp, not including additional space required for primer location.

Insertions and deletions

The most profound of the sequence variations described here, large-scale insertions and deletions, can have the most noticeable phenotypic effects. Insertions of DNA sequence within a gene can have the same deleterious effects on gene function that have been discussed earlier, ranging from changes in gene transcription rates to total elimination of gene function. An excellent example of the spontaneous insertion of DNA sequence is represented in the cytosine beta synthase gene, in which associations have been made between the insertion of a 68-bp segment of DNA sequence from a previous intron/exon junction and observed changes in plasma total homocysteine. The analysis of PCR fragment size has been commonly used for genotyping of this polymorphism by methods similar to that mentioned previously.

Deletion of genomic sequence can have substantial repercussions as well. The elimination of DNA sequence can vary in magnitude from single base pairs to entire genes. Various methods are capable of genotyping these variants; however, the deciding factor on their application lies in the conservation of the sequence surrounding the deletion junction. Pyrosequencing has been used successfully to interrogate deletions as long as 100 bp, and the analysis of changes in amplicon size of PCR products containing the deleted sequence has been used for detecting deletions up to a few hundred base pairs. A primary benefit of these two methods for the genotyping of deletions is the capability to detect heterozygosity in samples.

Types of Pharmacogenomics Studies

Early studies of pharmacogenomics focused on the assignment of Mendelian inheritance patterns to observed clinical phenotypes. This method was limited to finding mostly monogenic traits that showed simple inheritance patterns identifiable in relatively small treatment groups. Advances in the generation of genomic, functional genomic, and proteomic data have lead to the identification and classification of a wealth of gene ontology and pathway information. These resources have allowed for the identification of candidate genes that are likely to be involved in the observed clinical phenotypes. Methodologies for interrogation of these specific loci have made possible the study of more complex, multi-locus genetic interactions. This method of screening candidate genes has been successfully applied to Pharmacogenomic studies of drug metabolizing genes in a variety of diseases. These efforts have identified both associations between the variants and clinical phenotypes as well as the novel variants responsible for the functional changes.

Some studies in pharmacogenomics have taken a broader approach to the identification of significant genetic variants by scanning the entire human genome. The primary limitation for this technique is the need to do a large number of assays to get adequate coverage of the complete genome. Estimates of the number of markers necessary for this type of study are highly dependent on sample size, but can quickly exceed 50,000 markers necessary to have adequate power of detection. Because many studies have a predefined number of available samples, statistical analysis can be performed to estimate the detection capabilities of various numbers of maker within the study group.

These classifications are relative to one another and highlight the strengths of these different study designs. The whole genome approach requires a method that can efficiently process the larger number of assays that are required to provide sufficient power of detection and coverage of the entire genome. Although a greater number of assays may be required, the constraints on successful assay validation are relaxed in comparison with the candidate gene approach as a result of the prevalence of nonfunctional variants in the genome. If a robust assay cannot be validated for a specific polymorphism, it is likely that there will be another variant nearby that can be substituted. Additionally, the assays used for the whole genome approach are not required to be as robust because a slight drop in call rate for an individual polymorphism will not have as profound an effect on the data set as it would with the more demanding candidate gene study.

The current age of genotyping finds itself growing on the foundation of the human genome draft sequence but not yet at the point of cost effectively obtaining whole genome sequence information on an individual basis. This requires that genotyping methods exist to do both screening of known variants and identification of novel polymorphisms at levels of cost and throughput such that the data can be efficiently generated and effectively used in studies of pharmacogenomics.

The applicability of different genotyping methods changes as the demands of the genotyping project are defined. Important aspects for consideration prior to method selection are the type of variants that are to be interrogated and the type of pharmacogenomics study that the data will be integrated. Clear definition of these parameters will greatly aid in the selection and appropriate application of a genotyping method. Continuing improvement of genotyping methods, specifically reduction in cost and increases in both throughput and efficiency of template use, are central to continued advancement of genotyping in Pharmacogenomics studies.

Table 3.1. Implication of different types of pharmacogenomics studies on aspects of assay design

	Type of Study	
	Candidate gene	*Whole genome*
Number of polymorphisms	Moderate	High
Assay validation rate	High	Moderate
Individual assay call rate	High	Moderate

The following chapters cover in detail the application of several different genotyping methods currently used in pharmacogenomic studies. These meth-ods use a variety of different chemistries and platforms for the screening of genetic variants, and all have different advantages based on the constraints outlined in this chapter. Understanding of these constraints and their effect on the genotyping capabilities required of the project, combined with the thor-ough consideration of genotyping in the experimental design process, will greatly aid in the generation of high quality data.

4

PHARMACOGENOMICS AND GENOMIC TECHNOLOGY

The human genome project has generated data unprecedented in its volume and in the promise that it holds in providing a better understanding of the complexity of biological systems. With the ultimate identification of all of the genes in the human genome, a comprehensive understanding of life's organization at the molecular level becomes a rational scientific goal. Such information will ultimately transform the life sciences. It seems likely that the impact of these data will be felt most immediately in the pharmaceutical sciences because as compared to many complex, multifaceted health issues (for example, cancer, obesity, and cardiovascular disease), drug efficacy and toxicity are more tractable problems. This is owing to the fact that many drugs have relatively specific targets and are altered (transported and metabolized) by one or a few genes. In addition, there exists a wide body of pharmacokinetic and pharmacodynamic data for many drugs, which will aid greatly in interpreting the molecular and genomic data now being collected. In this article, we will discuss the role of these recent technologies in the pharmaceutical sciences. Specifically we discuss the application of genomic technologies in two major areas: (i) to assess the importance of human genetic variation in drug response and (ii) to identify networks of genes, which determine the efficacy and toxicity of drug therapies and to identify new therapeutic drug targets.

TERMINOLOGY

The genomic revolution in the life sciences has spawned a fair number of new terms representing not so much new fields of science as expanded opportunities in established fields. One of these, pharmacogenomics is a recently coined term encompassing the application of new genomic technologies and data to the pharmaceutical sciences. It can be understood to be similar to other fields spawned by the Omics revolution: proteomics (measurement and characterization of plasma proteins), toxicogenomics (structure and response of the genome following xenobiotic exposure), and metabolomics (analysis of the metabolites of an organism). All represent the infusion of genomic information and technologies into already well-established fields.

While pharmacogenomics as a discipline is recent, the application of genetics to pharmacology and the pharmaceutical sciences is not new. The term, pharmacogenetics, was coined by Vogel in 1959 following an earlier summary concerning the relationship of genetics (as understood to be the study of patterns of inheritance) and interindividual drug response. The first book titled "*Pharmacogenetics*" appeared in 1 962, with a number of books covering all aspects of pharmacogenomics and pharmacogenetics now available. Kalow provides an excellent historical review of the development of pharmacogenetics and pharmacogenomics. A simple literature search shows the rapid increase in scientific papers in the fields of pharmacogenetics and pharmacogenomics. The rapid increase in publications coincides with technological developments in DNA sequencing, DNA amplification using the polymerase chain reaction (PCR), and microarrays.

Pharmacogenetics and Pharmacogenomics

The terms pharmacogenetics and pharmacogenomics are generally used interchangeably, though pharmacogenetics has often been limited to examinations of genetic differences in single genes segregating in populations (polymorphisms) and the importance these differences have on individual variation in drug response. The term "*pharmacogenomics*" has come to include not only pharmacogenetics as defined above but also the interaction of all the genes present in an individual, a "whole genome view" of drug response. This includes not only the interactions of many polymorphic genes as they affect drug response but also the role gene interactions play in drug distribution, metabolism, and elimination.

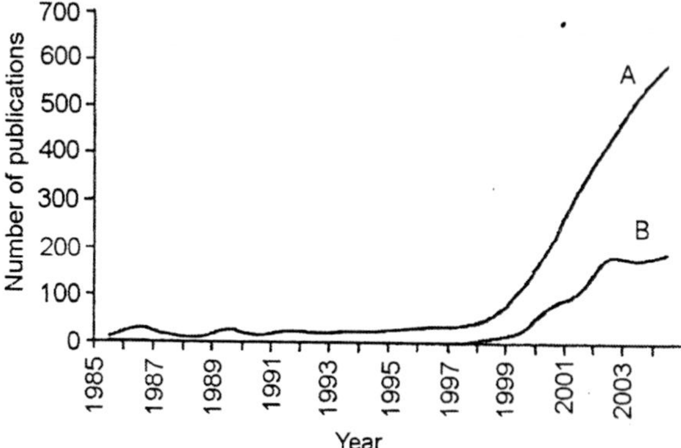

Fig. 4.1. Number of publications in pharmacogenomics and pharmacogenetics (A) and pharmacogenomics alone (B).

Any definition of pharmacogenomics should include the application of genomic technologies and information to the pharmaceutical sciences. Genomic technologies such as high-throughput DNA sequencing and gene expression studies using microarrays and quantitative real-time PCR are fundamental tools in the discovery and clinical assessment of genetic polymorphisms as well as identification of the network of genes and gene interactions that affect the efficacy and toxicity of drug therapies. Thus pharmacogenomics can be grouped into two relatively distinct, though interconnected, endeavors:

1. The use of genomic technologies to elucidate the molecular mechanisms underlying drug action, efficacy, and toxicity with the goal of producing improved therapeutic outcomes. The focus here is on conducting gene expression studies whether on the scale of the genome using microarrays or "*DNA chips*," or on a smaller more directed approaches using quantitative PCR technologies.
2. The examination of the role of human genetic variation in explaining interindividual differences in drug response. Much of research has been directed in identifying and assessing the importance of genetic differences (polymorphisms) in genes involved in drug transport (including drug receptors), and drug metabolism. The technologies here include microarrays and real-time quantitative PCR.

Drug Targets

The goal of this article is to examine the technologies that underlie discovery of molecular mechanisms and genetic specificity. Both endeavors are interconnected in that genes identified in gene expression studies that play an important role in drug response may prove to be useful targets for studies to examine how polymorphisms in those genes affect drug response. Similarly, genes implicated as playing a role in patient drug response may identify new pathways associated with the molecular response to a drug.

That different individuals respond differently to the same drugs is a longstanding observation. Factors such as diet, age, sex, concomitant diseases, and other medications are all known to alter how a patient responds to a drug. With the advent of the human genome project, it is now becoming possible to assess the role genetics play in patient variability in drug response. Specifically, how genetic differences in genes that code for proteins involved in drug metabolism, drug transport, or drug receptors determine drug pharmacokinetics and pharmacodynamics. Polymorphisms in humans (as is the case for most organisms) consist largely of:

1. Small insertions or deletions (indels)—usually 10s–1000s of base pairs.
2. Microsatellites (simple sequence repeats, simple tandem repeats)—regions of DNA composed of short two, three, or four nucleotides repeated 2–50 times.
3. Single nucleotide repeats (SNPs)—single base pair substitutions, estimated to occur every 100–300bp. Any two individuals differ at 3 million sites in a genome of three billion bp.

While all three types of polymorphisms have been identified in human genes responsible for drug response, SNPs are the most numerous and have become the target of intense study.

Large-scale programs are underway to identify all the SNPs segregating in human populations (SNP discovery) to discover and document their effects. This area of pharmacogenomics is progressing rapidly along a number of parallel research paths: (i) to identify new genes involved in drug response; (ii) to uncover polymorphisms in these genes and the many genes already known to play a role in drug response; and (iii) to assess the clinical relevance if any of discovered polymorphisms. These areas of research are expanding at a pace that makes just keeping up with the reviews difficult. The best source for timely information concerning genetic polymorphisms and drug response are the databases accessible via the internet. The two most comprehensive, up-to-date are the Online Mendelian Inheritance in Man (OMIM) maintained by the National Center for Biotechnology Information (NCBI) and the Pharmacogenomics and Pharmacogenetics Knowledge Base (PharmGKB). The OMIM database is the repository for all data concerning human genes and genetic diseases. OMIM has textual information and references with links to Medical Literature Analysis and Retrieval System (MEDLINE) and all the many additional related resources at NCBI including sequence data, genetic maps, and SNP data. PharmGKB is an integrated database providing clinical, pharmacokinetic, pharmacodynamic, genotypic, and molecular function data for human genetic polymorphisms and drugs. Both databases are open to the public and are the best source for up-to-date information concerning genes and drug response.

Genotyping

DNA sequencing is the predominant technology employed for the discovery of SNPs and other polymorphisms. Sequencing efforts are most often directed at exons and the flanking regions of specific genes or gene families, less so for the more difficult-to-define regulatory regions upstream of the gene. Once polymorphisms are identified, it is necessary to characterize their frequencies in human populations. This is often accomplished by sequencing some subset of the National Institute of General Medical Sciences (NIGMS) Human Genetic cell repository (the Coriell set) that includes samples for most of the distinct populations across the globe.

Genotyping techniques include older methods like restriction fragment length polymorphism (RFLP) analysis of PCR products and PCR amplification of microsatellites. For SNPs, several recent high-throughput technologies are available including (i) quantitative PCR using fluorescent probes; (ii) microarrays; (iii) pyrosequencing; (iv) invader assays; and (v) matrix- assisted laser desorption/ionization-time-of-flight mass spectrometry (MALDI-TOF). The technologies vary greatly in their speed, cost,, and limitations.

Gene Expression

Microarrays

Studies to identify and characterize patterns of gene expression provide insight into the underlying biochemical and molecular mechanisms of drug response. In that drug response, like most human traits, is the result of the interactions of multiple genes as well as environmental factors, and is necessary to examine actions of many genes simultaneously. Fortunately, the technologies now exist to conduct such studies. The genome-wide assessments of transcriptional events involved in drug response will provide the new foundations for more mechanistic-based studies of the molecular and physiological basis of effects and disposition of therapeutic agents.

Genomic technologies like microarrays and real-time PCR are quickly becoming standard exploratory tools in drug discovery, drug development, and clinical trials. Microarrays allow for the large scale and largely exploratory examination gene expression, which can then be followed by more quantitative measurements using real-time PCR.

Microarrays are now widely available from a number of commercial vendors and university core facilities. Densities of gene targets on a single array can range from 100s to well over 100,000 complementary DNAs (cDNAs) or oligonucleotides, providing an estimate of gene expression ranging from nearly the entire transcriptsome to smaller pathway-specific groups of genes. Arrays can be composed of either short (20–70 bp) oligonucleotides or longer PCR-generated gene segments. The trend is toward short oligonucleotides, as these can be chosen to be gene specific and therefore lessen the chance cross talk among genes having similar sequences (for example the P450 genes).

Gene-specific oligonucleotides can be synthesized directly on silicon chips using photochemical technology, printed on nylon membranes using ink-jet technology, or robotically spotted on glass slides or nylon membranes. Larger gene segments (cDNAs) are spotted onto glass slides or nylon membranes. These arrays are then probed simultaneously with labeled cDNAs reverse transcribed from the different mRNA pools of interest. For some formats (Affmetrix, SuperArray's Oligo GEArray), the cDNAs are used to synthesize labeled cRNAs as probes. Labeling can be done using isotope [P^{32} or P^{33} labeled Deoxycytidine Triphosphate (dCTP)], fluorescent dyes (Cy3 or CY5), or chemiluminescence (often biotin-labeled dUTPs). Results of these array experiments consist of image files containing intensity values (minus some assessment of background) resulting from the hybridization of labeled cDNAs or cRNAs to the "*genes*" on the array. Typical experiments result in the measurement of gene expression for 100s–1000s of genes replicated for each treatment, time point, dosage, etc.

The statistical methods applied to microarray analyses can be divided into two broad classifications reflecting two different desired outcomes. The first group of analyses concerns the identification of a subset of genes from the many thousands assayed in an experiment that exhibits significantly altered gene expression owing to the experimental conditions. The second broad group of analyses, often referred to as "*data mining*," use intensive computational methods (clustering algorithms, self-organizing maps, and principal component analysis) to identify patterns of gene expression. Within this second group, there are generally two different types of analysis representing distinctly different goals. In many cases, the goal is to classify or cluster genes into groups showing similar patterns of expression. Because these techniques do not provide any additional information to the computational algorithm other than the normalized intensities values, they are referred to as unsupervised approaches. Examples include cluster analysis, k-means clustering and self-organizing maps. In contrast to these clustering methods, researchers often seek to group samples into functional classes (for example diseased vs. normal tissues) based upon gene expression patterns.

The ultimate goal is to identify a subset of genes, which will allow the researcher to make predictions or assignments of unknown samples based upon gene expression patterns. Because the algorithms are provided with both intensity data as well as additional data in terms of classification groups, such methods are referred to as supervised approaches. The interpretation of microarray data is complicated by our incomplete knowledge of the complexity of biological systems (for example, the multitude of possible gene interactions) and our lack of a comprehensive understanding of life's organization at the molecular level. For example, the relationship between assessed mRNA levels as identified in microarray experiments and the concentrations of the respective proteins may be complex, or more often unknown. Further, the analysis and interpretation of the results from microarrays experiments are complicated by the lack of standardization of both the collection of these data and the statistical procedures used to assess significance.

This has resulted in reports of poor concordance of microarray data generated from different platforms (oligos and cDNA arrays) and manufacturers, though others have reported good concordance between different oligonucleotide array platforms and quantitative PCR. As is the case for any new technology, there is a need for caution in interpreting the data until uniform methods of data collection and analysis are standardized. Microarrays have become important tools in assessing gene expression responses in chemotherapy, development of drug resistance, pharmacodynamics, and transcriptional profiling to monitor patient outcomes and drug efficacy.

Quantitative Real-Time PCRs

Microarray experiments are, by their very nature, exploratory exercises. The extreme complexity of life's processes combined with the many sources of error associated with the microarray technology itself yields data, which even under the most controlled conditions are fuzzy. Microarray results should always be validated using more quantitative methods before conclusions are drawn for any specific gene. Recent technologies for assessing specific mRNA levels for individual genes are based upon the PCR. All procedures begin first with the use of the enzyme reverse transcriptase (RT) to convert the mRNA pool into a presumed representative pool of cDNAs. Through the use of intercalating DNA dyes or fluorogenic probes, the amount of DNA accumulating with each cycle of the PCR amplification process can be quantified.

Monitoring DNA quantities in real time allows researchers to estimate the initial, starting concentration of a given gene target based upon the amplification profiles. Thus from tissue samples as small as a few cells, it is possible to estimate the number of mRNAs present for a given gene. DNA dyes like SYBR Green are the simplest methodologies to implement requiring only the addition of the dye to an already optimized PCR protocol. However, DNA dyes are non-specific, thus any PCR product will result in a signal, and thus additional steps must be included in the protocol to insure that only the PCR product of interest is being synthesized and quantified. In contrast, fluorogenic probes can be designed to anneal to only a specific gene target. The design of fluorogenic probes generally consists of two dyes, one of which reduces or eliminates (quencher dye) the fluorescent signal of the second dye (reporter dye) when held in close molecular proximity to one another. This can be accomplished by placing the two dyes on either end of a single oligonucleotide that then hybridizes to the appropriate gene target within the region being amplified.

Fluorescence increases with each amplification cycle as the fluorescent probe is cleaved by DNA polymerase during amplification, thus freeing the dyes (TAQMAN assay) or when the probe assumes a hairpin loop conformation when not bound to the PCR product (Molecular Beacons). Other techniques incorporate the dyes into one of the PCR primers (Scorpion Primers) or incorporate self-quenching primers requiring with only one fluorophore (LUX Primers). Databases are now available with fluorogenic probe and primer sequences for a variety of genes in humans, mice/rats, and other species. Real-time quantitative PCR has been used to examine the kinetics of gene expression in response to specific drugs and to examine the role of drug transporters and/or metabolizing enzymes in drug distribution.

As noted above, this technology's real advantage is in confirming and extending the findings of microarray studies. Because PCR requires only minute samples, it is possible to assess gene expression for specific tissues or cells. The reduced costs of PCR assays also make it possible to monitor gene expression across many more time points under different dosage regimes. Finally, real-time PCR is also rapidly becoming an important means of genotyping for single nucleotide polymorphisms using allele-specific primers.

The technologies that are the driving force behind pharmacogenomics hold great promise in ultimately understanding the molecular mechanisms that underlie drug action with the dual goals of identifying new drug targets and improving the ones we have, and elucidating the role of genetics in interpatient variability in drug response. In early 2005, the technologies for collecting the data on genomic scales far outpace our ability to analyze them. Developments in data handling and statistics are desperately needed and are the basis for the growth of bioinformatics. It should be kept in mind that given our extremely limited knowledge of life's workings on the molecular level, the field of pharmacogenomics must be viewed as an exploratory endeavor with all the seemingly contradictory data that comes with nearly blind explorations. Hopefully continued work will provide the understanding needed to unravel the nature of medical therapeutics and the ailments that trouble humankind.

5

Regulatory Perspectives on Pharmacogenomics

Regulatory perspectives on pharmacogenomics (PGx) have been presented in the literature over the past several years to focus attention on an emerging technology that has the potential to make targeted treatments more widely available to physicians and patients. In this chapter, PGx will be used broadly to collectively describe all of the interindividual variations in the whole genome or candidate gene single-nucleotide polymorphism (SNP) maps, haplotype markers and alterations in gene expression or inactivation that may be correlated with clinical response. We intend that PGx encompass the more narrow science of pharmacogenetics (PGt), which refers to the study of interindividual variations in DNA sequence related to drug absorption and disposition (pharmacokinetics) or drug action (pharmacodynamics) including polymorphic variation in genes that encode the functions of transporters, metabolizing enzymes, receptors, and other proteins. We will use the term PGx tests to refer to an assay to study these interindividual variations in conjunction with drug development and therapeutics. It is well known that there is a major problem in the health care system in the United States related to providing new drugs that are effective and relatively safe in a wide diversity of patients with undifferentiated diseases whose individual dose–response relationship varies based on genetic, disease, environmental, and life-style factors. While many may argue over the magnitude of the problem or its root causes, few can deny that a problem exists.

There is increasing evidence for many drugs that genetic factors play a proportionally greater role in causing interindividual variability than other non-genomic factors. Advances in the technology to identify and measure genomic biomarkers related to the pathophysiology of diseases have led many to envision many more targeted drug/test combinations (e.g., HER 2neu coupled with trastuzumab) that are directed to specific patient subsets in the population as defined by their gene variants. From the perspective of the U.S. Food and Drug Administration (FDA), the pharmaceutical industry is facing a "*pipeline problem.*" This perception is based on the evidence that in 2002, the FDA received only 21 submissions for new molecular entities (NMEs) intended for marketing approval. This was more than a 50% decline from the NME submissions received in 1996 and the lowest number submitted over a 10-year period. Of serious concern, is the fact that this decline in NME productivity occurred despite a 2.5-fold increase in the U.S. pharmaceutical R&D spending over the same 10-year period. The same observations have been made regarding the productivity of the pharmaceutical industry in Europe and in other developed countries. Furthermore, it has been estimated that to develop a single, successful new chemical entity now costs in excess of 800 million dollars including opportunity costs: the average

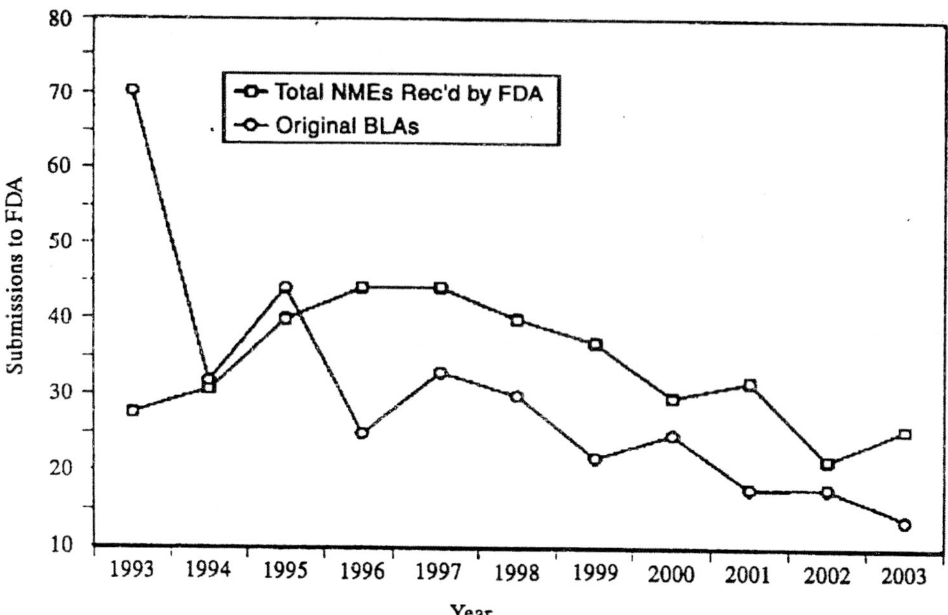

Fig. 5.1. The number of submissions of new drug applications (NDAs) for new molecular entities (NMEs) and the number of submissions of biologics license applications (BLAs) to FDA over a 10-year period.

time taken to do so is 8 to 10 years. The clinical component of the overall cost of new drug development is approximately 58% or 400 million dollars. A significant amount of these dollars go towards supporting the phase-3 randomized controlled trials (RCT) that provide the most convincing evidence of a drug product's safety and efficacy. However, from a recent report, one can estimate the failure rate in phase-3 trials to be approximately 50%, although the failure rate is dependent on the therapeutic area, being higher, for example, in oncology and lower in infectious diseases. The system for developing NMEs is not broke but it is in need of significant improvement. Until the drug development and regulatory process itself, and the translation of new discoveries into effective medicines, catches up with the rapid pace of technological advances in science, it is doubtful that significant improvements can be made.

Variability in Drug Response

Variability in drug response is a major barrier to successful drug development. As Sir William Osler said in 1892 about the practice of medicine, "if it were not for the great variability among individuals, medicine might as well be a science and not an art." PGx can provide the scientific tools that enable us to explore the pathophysiological mechanisms for these differences in drug response at the molecular level. We expect that there will be an increase in the public demand for more science and less art in the search for better and more effective therapies to reduce the morbidity and mortality of chronic diseases such as hypertension and cancer. In order to improve the "art" and the productivity of the drug development process, PGx can improve the predictability of preclinical safety studies and clinical safety and efficacy trials. A key to increasing R&D success is identifying failures early in the drug development process and reducing attrition in phase-3, before the high costs of late-phase clinical trials are incurred by a sponsor. This is an important achievement because the average size of a phase-3 clinical trial has nearly tripled in the last 20 years. It simply does not make much sense to wait until a phase-3 trial fails to try and figure out why and how to design the next trial; that is expensive and time-consuming. It's typical that each phase-3 trial is preceded by a much longer preclinical and early

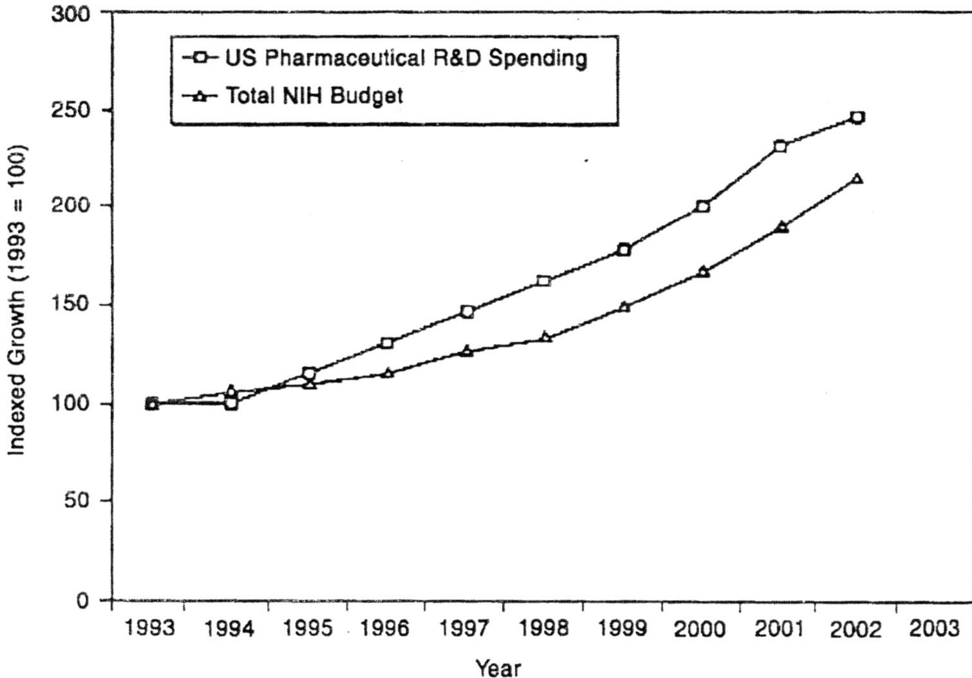

Fig. 5.2. The 10-year trend in biomedical research spending as reflected by the National Institutes of Health budget and by the pharmaceutical companies research and development investment.

clinical work-up of the drug, so what is needed is an increased ability to predict phase-3 success or failure, aimed at the preclinical and early clinical time period. For example, in terms of cost, a 10% improvement in predicting failure before large-scale phase-3 clinical trials begin could save approximately 100 million dollars in development costs.

Other opportunities for saving 12 to 21 million dollars in direct development costs can be attained by shifting only 5% of clinical failures from phase-3 to phase-1, or by shifting 1/4 of failures from phase-2 to phase-1. The major causes of attrition of drugs in late-phase clinical trials are either lack of efficacy or concerns about safety although drug development is also terminated for commercial reasons. In order to achieve increases in productivity and success, effective scientific development tools, such as PGx tests, are needed to predict product performance, whether it be success or failure, with a high degree of certainty, both early and reliably in the development process. For example, pharmacogenomic biomarkers can be used to identify potential responders. By stratifying patients by biomarker status in phase-2 clinical trials, populations with a high probability of response can be identified, thereby simplifying phase-3 trials and increasing their probability of success.

Clearly, modern innovative tools are needed to predict the performance and manufacturing quality of 21st century products. While it seems that everyone agrees with this premise, the problem is that the drug development process is no longer able to keep pace with the rate and scope of innovative basic science discoveries. For example, while imaging-based biomarkers are presently being used to develop drugs for Alzheimer's disease, there has not been a successful strategy to correlate imaging with primary clinical endpoints such of cognition and function in order to increase the success rate of new molecules intended to modify disease progression. The tools currently used in drug discovery and development--the so-called "*critical path*" tools—have not incorporated and linked the latest advances in biomarker technology, the basic and information sciences, such as the new knowledge and technologies provided by the rapid development of genomic research, and the clinical sciences to impact the success of drug development and improve the quality of public health substantially. While the reasons underlying failures of drugs in development (especially those failing in late-phase clinical trials), and inefficiencies in the development process in general, are not well understood, many suspect that a lack of understanding of variability in drug response between patients is a key part of the problem. Recent, and rapidly evolving, evidence is beginning to point toward genetic and genomic factors, alone and taken together with environmental factors, as playing a major role in interindividual variability.

The principle of genomic tests is that genetic variation among individuals causes, or correlates, with responses to drugs. Such variations occur frequent enough and that the differences in dose–response are large enough to justify testing before treatment, shortly after beginning treatment, or any time during treatment. It is important to point out that genomic tests are considered as adjunct tools to complement other forms of monitoring in order to better understand the causes of beneficial and adverse responses. Frequently genotyping can be used to more precisely define dosing for an individual patient.

From a clinical perspective, being able to predict failures in therapy or severe adverse events using PGx biomarkers and validated diagnostic tests for important polymorphisms in patient's receptors and/or drug metabolism genes, or in tumor and/or organism genes has the potential to optimize drug selection and/or drug dose *a priori* or much earlier in therapy to increases the probability of more effective therapy and decrease the probability of having a serious adverse event.

FDA's Approach to the Pipeline Problem

In keeping with its mission to advance the public health by helping to speed innovations that make medicines more effective, safer, and more affordable, the FDA issued a white paper on March 16, 2004 entitled "Innovation or Stagnation? Challenge and Opportunity on the Critical Path to New Medical Products". The white paper is a serious attempt by FDA to bring attention and focus to the need for targeted scientific efforts to modernize the tools, techniques, and methods used to evaluate the safety, efficacy, and quality of drug products.

The Critical Path document highlighted examples of the FDA's efforts to improve the critical path, and it discusses future opportunities as well. The public response to the critical path document was extensive and extremely positive, and many individual companies, as well as the trade associations representing the industry, provided many suggestions to FDA on ways to improve the efficiency and success of drug development. The critical path report also describes the urgent need to build coalitions between the constituencies, such as the FDA,NIH, the private sector, and the nation's universities, to modernize the medical product development process—the critical path—to make product development more predictable and less costly, and drug products more effective with greater safety by identifying key problems for targeted solutions.

The critical path is defined in the document as the path from candidate selection to product launch and it defines the potential bottlenecks in the process of bringing a product to market. The focus of critical path is to update the product development infrastructure for drugs, biologics, and devices and the evaluative tools currently used to assess the safety and efficacy of new medical products. Examples of evaluative tools include better pathophysiological cell and/or animal disease state models for preclinical screening of new molecules, and innovative scientific approaches such as the use of Bayesian statistics and adaptive trial design, validation of pathophysiological and/or descriptive biomarkers for clinical trial patient selection (enrichment) and/or as surrogate endpoints of drug effects, and the use of modeling and computer simulation to predict drug and device failures, and improve post-market reporting of implanted device adverse events, that could assist in developing more focused premarket trials. In addition, an important example of a critical path scientific opportunity is *pharmacogenomics* and *pharmacogenetics*, or more specifically, the identification of DNA-based biomarkers or RNA expression profiles that can provide insights into the stage of a disease, disease progression, drug response, and drug dosing requirements.

Advancement of Pharmacogenomics: Part of the FDA's Mission

The FDA's twofold mission includes protecting and advancing public health, and speeding innovations that make medicines and foods more effective, safer, and more affordable. With regard to PGx, the FDA has attempted to assure that the regulatory pathway for moving genomic biomarkers from discovery to clinical practice is articulated clearly. The Agency intends to promote high quality in PGx studies with regard to processes to demonstrate analytical validation, clinical validation, and clinical usefulness, respectively. Beginning in earnest in June 2001, FDA took the lead with several key initiatives in PGx intending to stimulate the exploratory use of PGx technologies in drug development and foster improvements in drug product safety and efficacy. After publication of a forward-looking paper providing a regulatory perspective on the opportunities and challenges of integrating pharmacogenomic in drug development and regulatory decision-making, the FDA has coordinated its efforts both between its own Centers, and with the pharmaceutical and biotechnology industries to convene a series of public PGx workshops. These workshops are a structured, modular approach to bring together stakeholders from industry and academia, and FDA scientists to openly discuss the status of PGx technology, the use of PGx in drug development and therapeutics, and what specific strategies are needed most for using PGx as a tool to facilitate more efficient and effective research along the critical path of drug development. Publications of the proceedings of these workshops are valuable references that lay out where PGx in drug development is currently and what is needed to continue to advance this critical path tool.

Guidances Related to New Drug Development

The culmination of many individual efforts within FDA and the public input derived from the synergistic FDA–Industry co-sponsored workshops led to a significant milestone in the advancement of PGx: the November 2003 publication of the Draft Guidance for Industry: Pharmacogenomic Data Submissions. This guidance was timely, in that there was considerable uncertainty and fear about what FDA would do with exploratory genomic data obtained during the new drug development process, and this was a stumbling block for many pharmaceutical companies. The major concern was that FDA would over-react to non-validated, exploratory genomic biomarkers, take them out of context, misinterpret them, cause delays in drug development, request additional clinical trials, and/or put clinical trials on hold. This concern led to a reluctance of the industry to introduce genomic studies into their drug development plans.

The FDA wanted to breakdown these real or perceived barriers and to motivate drug developers to consider PGx and PGt strategies seriously in their drug development portfolios. The PGx data guidance proposed a new pathway for industry and others to submit non-clinical and clinical exploratory genomic data during the IND period without it undergoing formal regulatory review, and describes the submission format and regulatory review of such data by the Interdisciplinary PGx Review Group (IPRG). It introduced some new concepts related to genomic biomarkers and defined categories of biomarkers, i.e., exploratory, valid, probable valid, and known valid biomarkers. By design, the guidance shied away from presenting very specific recommendations for biomarker validation and formats for submitting genomic data in order not to encumber progress in the field. The FDA recognized that the science is still evolving. Important components of the guidance are three decision algorithms or decision trees based on the categories of biomarkers and the stage of drug development. Generally, most genomic data submitted to FDA to date has been exploratory and not suitable for regulatory decision making.

Such data, e.g., derived from gene expression microarrays, have either no clear pathophysiological correlates, and/or are not critical to entering patients into clinical trials or supporting claims about safety, efficacy, and/or dosing.

Valid biomarkers are defined as those biomarkers measured in an analytical test system with well-established performance characteristics and with an established scientific framework or body of evidence that elucidates the physiologic, pharmacologic, toxicologic, or clinical significance of the test results. Known valid biomarkers are those accepted in the broad scientific community whereas probable valid biomarkers are those that appear to have predictive value for clinical outcomes, but have not yet been widely accepted or independently replicated. The decision trees elucidate when genomic data can be submitted voluntarily, and when submissions of the data are required by FDA regulations. In addition, the guidance describes the format (full report, abbreviated report, synopsis, or voluntary submission) for submitting such data.

It should be noted that the process for industry to submit VGDS to FDA was set up to be through the existing path for IND (or as a pre-IND in some cases) or NDA submissions, which assures the confidentiality of the data. The Genomic Data Submission guidance has been revised as of February 2005 and is awaiting final clearance through the Agency. Along with the finalization of the guidance, FDA has written SOPs to describe the operations of the Interdisciplinary Pharmacogenomic Review Group and the process for submitting VGDS documents. A web site will be available in spring of 2005 to which sponsors and the general public can refer for instructions and information related to VGDS. Since the draft guidance was published, there have been at least a dozen meetings between FDA and industry regarding VGDS. The agenda for these meetings have focused discussion on questions related to the validation of preclinical toxico genomics biomarkers, retrospective analysis of predictive biomarkers of drug safety and efficacy from phase-2 and phase-3 clinical trials, and the prospective designs of clinical PGx studies including study design and data analysis issues.

The FDA hopes that voluntary submissions will benefit both the industry and the Agency and will provide a rational scientific basis for future data standards and genomic policies. Information and knowledge gained from voluntary submissions will be shared publicly across submissions in a way that protects the proprietary interests of companies. The FDA is currently in the process of finalizing the Draft Guidance on Pharmacogenomic Data Submissions and writing two other internal documents that will describe the process for sponsors submitting voluntary genomic data submissions and the roles and responsibilities of the IPRG.

The most recent guidance initiative of the FDA is to articulate the principles and processes associated with drug or biologic and genomic test co-development. Several workshops will have been held to get public input into the key components of such guidance. The key elements of this guidance will focus on analytical performance standards for a genomic test, clinical performance attributes, and approaches to documenting clinical utility. The draft guidance, when released in 2005, will also provide a description of the regulatory pathway for submitting drug/test co-developed products and the framework for inter-Center cooperation to expedite review of such submissions.

Pharmacogenomics in the Process of New Drug Development

Over the past 5 years, PGx studies have become an increasingly greater part of drug development although the extent of inclusion of PGx data in NME submissions has not kept pace with the tremendous and rapid advances in genomic technology and the ability to generate extensive genomic and proteomic data profiles. Drug companies reportedly collect DNA samples from subjects in approximately 80% of clinical studies so that they can have the chance to identify genomic biomarkers of drug safety, efficacy, and dosing. The promise of PGx lies in its potential to identify sources of interindividual variability in drug response (both efficacy and safety) that arise from genomic differences in disease pathophysiology and/or genomic differences in drug pharmacology. The PGx biomarkers can serve many different purposes depending on the context and questions at hand, such as: (a) entry criteria for a clinical trial, (b) indicator of disease status, (c) patient stratification, (d) drug efficacy predictor test, (e) predictor test for adverse events, (f) test for monitoring drug response, and/or (g) guide to dose selection. PGx can also facilitate product differentiation in the marketplace by improving the benefit/risk profile compared with other similar products. Of course, whether or not to recommend mandatory or optional genotyping, which would be clinically useful, would need to be determined for each drug.

The current "*gold standard*" for evidence of drug efficacy is the randomized, adequate and well-controlled clinical trial. As mentioned previously, the number of phase-3 trials that fail to meet their prespecified acceptance criteria is around 50% as reported by PhRMA. So clearly, the current practice of controlled clinical trials is inadequate. Even when a study demonstrates an overall significant ($p < 0.05$) clinical effect, the efficacy signal often arises from a subset of patients, with other patients, in effect, being non-responders.

Two recent examples of this phenomenon from the field of oncology are provided below.

Gefitinib

Gefitinib is a tyrosine kinase inhibitor that targets the tumor protein, epidermal growth factor receptor (EGFR), and was approved by FDA for advanced non-small cell lung cancer in May 2003. The overall response rate in the United States was about 10% (n = 216). A subset analysis revealed apparent sources of variability in clinical responsiveness with greater responses observed in women and those with adenocarcinoma (17%) as compared to responses observed in men and smokers (5%). Furthermore, the response rate in Japanese subjects with NSCLC in Japan was approximately 25–30%. Impressively, individual patients of both genders demonstrated dramatic responses. A molecular mechanism underlying gefitinib efficacy was described as activating mutations in the EGFR in which specific deletions or amino acid substitutions around the ATP binding site of gefitinib increased EGFR signaling and susceptibility to inhibition by gefitinib. In a small trial, specific mutations were identified in eight of nine gefitinib responders and were not identified in any of the seven non-responders. Related to the variability in gefitinib, lung cancer cells with mutations were 10 times more responsive than normal cells to the medicine, and mutations were more common in tumor cells from Japanese patients. This may explain the higher efficacy response rate in Japan. It is not hard to imagine how a diagnostic test for EGFR positivity can be integrated into treatment decisions and as a guide as to when and in whom to use the drug.

Erlotinib

Erlotinib is an EGFR tyrosine kinase inhibitor approved by FDA in December 2004 for advanced or metastatic non-small cell lung cancer as second line monotherapy. The approved dose was 150 mg/day although doses of 25 and 100mg were also studied. From the clinical trial data, the median survival for erlotinib treatment (n = 488) was 6.7 months as compared to a placebo (n = 243) median survival of 4.7 months. The percentage of patients alive at 12 months was either 31.2% (erlotinib) or 21.5% (placebo). The median progression free symptom time was 9.9 weeks for erlotinib and 7.9 weeks for placebo. The medicine was clearly effective in the clinical trial general population compared to placebo. A subset analysis based on EGFR protein expression status found that the relative tumor response rate was 11.6% (EGFR + patients) vs. 3.2% (EGFR – patients), while the tumor response rate in placebo treated patients was similar to the response in the EGFR – patients. The survival hazard ratio for EGFR + patients was 0.65 demonstrating a survival benefit vs. placebo, while the survival hazard ratio for EGFR – patients was 1.01, indicating no survival benefit. However, the prevalence of EGFR positivity is thought to be approximately 50–55% so that it is likely that the positive response in the general population may have been due entirely to those patients who were EGFR positive. Had the prevalence of EGFR positive status been, for example, 10–20%, the trial in the general population may have failed. Erlotinib was approved for all patients, not just EGFR + patients, for several reasons: (a) the EFGR status was unknown in a large percentage of patients, (b) the EGFR assay was not validated appropriately, (c) the relatively small numbers of patients in the EGFR– subset, and (d) the confidence intervals for tumor response and survival overlapped. This example demonstrates how a differential disease diagnosis, based on EGFR protein expression patterns, can be used as a basis for future enrichment trials or as a diagnostic to identify those patients most likely to respond or not.

There are several other additional cases in oncology in which the efficacy response to medicines has been associated with genomic biomarkers, e.g., the well-known selective response to trastuzumab (Herceptin) in patients whose tumor overexpresses the HER 2 protein, the response in patients with chronic myelogenous leukemia to imatinib depends on the BRA/ABL trans- location, and the response to cetuximab in patients with colon cancer depends on the EGFR protein expression. Each of these examples demonstrates how a mechanistic knowledge of PGx–clinical phenotype relationships gleaned from earlier drug development projects can be used to improve the efficiency of development of second generation drug molecules, both with and without a diagnostic test.

There are also examples of the important role that genomic biomarkers can play in drug development outside of oncology such as the demonstration that the response to PEG-interferon in patients with hepatitis C depends on the virus genotype and the clinical response to certain CNS drugs and drug classes (selective serotonin reuptake inhibitors) depends on the receptor genotype.

Atomoxetine

A recent example illustrates the role that PGt played in the labeling of a new drug is the case of atomoxetine (Strattera). This drug was approved by FDA in January 2003 for attention deficit/hyperactive disorder with a fixed dose of 0.5 mg/kg to be titrated up to 1.2 mg/kg. The drug is metabolized by cytochrome P450 2D6 (CYP2D6) with a clearance of 0.35 L/hr/kg in extensive metabolizers (EMs) and 0.03 L/hr/kg in poor metabolizers (PMs). The ratio (PM/EM) of the area-under-curve (AUC) for plasma atomoxetine was approximately 10. The sponsor did a sensible analysis of adverse events in clinical trials by looking at a post-facto stratification of patient subsets defined by genotype. The frequency of adverse drug reactions (ADR), primarily insomnia and irritability, was 9% in PMs and 6% in EMs. There were no major differences in serious ADRs between PMs and EMs. The label of atomoxetine mentions CYP2D6 in seven different sections including those describing pharmacokinetics, drug–drug interactions, adverse events and laboratory tests. However, the evidence did not warrant recommending that a pharmacogenetic test for CYP2D6 status be done before prescribing the drug, but it did provide descriptive information that could be used along with other observations (e.g., an adverse event) to guide clinician decisions about an individual's need for dosing adjustment. This example demonstrates the value that pharmacogenetic information in a package insert can bring to the use of the drug, including knowledge related to genotype (e.g., CYP 2D6 alleles), phenotype (e.g., poor metabolizers), and clinical outcomes (e.g., adverse events) that can increase the quality of clinician's decisions about individualizing drug treatment.

Selective Serotonin Reuptake Inhibitors (SSRIs)

An emerging example of PGx being used to differentiate a chronic disease is in the field of depression with the development of new SSRIs. These drugs, along with supportive care, represent the standard of care of major depressive disorders (MDD). MDD are CNS diseases caused by underling complex polygenic traits. Genetic heterogeneity in the disease, and polymorphism in the 5-HTT receptor, which is the selective site of action of SSRIs, leads to high degree of intersubject variability in the clinical phenotype. Many clinical trials fail to either demonstrate a dose–response relationship and/or beat placebo partly because of the subjective and variable nature of the empirical clinical endpoints, the relatively high placebo response rate (~50%) and the variable duration of treatment needed to assess clinical efficacy response (~6 weeks). Clearly non-responders to SSRIs (~30–50% of entered patents) reduce the effective study power.

There are no valid or probable valid biomarkers to predict who will and who will not respond more favorably to SSRIs vs. placebo. Since the adverse event rate is relatively high (3.5%), patients who are non-responders have a different benefit/risk ratio than responders and it would be beneficial to differentiate between the responder and non-responder phenotypes. Recently genotypes were identified as having two forms of the 5-HTT gene, which regulates brain serotonin levels: either a short form (S allele) or a long form (L allele). In case control studies, clinical response scores (HAM-D and CGI-I) defined sequentially over time after dosing showed a significant difference in response between S/S and L/L groups. The L/L genotype responded more rapidly to model SSRIs such as sertraline, and a higher percentage of the L/L genotypes were classified as responders. The important implications of these findings are that clinical trials for new SSRIs may stratify patient populations on the basis of carrying either a S- or L-allele. Further, enriching trials with the L/L genotype will provide the maximum probability of a successful proof-of-concept study and greater success in phase-3 trials.

Revising Physician Labeling of Previously Approved Drug Products

Translating PGx from bench to bedside (or discovery to marketability) is a multidisciplinary problem, involving private and public sector philosophical, societal, cultural, behavioral, educational, drug development, scientific expertise, communication, and clinical practice issues. For drugs whose clinical activity is highly influenced by genetic factors, but were developed before the rapid growth of PGx, the Agency has decided it is worthwhile to question, if not change, the wording in drug labels. It recognizes that integrating PGx into therapeutics for previously approved drugs where there is an established history and practice of use represents a major challenge for regulatory agencies and other stakeholders in PGx. In addition, until recently, there were no FDA-approved tests for discerning the genotypes of CYP450 enzyme function.

Labeling regulations (21 CFR 201-57) related to tests to guide therapy are clear. If evidence is available to support the safety and effectiveness of a drug only in selected subgroups of the larger population with a disease, the labeling shall describe the evidence and identify specific tests needed for selection and monitoring of patients who need the drug.

The FDA has a long-standing interest in "*individualization factors*" such as those defined by intrinsic (e.g., age, gender, race, and renal dysfunction) and extrinsic factors (e.g., food, co-administered drugs, smoking, and alcohol). At best, these factors are crude differentiators of patient subsets at greater of lesser risk of toxicity or loss of efficacy. The Agency believes that an appreciation of controllable sources of variability in drug action and potential injury to patients should be achieved prior to the marketing of new pharmaceutical products. Information on these important co-variates influencing drug safety and efficacy are generally reported in various section of the product package insert and are in need of constant updating as post-marketing experience with the drug increases over time. The value of PGx in improving individualization of therapy depends on the ability to demonstrate a correlation between important clinical outcomes and individual genotype as expressed by validated biomarkers. It is unlikely that drug manufacturers of established drugs will be willing to subsidize prospective clinical trials to provide evidence of the clinical validity and utility of CYP 450 drug response predictor tests. Thus, the Agency has instead relied upon a systematic analysis of extensive literature data from case-control studies or prospective exploratory trials, and its own Med Watch reports, as well as prospective, randomized controlled trials wherever available. Understanding the strength, quality, and characteristics of the genotype–phenotype relationship is the first step towards developing a predictive test to optimize therapeutics on an individual basis.

In December 2004 a milestone in the evolution of clinical applications of PGx was reached. The FDA approved the first in vitro diagnostic test for CYP450 enzymes based on microarray technology (Affymetrix). The chip-based test provides a way for the physician to measure individual variations in drug metabolism genes for CYP 2D6 and 2C19. These CYPs metabolize approximately 25–30% of all clinically approved drugs including tricyclic antidepressants, CNS-active drugs, beta-blockers, and proton-pump inhibitors. The significance of this test is that approximately 25–30% of all approved prescription drugs are substrates for these enzymes. Several drugs metabolized by these enzymes are the frequent cause of adverse events thought to be related to excess systemic drug exposure following the administration of the usual doses. The chip can be used to analyze 29 polymorphisms for CYP 2D6 and two polymorphisms for CYP 2C19 and thus can be used to genotype nearly 100% of the global patient population. Physicians can get the genotype results within 1 day and can use the results of this diagnostic to help individualize treatment doses for individual patients receiving drugs metabolized predominantly through these enzymatic pathways. Genotyping for gene variants of 2D6 and 2C19 usually only has to be done once per patient and the results could be used to reduce doses of many drugs metabolized by the same enzymes.

An unknown issue is what will be the pace of physician and patient acceptance. It is well known that there is a gap between PGx research and physician prescribing decisions, and the best way to achieve knowledge transfer and translation is not entirely clear. Further, the additional information that PGx provides makes writing a prescription more complex. Models for translating PGx research results into applications in patient care are sorely needed. Uptake of new tests, genomic or not, typically must overcome significant medical, social, and cultural barriers to become established as a standard of care and in addition, reimbursement issues come into play. With the CYP 2D6 and 2C19 testing, the important considerations as to the decision to use a PGx test or not include the following:

1. What extent of intersubject variability dose–PK relationship, what percent of drug metabolism via the polymorphic pathway, and what shape of the dose–response curves for efficacy and safety should justify genotyping? Even with good genotype–phenotype associations, these basic questions will be made more complex by considering that the dose–PK relationship will be influenced by many demographic, environmental, and drug interaction factors. Dose–response considerations will also be affected by intended use of the drug (many drugs have multiple uses), the patient's concomitant drug therapy and disease subset (many disease have a range of clinical phenotypes), all of which have the potential change the dose–response relationship and influence the impact the genotyping will have on benefit/risk.
2. Why would genotyping tests be ordered and when? The intended use of the test is usually to reduce adverse events by more precise dosing in at risk genotypes defined by the tests. Possible scenarios include a priori testing followed by tailored initial dosing in patients at-risk, e.g., patients with heart disease who need a beta-blocker, or patients with atrial arrhythmias who need warfarin, testing only if unexpected toxicity occurs at a relatively low dose or if there is an overt lack of efficacy at maximum approved doses. Genotyping will provide complementary information to make better therapeutic decisions in these situations.
3. What dose is appropriate as defined by genotype? It is difficult to answer this question quantitatively because there are very little prospective clinical trial data on genotype-based dose–response relationships or prospective randomized, adequate and well- controlled clinical trials that have been

designed to answer the question about optimal doses for different genotypes. In lieu of controlled trials, dosing adjustment similar to other patient subsets, i.e., based dosing adjustment on the relative exposure in various genotypes using area-under-the-plasma drug level curve (AUC). However, it must also be recognized that often the dose suggested by increases in AUC is greater than the doses actually needed in patients titrated to desired dose based on clinical endpoints, an observation that points to the fact that many non-genetic factors contribute to variability in dose–response for most drugs.

The atomoxetine example presented earlier and the entry of the Amplichip into clinical practice settings also brings to mind several other challenges that face sponsors, regulatory agencies, and clinicians in translating genotype information from research to the clinic. Accurate tests for CYP enzyme alleles are effectively diagnostics of hepatic enzyme function and not clinical response. Medicines are used to treat symptoms, not enzyme function. Therefore, interpretation of the test results is critical to translate this PGx knowledge into wisdom as it applies to drug dosing requirements for individual patients. Some type of computer-assisted analysis to test results (i.e., a bioinformatics solutions) is needed to provide the physician some guidance on how to use the data similar to what has been used commercially with AIDS resistance diagnostic tests.

Specifically, with regard to physician labeling, there are some other complex decisions to be made. Some examples include:

1. What is the best way to define poor metabolizers in a research setting? The PM is a phenotype that can be also be determined in non-genomics ways by the urinary metabolic ratio, the observed AUC or plasma clearance of the drug in different genotype subsets. Frequently there is overlap between the phenotypes used to define poor (PM), intermediate (IM), and extensive (EM) metabolizers. For example, there are more than 40 alleles of CYP2D6 with about 25% of them having greatly decreased or null activity. There is also significant variability in the frequency of null alleles of CYP2D6, and other polymorphic enzymes such as CYP2C19 in different racial or ethnic groups. So, the open question is what alleles should be studied in drug development, and how should this information be translated into a product's package insert for use by physicians? Ideally, all common alleles should be studied in a way that includes patients of ancestral heritage in the general population that is expected to be prescribed the drug.
2. How should PGx information be reported in the label? The consideration are (a) whether or not to report only phenotype data (e.g., PMs and EMs), or specific alleles of CYP2D6 (e.g., *2, *3, and *10), and (b) how much information should be reported in light of who will interpret the significance of these data with respect to dosing, safety, and efficacy? Perhaps as commercial tests approved by FDA increase, there will also be an increase in clinical consultants (e.g., laboratory clinicians, clinical pharmacologists, and/or clinical pharmacists) who will interpret genotype information in the context of the total patient care. Perhaps point-of-care proprietary software will interpret the genotype data and classify the results as those coming from a PM, IM, or EM in the physician's office.
3. If PGx information is included in the label of a drug product in a way that gives physicians and patients an option to have a genomic test done as part of therapy, this raises other translational issues that include knowledge of the test availability, the quality of the test results, its turnaround time and costs, including reimbursement options, and as mentioned the proper interpretation of test results.

Despite a widespread recognition of the challenges above, and with all the reports of important gene effects on differential diagnosis and/or dose–response, there have been relatively little attempts to create models to translate of this information into drug development and even less into clinical practice.

The FDA believes that there is value in applying long-established drug response predictive genetic biomarkers to older, marketed drugs in the post-marketing period in order to improve their risk/benefit ratio by optimizing or individualizing dosing. Examples of older drugs that could benefit from PGx are 6-mercaptopurine (6MP), azathioprine, and 6-thioguanine, or 6TG, (each substrates for thiopurine methyltransferase or TPMT), irinotecan (a substrate for uridine diphosphate glucoronosyltransferase or UGT), and warfarin (a substrate for CYP2C9). Each of these drugs has a narrow therapeutic range, wide interindividual variability in pharmacokinetics, wide range of dosing requirements and frequent and serious safety problems.

The genes of each the enzymes mentioned above can exist in one of several isoforms (e.g., TPMT*2, UGT1A1*28 and CYP2C9*3) and these enzymes are mostly found in either red blood cells (in the case of TPMT) or the liver (for UGT and CYP2C9). Certain mutations in these isoforms, or gene variants, produce different phenotypes but most important to drug dosing is the poor metabolizer phenotype that results in heightened exposure to either the parent drug or a major metabolite, or reduced exposure to an active metabolite (e.g., morphine from codeine administration).

In July 2003, the FDA Pediatric Subcommittee of the Oncology Drug Advisory Committee (ODAC) was presented a comprehensive amount of relevant research data from the scientific literature and from FDA files to consider and asked to discuss whether or not the package insert of 6MP should be updated to include information on TPMT genotypes. 6MP was approved decades ago for use in children with acute lymphoblastic leukemia (ALL) and, taken orally together with methotrexate and/or other chemotherapeutic agents, is the backbone of continuation therapy. Dose intensity of 6MP is a major determinant of both event free survival (efficacy) and neutropenia (safety). The clearance of 6MP, and hence exposure, is dependent on its conversion to 6-TG which, in turn, is metabolized via the TPMT pathway. More than 11% of the Caucasian population is heterozygous or homozygous carriers of TPMT alleles. There are three major genotypes, each with a range of TPMT activity (high, intermediate, and low), and each with a different relative risk of developing neutropenia when administered the standard dose of 6MP (50 mg/m^2).

The poor metabolizer genotype, with an incidence of 1:300, accumulates excess 6-TG that is nearly certain to lead to severe and potentially fatal bone-marrow toxicity. It has been recommended that the usual dose of 6MP be reduced by 80–90% for the PM genotype to reduce the risk of neutropenia. Based on the evidence presented in July 2003, the Subcommittee considered the consequences of a label revision thoroughly, and in the end recommended that the label of 6MP should be updated with current information on TPMT genotypes, but stopped short of recommending that testing for TPMT status be mandatory before prescribing the 6MP. The experts on the subcommittee considered many factors in making their recommendation. Some important considerations that were discussed include: (a) the scarcity of prospective clinical trials to support specific recommendations about dose reduction in patients who were either heterozygous or homozygous, (b) the wide interindividual variability in TPMT activity in patients who had one variant TPMT allele, and the subsequent risk of reducing effectiveness if doses are reduced unnecessarily, (c) the potential benefit and cost of TPMT genotyping as compared to phenotyping based on TPMT activity in red blood cells coupled with measurement of neutropenia (drop in neutrophils), and (d) the widespread availability and cost of TPMT testing. As a result of the committee recommendations, the FDA and sponsors have negotiated updated label language to include the evidence of the genotype–phenotype correlation and the significance to clinical outcome.

More recently (November 2004), the FDA's Clinical Pharmacology Subcommittee (CPSC) met to consider the evidence supporting the clinical significance of UGT1A1 polymorphism in irinotecan treatment of colon cancer. Irinotecan is converted to an active metabolite, SN38, which is then metabolized by UGT1A1. Approximately 10% of the general patient population are deficient in UGT activity (UGT1A1*28 genotype) and because of elevated SN38 exposure, are significantly at risk for developing neutropenia and/or diarrhea. SN38 exposure is the main driver for neutropenia although the evidence for its causing diarrhea is less clear. At the end of the discussion, the advisory committee voted to update the label of irinotecan with additional information on UGT polymorphism and the need to be cautious in dosing irinotecan. The FDA is currently negotiating with the sponsor on the final wording in the label.

These illustrative examples demonstrate that PGx can, in fact, make a contribution to drug safety by guiding towards appropriate dosing. However, translating PGx information from research to clinic for older drugs is in some ways more challenging than for newer drugs for the reasons cited above. The three categories of issues or questions raised as challenges following the atomoxetine example above for new drugs still apply to older or previously approved drugs. However, in addition, there are additional issues or questions.

1. What is the best model to educate clinicians about the advantages and limitations of adopting a PGx test for a drug that they have been using, albeit not optimally, for decades, especially, as in the case of 6MP, where neutropenia or another test (e.g., TPMT activity in red blood cells) has been used phenotypically as a rough guide to reduce the intensity of dosing, or in the case of warfarin where two gene variants (CYP 2C9*2 and CYP 2C9*3) and other demographic, disease, and drug-drug interaction factors, when taken together, account for only 35–40% of intersubject variability?
2. How should the dosing of drugs like 6MP, irinotecan, and warfarin be adjusted, based on genotype, when there is an absence of randomized, controlled clinical trials to demonstrate the efficacy of the reduced dose as some experts have recommended? This is a pertinent question in the case of 6MP where the success rate of event free survival in childhood ALL is nearly 80–85% and evidence supporting the reduction of dose in patients with intermediate TPMT activity is not substantial. Patients with high TPMT activity relative to a given dose may not receive the maximum benefit from the drug because of rapid clearance. The problem of an appropriate reduced dose for irinotecan is complex because the optimally effective dose for the drug in colon cancer has not been well defined and many different dosing schedules are used in practice. On the other hand, prospective trials to determine effective reduced doses may take thousands of patients and many years, and would be costly. For previously approved drugs, especially those that are off patent, it is not clear who would pay for these studies.
3. When is the best time for genotyping patients administered 6MP for their TPMT activity status, irinotecan for their UGT activity, or warfarin for their CYP 2C9 status? Options include routinely genotyping prior to initiation of drug therapy, genotyping within the first week of receiving drug treatment or genotyping only in the case of overt toxicity, or lack of efficacy at the usual and/or maximum recommended doses.

However, as the Pediatric Subcommittee of ODAC pointed out in July 2003, and as the CPSC of the Advisory Committee for Pharmaceutical Sciences also recommended in November 2004, after careful consideration of the genotype-phenotype correlations for 6MP and irinotecan, genotyping is not a substitute for traditional monitoring of white blood cell counts in patients receiving 6MP or irinotecan, but as an adjunct to other clinical measures used to monitor for myelosuppression, or in the case of irinotecan, bilirubin measurements and genotyping, taken together are excellent predictions of a patient's risk for neutropenia. It is recognized that many other clinical factors (age, sex, indication, co-administered drugs, and body size) can influence maintenance doses of these drugs, but genotyping for TPMT or UGT1A1 testing, when combined with other tests and observations, can lead to higher quality decisions about drug selection and drug dosing that will further decrease the risk of severe and preventable bone marrow suppression, neutropenia, and possibly diarrhea (in the case of irinotecan). It is also known that genotyping alone cannot account for all of the observed toxicities of these drugs since there may be rare alleles that are not measured by the genotype tests. The FDA is in the process of revising the irinotecan label based on the recommendations of the CPSC and is deliberating all of these challenges in translating PGt data into useful information for practitioners and their patients.

The FDA has become a proactive and thoughtful advocate of PGx and believes, as a public health Agency, that it has a responsibility to play a leading role in bringing about the translation of PGx, as well as other emerging technologies, from bench to bedside to facilitate drug development and improve the benefit/risk of drug treatments in the marketplace. The FDA also realizes that it can hinder innovation and become a regulatory barrier in the translational process if it is not careful with its guidances, policies, label updates, and procedures.

The Agency hopes that pharmaceutical companies view advances in PGx as an opportunity in new drug development and one kind of investment in R&D that can help bring a fresh approach, and a partial solution, to addressing the "*pipeline*" problem outlined in the FDA Critical Path white paper. We believe that PGx has the potential to revolutionize the drug development process, making it more efficient through targeted enrichment trials, and bringing value to patient care, including more biomarker-based diagnostic or test products to individualize or target therapy with more precision. This may, in time, seem to have taken much longer than was anticipated but there are not an increasing number of examples of targeted therapies beyond Herceptin, and we expect that the pace of PGx will accelerate over the next 5 years.

Regulatory agencies, pharmaceutical companies, the clinical community, third-party payers, and patient advocacy groups are all interested in strategies that can improve the cost, quality, and time of drug development, and reduce the risks associated with drug therapy in patients for both new and previously approved therapies. Clinical guidelines for use of PGx tests or laboratory guidelines for the interpretation of PGx tests are needed, and the FDA is partnering with professional organizations to develop such guidelines. We do not expect that big changes in these areas will happen overnight with one seminal event or be straightforward, but rather will occur in a more evolutionary or iterative manner built upon one successful application of PGx after another, that now seem to be occurring at a rapid rate as exemplified by thiopurines, irinotecan, warfarin, atomoxetine, and the other examples illustrated in this chapter.

We acknowledge that there are and will be many different kinds of challenges in translating PGx from bench to bedside ranging from issues of historical clinical practices, concerns over cost effectiveness, test availability, and reimbursement by third party payers, to issues of biomarker discovery, analytical validation, qualification of clinical performance, health professional education, and adoption of PGx tests into routine clinical practice. But, as we have shown through examples with the promising results with gefitinib, erlotinib, SSRIs, and the tried and true examples of atomoxetine, 6MP, azathioprine, irinotecan, and warfarin, these challenges are being met and overcome to benefit both the science of drug development and the quality of public health. The FDA will be influential in a positive way and should play an important role in collaboration with others in translating the important discoveries of PGx from bench to bedside, and working with collaborators to interpret bedside findings in PGX to what might be needed in bench research to facilitate drug development.

But, regulatory agencies also need to be on guard. We are aware that drug development is a global enterprise, and we live in a small world, and thus international collaboration between regulatory agencies and other private (e.g., World Health Organizations) and national government organizations (e.g., National Institutes of Health), and international government agencies (e.g., EMEA) must continue to work more to harmonize guidance and policies in a way that facilitates and not complicates the drug development process and facilitates the benefits of PGx to patients worldwide. We must also strive more to engage the various stakeholders and constituencies (including Health Maintenance Organizations) in both the private and public sectors in conversation regarding effective strategies to advance PGx through cost-effective, well-conceived clinical outcome studies that can either be randomized, adequate and well controlled, legitimate case-control observational studies, or naturalistic studies with prespecified goals to address the questions of clinical utility of genomic tests. It clearly is in everybody's interest to streamline the pre-approval drug development process (in terms of cost, time, and early attrition), reduce the likelihood of toxicity in the post-approval period and to improve the use of established drugs that have a history of frequent and severe adverse events. We hope that others view the FDA's important initiatives and transparent strategies—the Critical Path white paper, and its advocacy of PGx—as a willingness to work together to link bench discoveries to bedside benefits, and vice-versa, and we look forward to continued involvement with the scientific, medical, and health care community.

6

Applied Pharmacogenomics

The statistics associated with drug development are astonishing. Historically, only one in 5000–10,000 chemicals screened successfully reach the market, only 30% of marketed drugs produce sufficient revenue to recover research and development costs, new drug development requires 12 to 15 years and a $ 500–800 million investment, and 30–50% of drug candidates fail due to toxicity. Each of these factors significantly contributes to the time and cost of drug development. Even incremental increases in the success rate would have favorable economic impacts for all stakeholders including patients, health provider organizations, and drug manufacturers. With ever increasing demands for cheaper drugs with predictable toxicities, pharmaceutical, and biotechnology companies are exploring alternative paradigms for the development of safer, more cost effective drugs. One emerging paradigm suggests that to fully assess the potential adverse health effects of chronic and subchronic exposure to synthetic and natural chemicals, and their interactions, a more comprehensive understanding of the molecular, cellular and tissue level effects is required within the context of the whole organism, its genome, proteome, and metabonome. This strategy, referred to as toxicogenomics, incorporates genomics, proteomics, and metabonomics into traditional toxicological practices, to further elucidate mechanisms of toxicity and the etiology of adverse effects elicited by exposure to drugs, chemicals, and natural products as well as their interactions.

The application of toxicogenomics into mechanistic research, predictive toxicology, and preclinical safety assessment has resulted in the accumulation of a torrent of data which must be accurately and efficiently indexed and archived to facilitate data analysis and the extraction of decision supportive information important to human health and drug development. Borne from this need, applied bioinformatics is the application of information and statistical sciences to the management and analysis of complex biological data sets to aid in the discovery of new information, the extraction of knowledge, and the development of solutions that enhance human health. This chapter reviews available bioinformatic resources relevant to pharmacogenomic studies elucidating mechanisms of toxicity and preclinical drug development.

Sequence Analysis

Sequence analysis is a core area of bioinformatics research. There are four basic levels of biological structure, termed primary, secondary, tertiary, and quaternary structure. Primary structure refers to the representation of a linear, hetero-polymeric macromolecule as a string of monomeric units. For example, the primary structure of DNA is represented as a string of nucleotides (G, C, A, T). Secondary structure refers to the local three- dimensional shape in subsections of macromolecules. For example, the alpha- and beta-sheets in protein structures are examples of secondary structure. Tertiary structure refers to the overall three-dimensional shape of a macromolecule, as in the crystal structure of an entire protein. Finally, quaternary structure represents macromolecule interactions, such as the way different peptide chains dimerize into a single functional protein. In general, analysis increases in complexity as one attempts to predict higher levels of structure. Primary structure is highly amenable to *in silico* analysis while quaternary structure is virtually intractable computationally. In this section the major methods of analysis at each level of structure will be reviewed. However, due to rapidly evolving computational capabilities, discussion will be limited to the underlying motivations for each type of analysis with a brief outline of the major software implementations.

Primary Structure

Primary structure refers to raw ordering of amino acids in a protein or nucleotides in a DNA or RNA molecule. The techniques for analyzing primary structure are largely derived from standard computer science algorithms for finding specific words within a long document. Primary structure analysis can be broken up into three phases: finding and formatting sequences, measuring the similarity between sequences, and detecting functional "*regions*", or domains, in a sequence.

Sequence alignment

A sequence alignment is a way of determining the similarity between two strings. This is a classical question in computer science, and has an exact solution referred to as the Smith/Waterman alignment. Unfortunately, this exact solution can be slow when analyzing large sequences, and therefore, approximate methods, such as Basic Local Alignment Search Tool (BLAST), have been developed to identify very similar sequences. There are two basic types of sequence alignment. Single alignments compare pairs of sequences to find the best match and would be used to locate a DNA sequence on the genome. In contrast, multiple alignments compare sets of sequences with one another to identify overall similarities, and have been used to compare sequence similarity within a superfamily of proteins such as the cytochrome P450 superfamily. In addition, sequence alignments can conduct global alignments which attempt to match two sequences against each other over their entire length when sequences are believed to be related, or locally in order to find small (local) regions of similarity. Although local alignments are more popular, the following discussion is also applicable to global alignments. All alignments—single or multiple; local or global—are predicated on some definition of what makes two strings similar, and are mathematically defined by a scoring system.

Scoring systems

The scoring system, the core of sequence alignment, assesses similarity by positively scoring matches and penalizing mismatches. In addition, any gaps between two sequences also receive a negative score. By tuning the scoring system, specific types of matches can be preferentially selected. For instance, some scoring systems are optimized for evolutionarily distant proteins while others are specialized for membrane proteins. The score/penalty assigned to a match/mismatch is dependent on the likelihood that this match/mismatch occurred by chance alone. If an event occurs randomly with a high frequency the score will be small, while very rare events will receive very large scores.

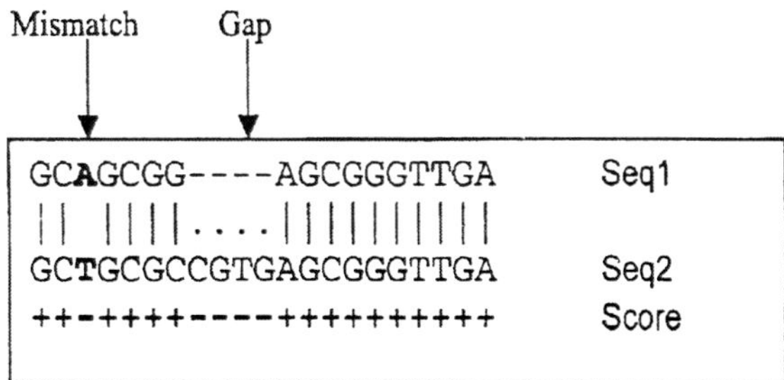

Fig. 6.1. Overview of alignment scoring system.

For example, a conservative amino-acid substitution will receive a very small penalty, while the introduction of a stop codon will be penalized heavily. A variety of scoring schemes have been generated based on factors such as the bio-physical character, evolutionary distance, and the subcellular localization of the sequences being compared. The presence of gaps in a sequence is a very important topic in sequence alignment, especially in phylogenetic applications. In general a large penalty is assigned for introducing a gap, and a smaller penalty is assigned based on the length of the gap. This gap-penalty often takes the form of a linear equation, and is called an "*affine gap penalty*".

Single alignment

A single alignment compares two sequences to determine the location and the quality of the best match. Single alignments can be used with nucleotides to identify unknown sequences within a database by searching for the most similar or to map novel sequences onto the genome and with peptide sequences in the identification of novel proteins, for phylogenetic comparisons, and to identify orthologous proteins.

Smith/Waterman. Smith/Waterman is a slow, computationally intensive method that finds the optimal alignment between a pair of sequences. It is based on the classic dynamic programming algorithm with run times proportional to the length of the sequence squared (n^2). For large databases or long sequences dynamic programming can become impractically slow, even on powerful systems.

Nevertheless Smith/Waterman alignment still has significant utility in practical applications when the need for sensitivity is paramount and the dataset to be analyzed is relatively small. Many evolutionary studies focusing on individual proteins use Smith/Waterman alignment. Several public servers providing access to Smith/Waterman alignment exist.

BLAST. To overcome the computational limitations of Smith/Waterman alignments, statistical approximations were developed by computational biologists in the early 1990s. These approximations do not guarantee that the optimal alignment will be found, but are overwhelmingly likely to identify the best alignments. More importantly, programs implementing these approximations generally run a full order of magnitude faster than full Smith/Waterman alignment.

Table 6.1. Versions of BLAST

Program name	*Sequence 1*	*Sequence 2*
BLASTN	Nucleotide	Nucleotide
BLASTP	Protein	Protein
BLASTX	Nucleotide	Protein
TBLASTN	Translated nucleotide	Protein
TBLASTX	Translated nucleotide	Translated nucleotide

The predominant statistical algorithm for sequence alignment is BLAST. The BLAST algorithm does not perform an exhaustive search of two sequences for similarity, but looks for short, exact matches called seeds or words, which are then extended on either side to find the overall best alignment. Short seeds will often be found by random chance, but longer seeds can miss strong-but-inexact similarities. Therefore, choosing a seed- length is an important factor, as it involves a trade-off between sensitivity and search speed.

Other alignment software. While Smith/Waterman and BLAST alignment are the most popular methods of performing single- alignments a host of other software has been developed for specialized pur-poses that attempt to improve execution speed by making simplifying assumptions about the types of matches that can be found.

Multiple alignment

Multiple sequence alignment involves the simultaneous comparison of several distinct sequences. If these sequences represent a single protein across multiple species, the alignment will indicate evolutionary relatedness. Alternatively, alignment of proteins within a single species may represent the series of gene-duplication events that led to the protein family. Multiple alignments are commonly used as the raw data input for the generation of phylogenetic trees. In contrast to single alignments, two basic classes of multiple alignment algorithms, progressive and iterative algorithms have been developed. Their performance varies with the characteristics of the individual alignments.

Table 6.2. Other Major sequence alignment packages

Package name	*Primary use*
FASTA	BLAST-like local alignments
REPuter	Maximal repeat identification
MUMmer	Suffice-tree algorithm
SIM	Linear space requirements
SENSEI	Very fast ungapped alignments
QUASAR	Suffix-array algorithm
BALSA	Bayesian-based alignment
PatternHunter	Extremely rapid large-scale alignments

Progressive algorithms follow a three-step path. First, pair-wise alignments are performed to rank sequences in order of similarity. The two closest sequences are then aligned together, and finally, the remaining sequences are added to the alignment one-by-one, in descending order of similarity. Therefore, this approach progresses by adding increasingly distant alignments to the analysis, and is the traditional approach to multiple sequence alignment. Common progressive multiple alignment software packages include CLUSTALX and GCG. Despite its age, CLUSTALX (and its graphical version, CLUSTALW) is the most common multiple alignment package.

In contrast, iterative algorithms use the entire set of alignments at once, but repeatedly iterate over the set until a stable alignment has been generated. Iterative approaches to multiple alignment are both newer and less popular than traditional progressive methods. Some common iterative multiple alignment software packages are DIALIGN and PRRP.

Motif detection

Motif detection involves searching for one sequence within another and is based on the assumption that one sequence is a part of another. Protein motifs are generally short sequences that represent conserved domains (CDs) or characterize protein families. Nucleotide motifs can range in size from full genes within the genome to short enhancer elements.

Protein motifs

Identifying protein function: Protein motifs are fragments ranging from a few to several hundred residues. Short fragments encode functions that evolved independently of their surrounding context, like glycosylation or phosphorylation sites. Moderate-sized fragments encode specialized functions, such as localization signals, while longer fragments constitute CDs with broader functionality. The CDs are usually thought to have occurred once in evolution, and were then transferred or swapped throughout multiple genomes. The total number of protein motifs is staggeringly large, with well over 15,000 motifs known, and new ones continuously being discovered.

Short sequences can be found by thoroughly scanning protein sequences for all possible occurrences. For example, localization signals and other targeting sequences are usually detected in this manner. Longer regions, like DNA-binding regions, enzymatic active sites, and protein–protein interaction domains are typically identified through sequence alignments, much as described above. A variety of databases and online tools exist to facilitate searches for protein motifs. The most comprehensive resource for the detection of large protein motifs is the Conserved Domain Database (CDD) provided by NCBI. The CDD includes all data present in the SMART and PFAM databases, along with some manually curated entries. All protein–protein BLAST searches performed through NCBIs web-service automatically perform a CDD search using Reverse Position Specific BLAST (RPS-BLAST).

Nucleotide motifs

Annotating the genome: Nucleotide motif finding occurs at three distinct levels: identification of coding sequences, identification of promoters, and identification of enhancers. At each level the core question is how to identify a signal from the underlying noise of genomic sequence.

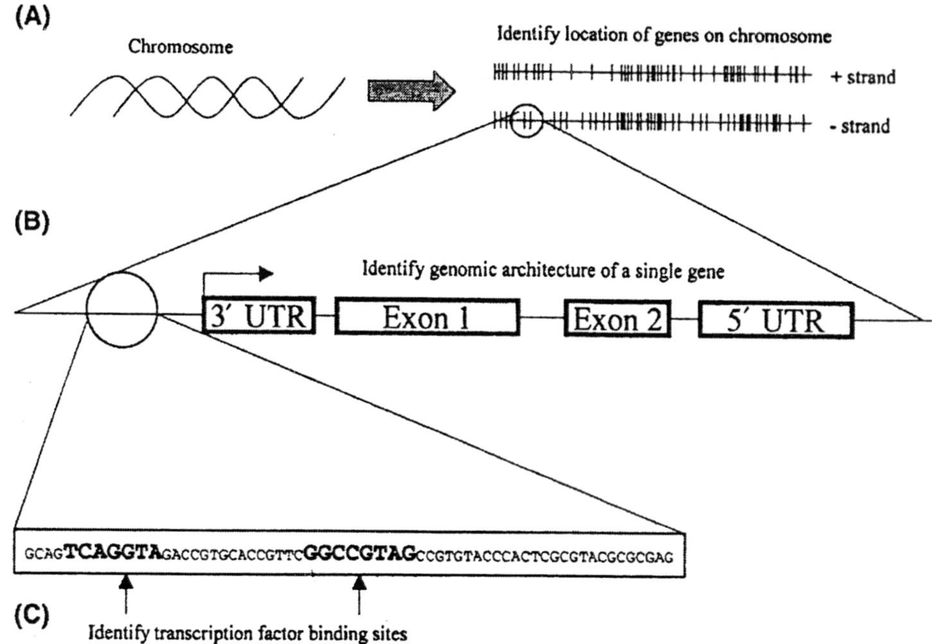

Fig. 6.2. Relationships between the three types of nucleotide motifs.

Finding genes. Gene finding is one of the most important genomic applications. Originally it was believed that the human genome sequence could be fully annotated using automated gene-prediction software. Instead, the identification of open-reading frames (ORFs) has turned out to be a challenging problem.

Even in simpler organisms, like yeast, ORF annotation has exhibited high error-rates. High-throughput proteomic and genomic studies combined with in silico approaches have corrected many mis-annotated ORFs in the yeast genome. With the greater complexity of the mammalian genome, it is not surprising that ORF prediction has had limited success.

Empirically, ORFs have been identified through the high throughput single pass sequencing of individual clones within a cDNA library to rapidly and inexpensively generate Expressed Sequence Tags (ESTs). The ESTs can then be mapped to the genome to identify representative genes. This approach has also been used to detect splice-variants. Unfortunately it is biased towards highly expressed genes, and requires that a particular mRNA be expressed in a given experimental sample. Further, the iterative computational assembly of multiple ESTs into "*clusters*" that represent putative gene-products is a challenging problem, which is error-prone. Coding sequences have characteristic features such as codon frequencies, start- and stop-codons, upstream TATA-boxes, and splice-sites, which can be used to annotate an ORF. While each piece of evidence is not, by itself, conclusive, the combination of factors can lead to firm identification of genes. Unfortunately this method is prone to a large number of false-positives, with at least 75% of predicted genes typically being artefacts.

The most reliable method of identifying ORFs is by identifying genes that share high sequence homology across species, which are also known as orthologs. Conserved genomic structure with comparable function in a closely related species can be used as a strong guideline for identifying ORFs. However, this method is inherently limited to genes with high homology in closely related species. For example, annotating rat genes through comparison with their mouse orthologues will miss genes that are unique to that species. Nevertheless, this approach does not suffer from the excess of false-positives associated with gene-structure-based algorithms, nor the very high computational burden associated with EST-based predictions.

Finding promoters. The promoter is a region proximal to the transcriptional start site (TSS) that contains cis-acting motifs for transcription factors that regulate gene expression. Finding the promoter of a gene is usually significantly more difficult than finding the coding sequence for a gene since there are no absolutely conserved elements that define the promoter. In contrast, identifying coding sequence requires identification of conserved elements such as the start codon, splice-sites, and the stop codon. Two basic methods for identifying promoter sequences have been developed: signal-based approaches and content-based approaches: signal- based and content-based approaches.

Signal-based approaches involve searching for elements like the TATA and CCAAT boxes used by the basal transcription machinery. Often these elements occur with conserved spacing patterns which can be used by techniques like support vector machines and genetic algorithms to identify putative promoter regions. Content-based approaches leverage the underlying structure of DNA to identify promoters, rather than the presence of conserved elements. In contrast, content-based algorithms will look for features such as base-pair triplet frequencies, the presence of CpG islands, or a randomness characteristic to non-coding sequence.

Alternatively, promoters could be identified by mapping mRNA sequences directly against the genome. If the mRNA transcript sequence is complete, the region immediately 5′ to the genomic location will be the promoter location. This approach, often used in combination with signal- or content-based algorithms has proven to be up to 80% accurate and 50% sensitive.

However, the identification of alternative promoters and splice- variants continues to be a challenge. A recent study showed that at least three-quarters of multi-exon human genes exhibit alternative-splicing, usually in tissue- and cell-type- specific patterns. No computational approaches have been developed to rapidly predict and screen potential alternative promoters for a single gene.

Finding enhancers. In general, the proximal promoter of a gene contains the binding sites for components of the basal transcription machinery. Upstream of this region is the distal promoter, which contains binding sites for a variety of cis-regulatory elements. These cis-acting elements act as binding sites for transcription factors. Transcription factors regulate aspects of gene-expression such as tissue-distribution, response to signalling pathways, and temporal specificity. This regulatory function is achieved in several ways, including direct recruitment of the basal transcription machinery, recruitment of complexes that modify the histones, and recruitment of co-activator proteins that specialize in enhancing transcriptional initiation.

Enhancer sequences are short 5 to 25 bp motifs may randomly occur many times in the genome. For example, a 10 bp motif would be expected to occur approximately once every million (4^{10}) bases by chance alone. Accordingly a major challenge in searching for enhancer elements is determining the functionality of an element. At present no current in silico search algorithm can definitely identify a functional cis-regulatory element. Statistical analysis can indicate whether a given promoter is likely to be active, but predictions must be empirically confirmed. More effective in silico prediction of enhancer elements may utilize comparative genomic approaches and will require a better understanding protein and DNA interactions.

The consensus binding sequence for a known transcription factor is usually encoded in a weight-matrix. This matrix indicates what base each position of the binding-site is likely to contain, and is generated from transcription factor binding specificity data. The most comprehensive listing of transcription factor binding sites and their associated weight-matrices is in the TransFac database. A less extensive free database, JASPAR, is also available.

Alternately, an analysis of co-regulated genes can identify conserved motifs for novel transcription factor binding sites. This involves identification of a set of co-regulated genes that have similar expression profiles in response to some stimuli. The distal promoters of these genes are then analyzed for sequences that occur more often than would be expected by chance alone. These over-represented sequences are putative binding sites, which can be compared to the consensus sequences of known transcription factors and empirically tested using DNA foot-printing, reporter gene and band shift assays.

Phylogenetic foot-printing is a technique that is gaining popularity in enhancer searches. The underlying premise is that regulatory sequences will be conserved across species. In other words, it is assumed that non-coding regulatory sequence is evolutionarily conserved, and that regions of non-coding DNA that are highly homologous across species are likely to contain important regulatory motifs. A study in skeletal muscle showed that 19% of the best conserved regulatory DNA contained 74 of the 75 known transcription factor binding sites. Accordingly, a transcription factor binding site that is observed in a conserved position in multiple species is much more likely to be functional than one that is only present in a single species. Both the weight-matrix scans and sequence-representation searches described above can be supplemented by phylogenetic foot-printing.

Higher-Order Structure

While the primary structure of proteins and nucleic acids can be experimentally determined in a straight-forward manner, their higher-order structures are much more difficult to elucidate. In general, computational methods dealing with primary structure focus on interpretation of the structure–function, as in promoter analysis. By contrast computational methods working on higher-order structure instead focus on the prediction of structural details. Further, most techniques are limited to the prediction of RNA and protein structures—sugar-, fatty-acid-, and DNA-structural prediction methods are in their infancy. We consider higher-order structure for both RNA and proteins. Surprisingly, the folding problem is quite different for each of these two heteropolymers at all levels of structure, with RNA folding being more tractable, both theoretically and computationally.

RNA folding

The RNA secondary structure can be defined as a state where all bases are mapped into one of two states: pairing or non-pairing. The RNA base- pairs include both Watson–Crick associations and weaker "wobble" pairs like G:U associations. These pairs of associated bases are usually adjacent with and anti-parallel to other associated pairs, creating regions with complex three-dimensional structure. These well-folded regions are islands, separated by stretches of single-stranded, unstructured RNA. There are four basic types of RNA secondary structure—helices, much like those found in DNA; loops, like the hair-pins found in tRNAs; bulges and junctions. Of these four basic forms, only helices are made up primarily of Watson- Crick base-pairs. The latter three structural types are largely comprised of aberrant base-pairs, terminated by helical regions.

While there are several different approaches to predicting RNA structure, it should be emphasized that RNA structure prediction remains a challenging, but tractable task. All the algorithms and software packages discussed here are capable of predicting RNA structure with 70% or greater accuracy. The four major approaches to RNA structure prediction are: thermodynamical, naïve, homology-based, and empirical.

Thermodynamical approaches assume that a folded RNA molecule will adopt its most stable conformation. These algorithms model the free energy of the molecule as the sum of the individual base-pairing and base- stacking interactions. The best-known implementation of this approach is the mfold web-server, which has been available for nearly a decade. The web-server provides access to a wide-range of tools, including RNA- and DNA-folding, melting-point determination, and structure-viewers. This server is being continually maintained and upgraded with new tools and enhanced implementations.

Naive approaches avoid theoretical assumptions and instead focus on statistics about solved RNA structures, using these to probabilistically align new sequences with solved structures. One elegant approach to this problem has used an rRNA database to generate a novel RNA-specific substitution matrix. The advantage of this approach is that it makes the whole spectrum of primary-structure sequence-analysis tools available for secondary-structure prediction.

Homology-based approaches to RNA-folding are conceptually similar to the phylogenetic foot-printing methods used for transcription-factor binding-site analysis detailed above. The assumption underlying both methods is that evolutionarily conserved sequences will be functionally relevant. Phylogenetic foot-printing assumes that such conserved sequences contain transcription-factor binding-sites. Homology-based RNA-folding methods assume that these conserved sequences contain regions of secondary structure, rather than unfolded regions of primary structure. Unfortunately this is a stronger assumption for folding methods than for motif-detection methods because it is now postulating linkages between both primary structure and secondary structure, and between secondary structure and function. Despite the strength of this assumption, homology-based methods have proved useful, and some methods have even been developed that achieve >80% accuracy from aligned sequences.

The final method of RNA structure prediction, empirical algorithms, are also analogous to primary-structure motif detection methods. Known RNA structural motifs are extracted from structural databases, and the primary-structure patterns underlying these motifs are identified. Novel RNA sequences are then scanned for these primary-structure motifs much like a novel protein sequence might be scanned for CDs. In essence, these methods search the primary structure of sequences for conserved motifs that indicate secondary structure. One of the most flexible and powerful empirical tools is RNAMotif, which is freely available for download, but does not have an associated web-server.

Protein folding

The process through which a linear string of amino acid residues newly synthesized at a ribosome folds into a complex, three-dimensional, biologically active protein structure remains poorly understood. Consider how protein-folding contrasts with RNA-folding. Proteins have 20 distinct monomeric units, RNA only four. The amino acids include aromatic, hydrophobic, cationic, and anionic chemical properties compared to four comparable RNA nucleosides. Moreover, secondary and tertiary structures were fundamentally inter-linked in proteins, but are essentially distinct in RNA molecules.

An enormous body of research into protein-folding has led to the development of several computational methods for predicting and understanding the lowest level of three-dimensional protein structure. While high-resolution (1Å) crystal structures are the gold standard for elucidating three-dimensional protein-structures, this level of accuracy is not necessary for many applications. For example, virtual screening of ligands through docking simulation can be done with lower resolutions. Site-directed mutagenesis studies can be motivated by structures with resolutions of only 4 Å and three-dimensional motif-scanning can be performed at even lower resolutions. In short, low-resolution predictions of structure still have utility.

Computational approaches

A major problem in predicting protein structure is the computational intractability. A short, 100-residue protein will contain at least 100 side-chain-to-side-chain or side-chain-to-solvent interactions. The orientation of each of these interactions will lead to cascading effects throughout the protein. Comparative modeling, threading algorithms, and de novo predictions seek to predict protein structure in reasonable execution times.

Comparative methods leverage primary-structure similarity between the sequence of interest and a protein with known structure. Sequence homology is then assumed to result in structural homology, and is used to develop an all-atom structural model. Of the four basic steps in homology modeling, it has been shown that template-target alignment is the most critical for development of a reliable model. When the target and template have sequence identity of at least 50%, the leveraging of a homology relationship becomes very powerful, and comparative methods are the most accurate protein structure prediction tool. When target-template identity is low, heuristics and user-input are required to generate a model of any reliability. Threading algorithms, like comparison methods, leverage known structures to help identify the correct fold for a new protein sequence. Rather than employing sequence-level homology as a screening tool, threading methods attempt to fit the new sequence to every known crystal structure. These algorithms essentially "thread" the new sequence through each of the known structures. The energetic stability of each conformation is calculated, and taken as a measure of how well the known structure matches the new sequence. While threading methods are successful as comparative methods, they are very computationally intensive, and are inherently limited to previously characterized folds. As novel protein folds are continually discovered, this limitation is decreasing.

De novo algorithms predict three-dimensional structure directly from the primary sequence, without any leveraging of known structures. While predictions are often of poor accuracy (low-resolution), it remains the only way of determining structures for families with no known members. The sole assumption is that the native conformation is the most energetically favorable. This may not be true for proteins that undergo chaperone- mediated folding, but is a reasonable assumption. Most de novo algorithms walk along a sequence in words varying in length between 5 and 27 residues. For each word, the most probable set of secondary structures is predicted. Finally, the protein is allowed to vary over the possible combinations of secondary structures, with the lowest energy structure being selected as the prediction. One major implementation of this algorithm is the ROSETTA software, for which a web-server is available.

Protein-structure prediction methods are routinely compared and contrasted in a public competition called the Critical Assessment of Techniques for Protein Structure Prediction (CASP). These large-scale events allow for a comparison of the state-of-the-art tools and algorithms on a variety of target sequences. The results of each event are scrutinized. There have been five such events thus far, with CASP5 being the most recent.

Data Management

Introduction to Bioinformatics Data Management

Data management refers to the storage, sorting, and retrieval of data. While not traditionally an important part of bioinformatics, the explosive growth in high-throughput technologies has generated large complex data sets requiring a need to archive, process, integrate, and search data for biological meaning. Consequently, data management is becoming an increasingly important part of applied bioinformatics.

Why is data management needed?

The sheer magnitude of modern biological datasets is daunting. Consider the publicly accessible GenBank sequence database currently comprises 591 distinct files, with a cumulative size of dozens of gigabytes. Even the largest available hard-drives available for a personal computer can barely store this entire database. In comparison, a standard two-color microarray experiment will generate two image files (≈30 MB each), one quantification file (≈5 MB), a normalization file (≈5 MB each), and one final gene-list (≈1 MB). A single array can generate up to 70 MB of data, and even a simple experiment can easily require 20 arrays resulting in over 1 GB for this simple experiment. This data must be stored securely so that it remains accessible after publication, and for future researchers looking to explore the data in greater detail, possibly with newly developed methodologies.

Table 6.3. Relative size of standard bioinformatics resources

Resource	*Size*	*Best comparison*
One Microarray Slide	~40 MB	One full length music album
One Human Chromosome	~250 MB	One full installation of Microsoft Office
All SNPs on a Chromosome	~2 GB	One full length movie
All ESTs on a Chromosome	~50 GB	Every complete Simpson's episode

Fortunately, microarray experiments generate highly ordered data, and therefore the challenge is not simply the data storage but the intrinsic relationships within these highly structured datasets, which must be preserved and enforced. Each microarray in an experiment has very specific samples hybridized to it, and each sample must be associated with a microarray. Each feature on the microarray contains a specific sequence, and has associated with it a variety of intensities, quality metrics, and ultimately expression measures. These different types of data must be integrated and co-ordinated, so that a researcher can look at a single gene, and see how that gene has behaved across a set of microarray experiments, and what annotation has been ascribed to that gene. The user-friendly integration and storage of large datasets is a long-standing challenge for bioinformatic researchers.

Role for databases

Storing and organizing large datasets is typically performed using relational databases. Tuned to optimize storage efficiency and retrieval speed, relational databases were first used by government departments and large corporations. As their broader applicability became apparent, relational databases were deployed across a broad spectrum of industries and groups, and standard office software packages now come with a rudimentary relational database included.

The term "relational" is derived from the way the software leverages known relationships between different types of data to optimize storage space, to speed data access, and to enforce rules that maintain the underlying coherence or integrity of the data. A typical relationship may be expressed as: every polymorphism in a coding region must be either synonymous (silent) or non-synonymous, or every microarray slide must contain one or more spots. The underlying design or schema of a relational database is the specification of a large number of data associations of this sort.

Genomic Data Standards

A great deal of interest has been generated by many for sharing genomic data. However, without data standards in place to govern protocols for sharing data, exchanging genomic data will be fraught with difficulties. Recently, the Microarray Gene Expression Data Society proposed the Minimum Information About a Microarray Experiment (MIAME) standard to provide guidance in determining the minimum amount of information required to independently replicate an experiment or reanalysis a deposited data set. Others have since began exploring other key issues in standards development, including the development of controlled vocabularies and ontologies, to harden terms and definitions, thereby creating a standard language for describing genomic experiments.

This section will discuss the standards for sharing and discussing micro- array experiments, including the ontologies and controlled vocabularies. A non-technical description of the sharing process will be provided, as well as an introduction to the pharmacology/toxicology focused version of the MIAME standard, MIAME/Tox, which is currently under development.

Ontologies and controlled vocabularies for genomic data

In order for investigators to effectively share their data, they must ensure that the language they use for describing the experiment can be understood by others. The first step in sharing data is the creation of a controlled vocabulary or an ontology. Once the community is speaking the same language, they can begin sharing data.

A microarray generally consists of a glass slide with some material affixed to it, and some other labeled material hybridized to the array. When investigators use the term "probe," to which material they are referring? The term probe has been used to describe both materials in the past, and may be a source of confusion. The solution to this kind of terminology problem is for the community to agree on a common language, called a controlled vocabulary or an ontology. A controlled vocabulary is a set of descriptors that a community agrees to use when describing an experiment. Definitions are not explicitly given with the vocabulary as they are expected to be understood. One example of a controlled vocabulary would be the National Toxicology Program's Pathology Code Tables for describing pathology lesions. The terms used in the vocabulary should be definite and distinct, such that any lesion should only be identified by one term in the vocabulary list. If controlled vocabulary terms are associated with a specific definition, then an ontology is created. Generally, a true ontology should be a complete specification of a concept, in this case a microarray experiment. Currently, the MGED Ontologies Working Group is assembling a microarray experiment ontology.

MAGE-OM and MAGE-ML

The emerging method for sharing genomic data between databases is the Microarray Gene Expression Object Model (MAGE-OM) and MAGE Markup Language (MAGE-ML). The MAGE-ML is derived directly from the MAGE-OM, a data representation standard approved by the Object Management Group (OMG). The MAGE-ML is built in the eXtensible Markup Language (XML), and is the preferred data sharing method. As part of the MAGE-ML development, documents are generated that are used by computers to decode the MAGE-ML documents. The MAGE compliant software and databases use these decoding documents to properly interpret the MAGE-ML encoded data, and to populate the appropriate database tables or data structures within the application.

The MAGE has built within it a controlled vocabulary that is used to standardize communication between data providers. However, MAGE can also be extended to encode other types of "omic" data beyond genomics, such as proteomic data, so long as a reference to the ontology or controlled vocabulary is provided. Although a description of the extension mechanism is beyond scope of this book, practitioners must become familiar with it in order to ensure their software products and applications will be able to accept any and all annotation data that may be submitted with the genomic data.

Minimum information about a microarray experiment standard

The MIAME standard defines the minimum information investigators must report for a microarray experiment to be reproduced. The MAGE standard was born partially from MIAME, and the European Bioinformatics Institute used MIAME and MAGE to guide the development of ArrayExpress, their public genomic data repository. Sample annotation lies at the heart of MIAME, underscoring the need to understand as completely as possible the experimental conditions that may influence the microarray data. Many journals that publish microarray data require the submission of MIAME-supportive microarray data to a public genomic data repository as a condition of publication. These typically include submission of protocols; species, strains, and sex used for in vivo studies; cell line name and culture conditions for in vitro studies, and other relevant information. To assist investigators in meeting the requirements of the standard, the MGED Society provides a MIAME-checklist. The checklist outlines the most pertinent points of the standard to facilitate data submission compliance. The MIAME standard includes a glossary of the controlled vocabulary used throughout the MIAME document to assist data for submission.

MIAME/Tox—A MIAME specific for toxicology and pharmacology

Although the MIAME standard will suffice for many experimental paradigms, it is not complete enough for the purposes of the regulatory toxicology and pharmacology communities. The MIAME standard does not include reporting requirements for toxicological or pharmacological endpoints or measures to place the genomic data within proper context. The MIAME/Tox standard is being developed to address these concerns. Additional reporting requirements of the MIAME/Tox extension include (1) clinical pathology, (2) chemical mixtures and constituents, (3) chemical exposure protocol, (4) husbandry details, and (5) histopathology data. It is unclear at this time what the actual reporting burden will be, and whether or not differences will exist between academic research and industrial regulatory submissions as the standard is still under development by MGED Society's Toxicology Working Group.

Microarray Data Analysis

Analysis of microarray experiments spans many subjects including study design, quality control, normalization, data filtering, and result.

Microarray Experimental Design

Prior to any experiment, study design considerations must be considered in order to ensure the study addresses the question of interest and has sufficient technical and biological replication to support data analysis using appropriate statistical methods. A technical replicate is a sample from the same source that is hybridized to more than one array and is expected to have less variance. Biological replicates are samples from independent experimental units (e.g., animal). For example, total RNA from the right lateral hepatic lobe excised from individual Sprague–Dawley rats receiving the same treatment would constitute biological replicates. Whereas a technical replicate allows for better estimation of the precision for gene expression assay, biological replicates provide an estimate of assay variation and biological variation. In general, biological replicates are more informative than technical replicates, however, technical are still important to assure competence and consistency with the assay. Other factors that will influence study design and the degree of replication include the type of study (e.g., time-course, dose-response, and class discovery), available resources (e.g., number of slides and expense), and the amount of sample. For two-channel microarrays, conventional wisdom suggests that comparisons of greatest interest should be paired on the same microarray.

Microarray Data Normalization and Transformation

Normalization attempts to remove technical variation in the data that is not attributed to biological or treatment related variation. Examples of technical variation include differences in dye incorporation, physical differences in fluorescence efficiency of incorporated dyes, print-surface irregularities, and print tip effects, although there are several methods, most investigators use global or local normalization methods. Global methods normalize across the entire dataset whereas local methods perform the normalization across a subset of the data. Local methods have the advantage of correcting for spatial biases.

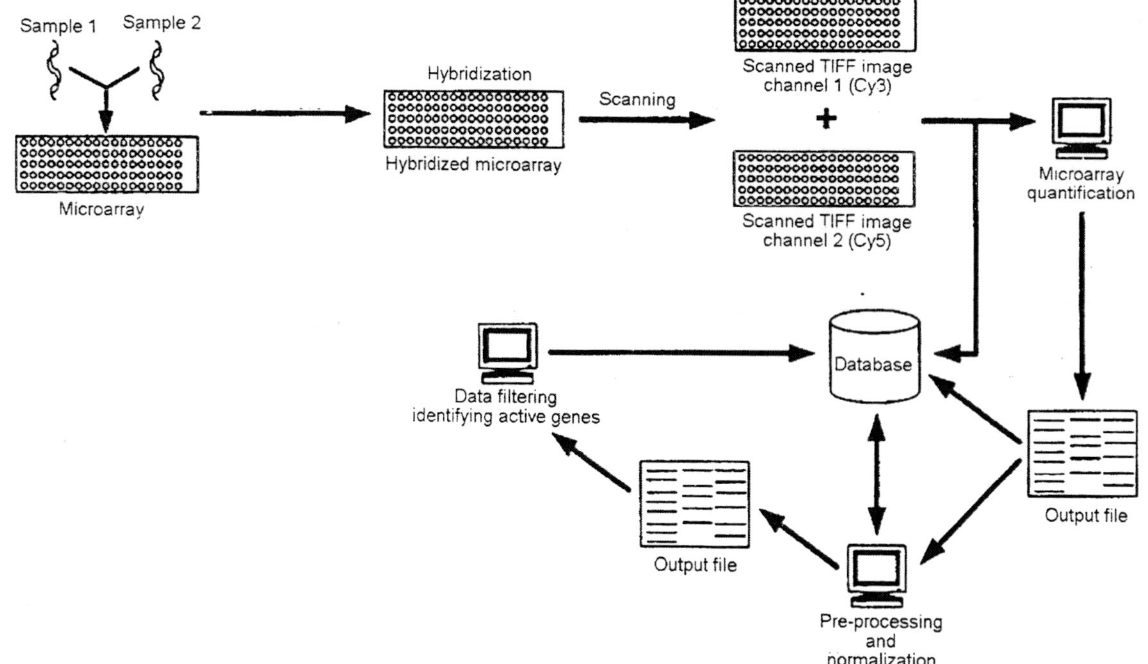

Fig. 6.3. Microarray data flow.

Microarray data may require transformation to stabilize the variance by applying a global logarithmic transformation prior to normalization and further analysis. This may unpredictably skew the measurement, making further analysis difficult and unreliable. As many of the techniques used for the analysis of microarray data are not robust to the equal variance assumption, a family of variance stabilizing transformation (VST) methods for microarray data have been proposed.

Normalization factor calculation methods

One common microarray data normalization method is to calculate a normalization factor on a per array basis or across an entire experiment. The primary assumption for using a singular normalization factor is that the volume of labeled sample is comparable across the two channels. Thus, due to the large population of labeled cDNA within the uniform volume it is assumed that the same number of labeled cDNAs exist in both samples. Ideally, the overall intensity in the two channels will be the same. Furthermore, any increases in labeled cDNAs, due to increases in mRNA, must result in decreases of some other labeled cDNAs. Typical methods include mean- or median-centering, where the mean/ median values are centered within the data distribution, and z-score normalization which adds a scaling factor to mean-centering.

The drawback of these approaches is their failure to compartmentalize sources of variation. Thus, in studies where biological and technical replicates both exist, there is the possibility that the normalization method will inappropriately remove biological variance, such as the treatment effect itself. This can lead to a reduction in the overall treatment related response. Other sources of variation include replicate effects, where the timing of hybridization and scanning, may cause persistent trends in the data.

Lowess normalization

Lowess normalization methods are based on lowess (loess) scatterplot smoothing algorithms. The lowess smoother attempts to smooth contours within a dataset. Typically the lowess will be robust to genes which are active in treatment as they will be observed as outliers. Some normalization methods include a print-tip normalization, since physical location on the array and the print-tip may contribute some effect and variance beyond the biological and treatment variation.

The lowess normalization method is typically coupled with scatter- plots (e.g., M vs. A) illustrating the relationship between the two dye channels, as a function of the overall intensity (i.e., geometric mean of the intensities). The lowess normalization smooths the microarray data in the scatter plot to correct for data artefacts. The normalization is performed on a per-array basis, and does not account for temporal effects, such as the date the assay was performed.

Microarray Data Ranking and Prioritization

Normalized data may be compared across the experimental variables of interest, such as dose, time, or chemical exposure. However, analysts are interested in grouping features into changed or unchanged groupings compared to some metric or control. Numerous methods abound for identifying significant changes in gene expression including (1) arbitrary fold-change cut-offs, (2) model-based *t*-test, and (3) ANOVA with post hoc test. The fold-change method, which historically was the primary method for filtering, has generally been replaced by more robust statistical means. All of the methods discussed or presented may be coupled with an empirical Bayes method to either adjust the false discovery rate (FDR), or define the cut-off level.

Ratios of normalized values vs. not using ratios

For two-channel microarray data, ratios are commonly used to compare genes based on their fold-changes. However, use of ratios requires the proper propagation of error between the divisor and dividend, which can become complicated if the samples or measures are not statistically independent. Furthermore, ratio values generally do not follow a normal distribution, a requirement of parametric tests. Although it is true that most populations will begin to follow a normal distribution as the population size approaches infinity (due to the Central Limit Theorem), this assumption must be tested prior to appropriately using a parametric analysis technique. Therefore, ratios or the normalized values for data filtering, as the techniques discussed below will work for both types of data provided these assumptions are met. Note that performing multiple hypothesis tests (e.g., Student's *t*-test) may inflate the false positive rate. That is, the number of genes detected as active by chance alone will increase with the number of genes tested. For example, a microarray with 7000 features would require at least 7000 hypothesis tests per treatment comparison. Several methods have been developed to control the false positive rate, such as the conservative Bonferroni correction and the FDR control method.

Student's t-test

The t-test is a popular method for comparing measures from two samples exposed to different conditions, or from different time-points. The hypotheses that may be tested include: (1) does treatment cause a change in gene expression compared to vehicle treatment and (2) does treatment cause a change in gene expression relative to the control after H hours? The key to using the *t*-test is that a comparison is being made between two samples. As with all hypothesis tests an alpha value is chosen, typically thought of as a cut-off value for significance, which determines the false positive rate (the rate of finding something significantly changed due to chance alone). Alpha values for most scientific studies are set to $\alpha = 0.05$, meaning the study accepts a 5% false positive rate, regardless of the *p*-value.

The *t*-test also assumes that the data have equal variance and follow a normal distribution. If the data violate the equal variance assumption, VST methods, or a modified t-test that is robust to the assumption of equal variance (present in most statistical software packages) can be applied.

Data filtering can occur using either the *p*-value or the *t*-statistic. Use of the *t*-statistic avoids complications due to arguments concerning estimation of the degrees of freedom, but the false positive rate becomes much more difficult to calculate. The *p*-value is confounded by false positive rate inflation and arguments concerning the degrees of freedom.

The Wilcoxon's Rank-Sum Test (WRST) is a non-parametric alternative. The WRST is robust to the normal distribution assumption, but not to the assumption of equal variance. Furthermore, this test requires that the two groups of data under comparison have similarly shaped distributions. Non-parametric tests typically suffer from having less statistical power than their parametric counterparts. Similar to the *t*-test, the WRST will exhibit false positive rate inflation across a microarray dataset. It is possible to use the Wilcoxon test statistic as the single filtering mechanism; however calculation of the false positive rate is challenging.

Pattern Classification

Following the identification of significant changes in gene expression, the formidable challenge of interpreting the biological relevance of these changes. Borrowing from other large data fields, a common practice is to subject the data to one or more visualizations in order to group similar gene expression change patterns, which may shed light on shared mechanisms of co-regulation and co-ordinated biological function that is involved in the etiology of the observed pharmacological or toxic response. All pattern classification methods listed group items by similarity. Measurement of similarity differs depending upon the method, and therefore different methods yield different results.

Ultimately, the underlying question dictates the pattern classification method. Sample classification methods are most appropriate where the goal is to classify different samples based on expression. These methods are also known as supervised methods because there is prior knowledge of which samples should cluster and are useful for generating mathematical models that can be trained and validated for the assignment of chemicals based on gene expression fingerprints. If instead the question concerns identifying patterns for individual genes then an unsupervised, or clustering, method would be more appropriate.

A common misconception about clustering methods, especially unsupervised methods, is that all genes within a cluster are co-regulated by the same mechanism. Although genes

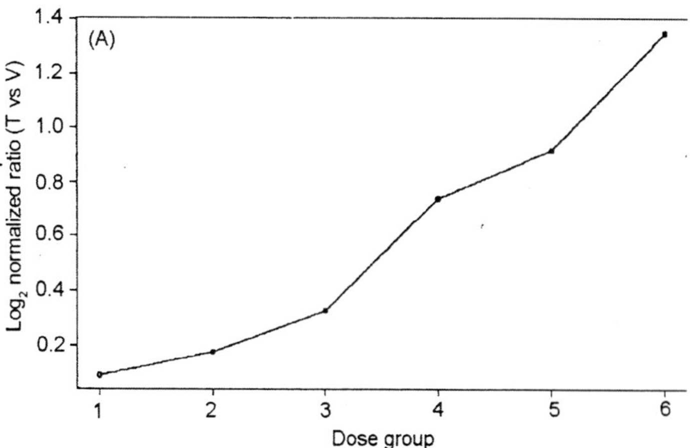

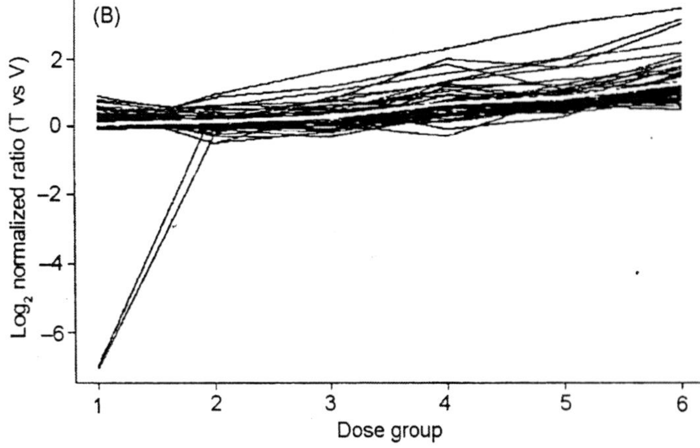

Fig. 6.4. Clustering of genes by expression pattern by k-means clustering. A–The overall pattern exhibited by this cluster illustrates a dose-response where the response increases with increasing dose. B–Examining the plot of all genes within the class makes it difficult to discern the overall pattern of the cluster.

within a cluster exhibit comparable expression dynamics, their regulatory mechanisms may differ. The simplest conclusion is that these genes follow similar dynamics due to a comparable regulatory mechanism that governs their dynamic expression. However, clustering methods only identify genes that are highly correlated in their expression, not by their mechanism of regulation, which can only be definitely elucidated through empirical studies.

Practical Examples in Pharmacogenomic Analysis

Each of the tools and databases discussed previously is grounded in a significant amount of both technical and theoretical detail. To illustrate the utility of these tools, practical data-analysis examples are provided that outline how a microarray experiment can be designed and analyzed. In addition, the annotation of an uncharacterized EST is defined and mapped to the genome. These examples also demonstrate how to assign annotation to microarray analysis, when the identify of a EST represented on an array may be unknown.

Designing and Analyzing a Microarray Experiment

Dose-response: Reference design

The goal of a dose-response experiment is to identify significant changes in gene expression following exposure to different doses of some treatment. Although gene expression can be compared from dose-to-dose, it is imperative that vehicle gene expression profiles be taken into consideration. Thus, the best design would be the common reference design with dye-swaps to take into consideration dye biases, where every microarray hybridization contains at least one labeling from the pooled reference vehicle sample. Although, the reference design takes many more measurements of the relatively biologically uninteresting vehicle sample, the increased technical replication of the vehicle sample is not a weakness, but instead a strength, due to the importance of establishing vehicle effects within the model. This design should include at least three biological replicates.

Normalizing the raw data

Our normalization method is based on a combination of a non- parametric loess smoother and a parametric General Linear Mixed Model (GLMM). As the goal of normalization is to ensure data are comparable across microarrays, that is a value of x represents the same biological concept across all arrays, and the underlying assumption is that most genes on the array will be unchanged, normalized microarray data will typically exhibit the same distribution.

Ranking and prioritization of data

The most robust method for identifying alterations in transcript levels is the WRST. This method does not make assumptions concerning the distribution or the variance of the data to be compared. However, many investigators use the t-test due to its simplicity. Alternatively, a model-based t-test from the GLMM could be used which performs contrast tests between two groups of interest, such as an effect at a particular dose vs. a vehicle effect, much like a *t*-test. The values for the test come from the model fit to the data, and provide a

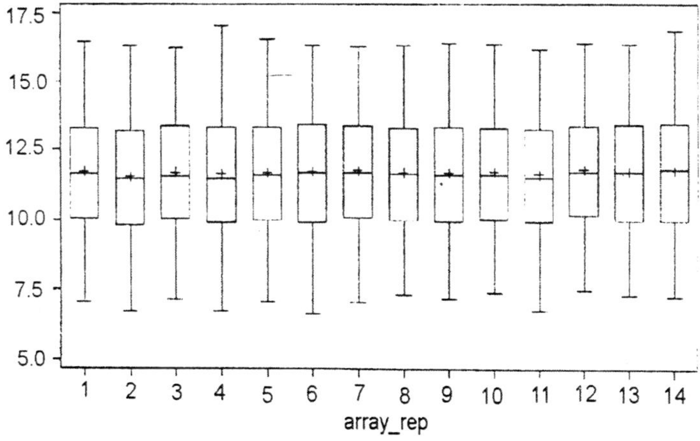

Fig. 6.5. Boxplots of normalized intensity values across arrays, boxplots facilitate comparison of sample distributions and dynamic range across microarrays.

better estimate of the difference between the two groups, as other data are used to better constrain the real effect of the dose and vehicle under consideration.

When constructing the GLMM to perform the model-based *t*-test, the terms within the model include the dye (to model dye-effects), the microarray (to model any random microarray-specific effects), and the dose (including vehicle, to model dose/vehicle effects).

Data interpretation and mining

Following the identification of active genes, and their ranking and prioritization, the resulting subset is subjected to clustering to identify common patterns of expression using, for example, agglomerative hierarchical clustering. This method results in a dendrogram relating genes by their expression pattern. Alternatively, for a dose response study, a two-way agglomerative hierarchical clustering, where the doses are also clustered based on expression, could be used to assess which doses are more alike based on gene expression, which may identify subtle changes in target specificity across dose.

Due to the difficulty in identifying the boundaries of clusters in a dendrogram, k-means or fuzzy c-means are also useful. These methods generate a predefined number of clusters where a consensus pattern may be determined and a gene can only belong to one cluster. Although the genes have been clustered, a cluster is of little biological significance. It is difficult to assign a single function to a cluster, as genes with common expression profiles do not necessarily reflect genes with similar functions. Further, clustered genes may or may not represent genes with similar regulatory mechanisms.

In order to identify common functional themes, genes may be clustered by using the Gene Ontology (GO), specifically GO Slims. The GO is an ontology, which can be thought of as a controlled vocabulary with term definitions for defining gene functions, cellular locations, and biological processes. The GO is a directed acyclic graph, where a term, and a gene, may be associated with several other "*higher level*" GO terms representing a broader category, such as "*protein kinase.*" The GO Slims are a "slim" version of the GO, providing slightly higher-level mappings of genes to ease clustering and functional annotation. By clustering the filtered dataset by GO entries it may be possible to identify "*over represented*" functions within the cluster. The GO clusters can be further mined for interactions; places where two GO terms share the same genes. The GO numbers with a high degree of interaction may represent functional annotations that are of more importance in the mechanism of action/toxicity.

Assigning Putative Function to an Uncharacterized EST

Consider this scenario: you have recently designed, executed, and analyzed a complex microarray experiment. With the help of a biostatistician, you have analyzed the results, and now have a list of genes believed to be significantly differentially regulated in your experimental system. However, one of the interesting candidates exhibiting an intriguing expression profile has a UniGene cluster number of Hs.482760, and is annotated as:

Transcribed sequence with weak similarity to MOST-1 Protein

What can you do with this information? Is it possible to link a function to this hypothetical protein? How much trust can you even have in this sequence? Is it really a gene, or could it just be an error on the array?

What is the raw sequence?

The UniGene database operated by NCBI clusters full-length mRNAs from short, single-pass sequencing reads called ESTs. While ESTs are inexpensive to sequence, their error rat is typically 3–5%, leading to a large quantity of moderate-quality data. The UniGene database is an attempt to organize ESTs into a set of putative gene products. The first task is to identify a sequence with this cryptic gene name. The UniGene cluster number is a unique identifier that facilitates retrieval of the record for this cluster. The record provides weak homology information to another human protein, MOST1, with a region of 63% identity between the two proteins covering 36 residues. In addition, there are no mRNAs matching this set of ESTs, and most importantly, all ESTs that have been grouped together in this cluster are listed. This can be used to select a representative sequence to assess the gene based not only on sequence length, but also the presence of a poly adenylation signal, which provides evidence that of a transcribed gene. For this clusters an EST with accession AA004311 of >500bp was selected for further analysis.

Does this sequence match any known mouse genes?

While this appears to be a novel gene in human, it is possible that it has already been characterized in another species such as the mouse. Annotation of the mouse genome is nearly complete, and in many cases share similar biology with its human ortholog. The BLAST sequence-alignment tool is used to characterize the homology of this sequence across species by using the novel sequence as a probe and searching a database of all mouse sequences. The E-value shows the "expectation" of this match occurring by chance in the database. For example, an expectation of one indicates that an alignment of this strength would be expected to occur by random chance once. Lower E-values indicate stronger the alignments. The sequence was found to align with moderate strength (E= 0.015) to two sequences on chromosome 18, making this the likely location of a mouse homologue. This potential homologue does not appear to be identified and the length of this match (26 bp) is short.

Where does this sequence match to the genome?

If homology assessment fails to provide insight, it is still possible to map the sequence to the human genome using the BLAST tool offered at the University of California, Santa Cruz. The BLAST is an efficient sequence-alignment tool that specializes in locating the best match between genes and the genome, taking into accountant potential splicing. There is only one strong match, on the + strand of chromosome 5. This mapping is 97% accurate, fitting well within the 3-5% error-rate typical of EST sequences, and encompasses nearly 500 of the ~580 base sequence.

What protein does this gene encode?

To see what the genome looks like in this region, the "browser" link can be used show EST alignment to the genome in this region, thus providing evidence for a real gene-product. Even more encouragingly, several full-length mRNAs aligning in this area are also shown, and gene-prediction software packages predict a full-length protein in this area that includes the initial sequence used for further analysis. While there are several protein predictions that could be used, all of which might differ by a few residues, the sensitive TwinScan prediction software package identified chr5.87.001 .a, and provides further information regarding the putative protein product.

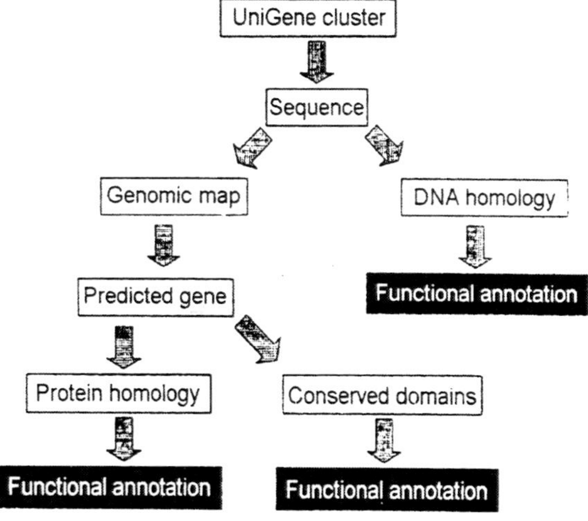

Fig. 6.6. EST-identification pathway.

What is this protein's function?

Putative functional domains within the uncharacterized protein can be identified using the CDD search tools while performing protein-protein BLAST (BLASTP) alignments to obtain insight into possible functions of the predicted protein. The predicted protein sequence is used since amino-acid sequences are more evolutionarily conserved than nucleotide sequences, and therefore a broader search across all available sequence information from a variety of organisms can be conducted to identify potential functionality. Results from the BLASTP and CDD analysis have identified three KOG3508, GTPase-activating protein domains with Expectation- Values below 10^{-10}. In addition, an SH2 domain and a RAS-like GTPase domain are also detected. Collectively, this provides strong evidence that the protein is a RAS-interacting GTPase.

Table 6.4. Assessment of genomic mapping through BLAST analysis

Score	*Identity (%)*	*Chromosome*	*Strand*
497	97.1	5	+
33	100	1	+
25	100	9	–
21	100	9	–

The actual BLAST results provide a graphical depiction of the alignments. The strongest alignments (E-values below 10^{-50}) are to RAS-like GTPase proteins, with homology to a protein called RAS p21 protein activator (GTPase activating protein) 1. Investigating the biology of this protein through the LocusLink indicates that it is a close neighbor of our target sequence on chromosome 5, and plays a critical role in neuronal differentiation.

What have we learned about the gene from all this?

This example demonstrated the ability to characterize an unknown DNA sequence of questionable validity using publicly available resources. Although cross-species homology searches bore failed to identify an ortholog, further information and putative identification of the sequence was achieved by aligning it to the genome. Moreover, the genome alignment spanned a region covered by other ESTs, supporting the presence of an actively transcribed gene, rather than a pseudogene.

Using the genomic sequence, a predicted protein was examined for functional domains identifying several protein regions with high homology to RAS-like GTPase, which was further supported by the strong protein-level homology to several human RAS-like GTPases. In addition, the presence of this protein in relative proximity to its closest homologue strongly suggests a gene-duplication event. Empirical studies can now be designed to test the predicted functions, and elucidate the significance of its change in expression in the original microarray experiment.

Computational Future of Pharmacogenomics

Emerging technologies, novel computational approaches, and the availability of human, mouse, and rat genome sequences continues to provide unprecedented opportunities to investigate the mechanisms of action of drugs, toxicants, natural products, and their mixtures that can significantly contribute to safety and risk assessments. The next challenge is to translate this information into decision supportive knowledge by integrating all available disparate data into the assessment process in order to make scientifically sound decisions that minimize potential negative impacts on patients, health provider organizations and the allied health care industry.

The current biomedical research "*build and test*" paradigm that is fueled by combinatorial chemistry, genomic mining for drugable targets, broad coverage omic technologies, and high throughput screening will need to evolve and adopt simulation strategies that have been used in other data and knowledge rich enterprises such as model simulations in the aeronautical field. Central to this objective is the growing importance of computational biology in safety and risk assessments which will not only provide a richer and more refined understanding of the elicited adverse effect through the management and analysis of large, complex data sets, the extraction of knowledge through the integration of disparate data, and the development of solutions that enhance human health, but will also produce models that are based on empirical data and can accurately predict outcomes. In anticipation of biomedical research becoming more computationally intensive, the National Instutite of Health established the Biomedical Information Science and Technology Initiative (BISTI), which was charged with identifying potential impediments in the application of computational approaches in biomedical research.

In parallel, the new field of systems biology emerged which can be defined as the iterative development of computational models that integrate disparate biological and other relevant meta data which can be used to predict adverse health outcomes. More recently, similar efforts have been initiated in pharmacology, toxicology, and risk assessment in order to more accurately predict adverse health effects following exposure to drugs, chemicals, contaminants, natural products, and their mixtures. It is widely believed, as demonstrated by the examples provided above, that applied bioinformatics and computational biology will play an ever-increasing role in pharmacogenomic research.

7

TOXICOGENOMICS

Toxicogenomics is a relatively new discipline within the field of toxicology. The phrase was first coined in 1998 at the first Toxicogenomics Workshop held as part of the U.S. and European Community Consortium on Molecular Toxicology in Palo Alto, California. In its broadest sense, it is defined as the use of OMICS technologies to investigate issues of toxicity. In its narrowest sense, it is defined as investigating the safety of compounds by using only cutting-edge gene expression technologies. Toxicogenomics is the use of OMICS technologies to assess the safety of new chemical entities or other compounds used in diagnostics or therapeutics.

OMICS technologies encompass genomics, proteomics, metabonomics, and pharmacogenomics. Other descriptive terms (for example, transcriptomics, toxicoproteomics, and toxicogenetics) have been used intermittently. Genomics is the study of gene expression through the use of high-throughput screening techniques, such as gene expression microarrays. Other gene expression techniques have been added to this category, and these methods include gene reporter assays, branched DNA amplification assay, scintillation proximity assay (SPA), rapid analysis of gene expression (RAGE), serial analysis of gene expression (SAGE), and various polymerase chain reaction PCR-based assays (e.g., real-time, quantitative, representational difference analysis, differential display) as has already been reviewed. However, in some cases, it may be a stretch to qualify the method as "high-throughput" because several of these technologies either address gene expression more indirectly, such as SAGE, or can only address a few genes at a time, such as PCR.

Proteomics, on the other hand, is the study of protein expression using either two-dimensional polyacrylamide gel electrophoresis (2DE) annotated by mass spectrometry (MS) or protein expression microarrays. Metabonomics is the use of high-resolution combinations of nuclear magnetic resonance (NMR), chromatography, or mass spectroscopy to evaluate metabolite profiles of body fluids or cells. Finally, pharmacogenomics is the study of genetic variability to explain the adverse effects caused by compound–cell interactions. Most pharmacogenomics studies have focused on single nucleotide polymorphisms (SNPs). This chapter will describe all of these OMICS methods and show how they can be applied to studying toxicity in pharmaceutical development. Case studies will be presented from very early citations to examples of current applications.

GENOMICS IN TOXICOLOGY

The applications of genomics to toxicology will be discussed with the focus on gene expression microarrays and how they have been used to investigate toxicity. Briefly, they are manufactured by attaching pieces of DNA or RNA molecules to a nitrocellulose filter, a glass slide, or a silicon wafer. Although early forms of arrays used nitrocellulose filters (now referred to as "macroarrays"), the most common substrate used today is a glass slide. Once the arrays have been printed with portion(s) of DNA or RNA ("probes"), they can be stored for further processing. The next step is to make the "targets" or isolated RNAs from both control cells and treated cells. These RNAs are labeled with a tag (most commonly fluorescent) and hybridized to complementary probes on the printed arrays. The microarrays are washed, scanned, and image analyzed to derive quantitative values for each probe signal. The remaining steps include data analysis of this raw information yielding (1) statistical analysis of replicate arrays and a measure of the variability in the processing steps, (2) similarities between gene expression patterns of control and treated samples, (3) identification of significantly expressed genes that may be biomarkers, and (4) patterns of gene–gene and gene–cell interactions.

Microarrays have been used as a screening tool in drug discovery and development. However, the focus and application of arrays in toxicology differs from discovery in several aspects. The emphasis in discovery is feasibility: to ascertain the interaction of the compound and drug target rapidly. The emphasis in toxicology is development and validation: to understand this interaction more fully and, more importantly, to assess if any adverse effects are occurring. The focus here is on (1) validation of the compound–target interaction, (2) the prediction of adverse effects, and (3) the discovery of any alternative mechanisms of action resulting in "off-target" effects and aiding in the redesign of the candidate to a less toxic substance.

One of the most significant factors in microarray experiments is the experimental design. The overall design is dictated by whether a one-color (one label) or two-color (two labels) array system is being used. A one-color system requires that the control and treated samples are run on separate arrays, and therefore, intra-array as well as interarray variability needs to be considered. A two-color system requires that both the control target and the treated target compete for a complementary probe molecule on the same array. In this system, the importance of the intra-array variability is lessened. This aspect is the same whether a discovery approach or a toxicology approach is being used.

However, several aspects of the experimental design do differ between microarray screens used in discovery or toxicology. In toxicity assessments using microarrays, the emphasis on validation is an essential requirement of the experimental design. Particular attention needs to be paid to (1) types of species; (2) gender; (3) cell or tissue system; (4) treatment scheduling, dose, and route; (5) appropriate controls; (6) numbers of replicates, and (7) correlation with independent morphological and pathological toxicity assays. Making these choices is critical for minimizing the process variability in order to maximize and visualize the biological variability. In 2001, The Microarray Gene Expression Data (MGED) Society proposed a list of guidelines for microarray work, known as the Minimum Information About a Microarray Experiment (MIAME) guidelines. These guidelines are recommended requirements for how experiments are designed and reported. A set of guidelines specifically for toxicogenomics applications was drafted, but this draft has not yet been agreed to.

Another aspect unique to toxicology research is the emphasis on analyzing the activity of annotated genes as opposed to unannotated genes. Annotated genes are genes whose sequence and function is already known. Unannotated genes are genes whose sequence is known but have not been assigned a function. As the focus for toxicology is validation, one priority is correlating significant expression of annotated genes observed in the data with their previously published values. A secondary priority is discovering which annotated genes or proteins are involved in any adverse or "off-target" effects. The final priority is discovering whether any unannotated genes are involved in these adverse effects and what their function or role may be.

Therefore, when selecting microarrays to use, arrays that have the most annotated genes are preferred. Two exceptions to this recommendation are (1) whole genome arrays and (2) focus arrays. The availability of whole genome arrays, or arrays containing the entire complement of genes for that organism, make the selection of arrays biased toward annnotated genes a mute point. Focus arrays are sets of a smaller number of genes printed several times on one substrate. These arrays allow for profiling different samples using one array and, conceivably, hundreds of compounds could be screened in a high-throughput manner.

A third aspect of the experimental design that differs is the use of control or untreated samples. Discovery-focused experiments have emphasized the use of pooled samples to maximize consistency and minimize cost. Pooled samples are individual samples from a cell or tissue system within a species and from the same treatment group that are pooled together to make one sample. In some cases, the control samples (from normal, non-diseased individuals) are pooled to make a "universal". However, the concerns are that (1) the resulting gene expression is an average of the group of samples, (2) the whole range of expression for the individuals within the group is not observed, and (3) pooling can only take place if the biological variation is greater than the process variation. One proposed method to address some of these concerns is "sub-pooling" where only subsets of samples are pooled and there are still replicates run for each group.

Toxicology-focused experiments may also include different sets of control samples. One set of control samples includes untreated samples both at the initial time point as well as at subsequent time points. If sufficient activity is found in the untreated control curve, this activity may need to be subtracted from the activity of the test curve. Another set of control samples includes samples from treatments using both positive and negative control compounds. Investigating the gene expression of the test compound is done by comparing it with the gene expression of the known control compounds. All of these controls need to be woven into the data analysis scheme.

As the focus is on validation, part of the evaluation is to determine how much the individual samples from a group vary in their gene expression. If the samples are pooled, the differences between responders and nonresponders will not be seen.

To understand toxicogenomics, it may be important to understand how microarrays evolved. An ongoing effort for developing more efficient sequencing by hybridization methods led to various initial microarray efforts where large numbers of genes could be screened at a time. The first use of a microarray was in 1987 by Augenlicht et al., where macroarrays were used to differentiate a disease state. In this case, cDNAs from a reference polyA mRNA library of the human colon carcinoma cell line, HT-29, were inserted into bacterial plasmids. Over 4000 clones were isolated and gridded onto several nitrocellulose filters.

Radiolabeled cDNA probes from several biopsy samples (ranging from patients at low risk for colon cancer to familial adenomatous polyposis [FAP] patients to colon cancer patients) were then hybridized to the filters. The amount of radiolabel was scanned and analyzed. The amazing fact from this experiment was that a high percentage (20%) of FAP biopsies (in which the cells had not yet accumulated into adenomas) was upregulated as compared with the low-risk biopsies. These results suggested that increased gene expression seemed to correlate with early stages of the disease.

Initial toxicology studies using microarrays focused on screening and prioritizing lead compounds. Gray et al. designed a combinatorial library of protein kinase inhibitors used in cancer therapy and initially screened the compounds through an *in vitro* toxicity activity assay. Then, three compounds were selected, and their interactions with yeast were investigated with oligonucleotide microarrays. The microarray results confirmed the diminished activity of one compound observed in the *in vitro* assay. Another collaborative study between Incyte and Tularik screened several lead compounds for efficacy and toxicity using two-color microarrays. The result was that the optimized lead compound had a similar profile to a known toxin, which led it to be redesigned to a better nontoxic lead compound.

One early study focused on discovering alternative modes of action. Karpf et al. used microarrays to broadly screen for genes expressed when a colon adenocarcinoma cell line was exposed to 5-aza-2′-deoxycytidine. Several genes were significantly expressed. When investigated further, an alternative pathway was discovered and linked to the signal transducer and activator of transcription (STAT) genes.

The first comprehensive gene expression profiling time-course study using microarrays was first cited in 1998 by Cunningham et al. Using an acute short-term exposure regimen, rats were treated with toxic doses of three known hepatotoxins: benzo (a)pyrene (BP), acetaminophen (APAP), and clofibrate (CLO). mRNA isolated from the livers were analyzed using a cDNA microarray containing 7400 rat genes. Significant gene activity was observed at the early time points (12 hours, 1 day, and 3 days), and less activity was observed at the later time points (7, 14, and 28 days). All three compounds resulted in different expression profiles. Several cytochrome P450 genes and genes involved in phase II reactions were expressed over all six time points; however, the genes were induced at different times depending on the compound used. Three different data analysis methods were compared. It was hypothesized that both nongenotoxic (causing damage by a non-DNA mechanism) APAP and CLO would have the most significantly expressed genes in common compared with genotoxic (damage caused by a DNA mechanism) BP. However, with all three analysis methods, APAP and BP showed the most overlap of significantly expressed genes. Interestingly, both APAP and BP have their primary metabolic pathway involving cytochrome P450, whereas the metabolism of CLO involves both cytochrome P450 and β-oxidation.

Since these early citations, the use of gene expression microarrays as a tool for predictive toxicology has progressed. An early emphasis was to use microarrays to classify compounds based on their resulting gene expression profiles. More recently, specific "*sets of genes*" giving rise to a gene expression profile have been used to distinguish classes of compounds. For example, Hu et al. showed through hierarchical clustering that distinct differences were observed between the gene expression profiles of direct- and indirect-acting genotoxins. When an array of over 9900 probes was used, a set of 58 genes could distinguish between these classes of compounds.

Another emphasis was to use gene expression microarrays to investigate mixtures. The profiles of the cellular interactions of mixtures were compared to the profiles of each component of the mixtures. Nadadur et al. compared the profile of residual oil fly ash (ROFA) in rat lung to the single profiles of vanadium sulfate and nickel sulfate, which are known components of ROFA. ROFA is derived from the exhaust plume of a power plant and is used as a model mixture to investigate the effects of air pollution. Using a focus macroarray, 12 genes were found to be significantly expressed in all three treatments. In a more recent study, arrays were shown to be able to distinguish toxic components of another type of mixture, wastewater effluent. From this study, Wang et al. found 11 genes that may ascertain the presence of endocrine-disrupting compounds in the environment.

A third emphasis was to match gene expression profiles to phenotypic changes. This correlation is the current goal for toxicogenomics. It will help toxicogenomics to be established as a tool in the regulatory arena. Early investigations focused on correlating gene expression from *in vivo* biological systems to gene expression from *in vitro* systems. Taking this concept further, attempts were made to correlate gene expression with specific organ regions exhibiting toxicity. More recent studies have focused on anchoring specific cellular histopathological changes to gene expression. To identify these changes, investigators have used laser capture microdissection (LCM) to extract specific cells exhibiting the phenotypic changes and then comparing the gene expression profiles of these cell populations with "normal" cell populations.

Finally, the most pressing issue in toxicogenomics may be the relevance of gene expression to toxicity. In other words, how does both the qualitative and the quantitative expression of a gene relate to toxicity? Several studies, including most of the papers already cited, have attempted to find this answer. Investigations by Heinloth et al. and Zhou et al. reported seeing gene expression changes before the observance of the overt toxicity. In each paper, *subchronic* doses of a toxicant were used and links of their expression with phenotypic changes were attempted. Today, research is ongoing, with the ultimate goal, to define a set of biomarkers that can predict toxicity earlier than the occurrence of phenotypic changes.

Proteomics in Toxicology

Two new words, *proteome* and *proteomics*, were coined a decade after classic terms such as *genome* and *genomics*. Here *proteome*, the complement of a *genome*, refers to the expression of all proteins in an organism, organ, or cell line at any given time. The study of the proteome, its interactions, and its post-translational modifications (such as glycosylation, phosphorylation, etc.) that may be associated with a specific disease or toxicant is defined as *proteomics*. One advantage of proteomics is the ability to profile several thousands of proteins on a single platform and provide insights into post-translational modifications. Another advantage is that because proteins govern the normal physiology and disease processes, a more accessible endpoint of any changes in gene expression can be determined by direct analysis of proteins. Also, unlike genomics, proteomics offers the advantage of readily assaying both tissues and body fluids (e.g., plasma and serum) to investigate the molecules correlating with disease and drug action. The proteomic analysis of body fluids is of particular interest as it can provide a noninvasive method for biomarker identification.

In the realm of toxicology, proteomics is one of many new technologies being used today to identify novel protein biomarkers and signature patterns in protein profiles that measure sensitive cellular changes in response to xenobiotic exposure. The most widely used technique to date for proteomic science is high-resolution 2DE coupled with MS. First developed in 1975, it separates proteins in the first dimension based on their isoelectric points and in the second dimension by molecular weight. Typically, 2DE can resolve hundreds to thousands of proteins from a single sample. To avoid overcrowding on a single gel, researchers now run multiple "zoom" gels that cover narrow pH ranges (e.g., covering 1 pH unit).

In the mid-1990s, 2DE was coupled to MS allowing for annotation of the resolved spots. Proteins resolved using 2DE are analyzed by MS to give mass spectra. Subsequently, individual spots are excised from the gel and trypsin-digested to give shorter peptide fragments for sequencing. With the help of software programs and sequence databases, the peptide mass spectrum is compared with known partial gene and protein sequences and is then assigned an annotation. Recent developments in MS techniques, such as "tandem MS" (MS/MS), allow for better analysis of protein sequences, by avoiding ambiguity arising when MS data match more than one protein sequence.

The use of proteomics in toxicology can be divided into two classes: (1) investigative studies and (2) screening/predictive toxicology. The mechanism of toxic damage in several model systems has been elucidated with proteomics. But proteomics offers the prospect of identifying new toxic mechanisms along with traditional toxicology methods. Such insights may provide valuable information about specific effects caused by a specific group or class of compounds. In addition to supporting investigative studies, proteomics promises to provide insight into screening and predictive toxicology. The screening of new compounds for toxicity can be possible by following specific signatures of protein expression, thus identifying them as predictive biomarkers of toxicity.

The sensitive nature of proteomics offers the detection of toxic effects at low dosage levels, which escape conventional screening methods, such as histopathology and clinical chemistry. In addition, proteomics provides a method for the early detection of potential toxicity and the opportunity of ranking compounds during drug development. A recent review lists publications that use proteomics in toxicology studies, with the most popular application being biomarker identification. The issues surrounding the experimental design and the emphasis on development and validation covered in the previous section for genomics applies to proteomics as well.

As an investigative tool, proteomics has been used to determine the failure of several drug candidates due to adverse drug reactions. In an early study, Anderson et al. developed a rodent liver proteomic toxicity database. This database, containing profiles of effects of 43 compounds on liver, was among the first available for the detection, classification, and characterization of a wide range of hepatotoxins. The development of such a database has considerable implications for predictive toxicology. The potential hepatotoxicity of a new and unknown compound can be determined by comparing its effects on the proteome against known toxins from the database.

New biomarker discovery from such studies can lead to early detection of deleterious effects. In a more recent study, researchers validated toxicological protein markers from an *in vivo* system (rat liver) as well as from an *in vitro* system (human HepG2 cell line). They reported a total of 11 protein markers with reactivity toward multiple toxic compounds and no reactivity toward nontoxic compounds. An important conclusion from this work is that cells in culture can be used as an *in vitro* toxicity testing system to assess hepatotoxicity. However, in the future, a much more extensive study may be required to identify a larger group of toxicology markers to detect more diverse types of toxic reactions.

Toward understanding the mechanistic action of toxicology using 2DE, Fountoulakis et al. showed the hepatotoxic effects of paracetamol (aceta minophen) overdose in human and rodent liver. They found that the expression of 35 proteins was altered after treatment with paracetamol or its nontoxic regioisomer 3-acetamidophenol. Paracetamol selectively increases or decreases the phosphorylation state of proteins. This effect translates to a decrease in protein phosphatase activity. The control of cellular functions of cells may be lost as a result of the dephosphorylation of certain regulatory proteins due to paracetamol overdose.

A dose- and time-dependent proteomics study with gentamicin confirmed the histopathological findings of renal toxicity at high doses and renal regeneration during the recovery phase. Gentamicin, a known renal toxicant, represents a class of aminoglycosides. The effects of gentamicin treatment were observed after proteomic evaluation of rat kidney cortex samples. Examination of rat serum samples exposed to varying doses of gentamicin identified a protein being consistently overexpressed. Surprisingly, this particular protein marker was present both at the low treatment dose as well as at early time points before changes were observerd by routine clinical pathology. Intriguingly, during the recovery phase, the marker returned to control levels, thereby highlighting the sensitive nature of proteomics. Such protein markers are of great interest as they provide a non invasive means of monitoring the onset of toxicity before any evident cellular damage.

Although 2DE offers a high-quality approach to proteomic research, it has certain limitations: Only major components of protein mixtures are visualized, the detection of low and high molecular mass of basic and hydrophobic proteins is inefficient, and it is a highly laborious technique. Alternative technologies, such as the protein microarrays, allows investigators to control conditions, such as pH, temperature, ionic strength, and different stages of protein modification, while monitoring the protein–protein interactions of thousands of proteins spotted on an array. Protein microarrays not only provide a technique for high-throughput screening but also a method to study interactions of proteins with non-proteinaceous molecules. Zhu et al. have developed a protein microarray of the yeast proteome from 5800 open reading frames. The expressed proteins are purified and printed on glass slides with high spatial density to form a yeast proteome microarray. They were used to screen for interactions with proteins and phospholipids. The researchers identified many new calmodulin- and phospholipid-interacting proteins. Thus, protein microarrays can serve to screen for several hundreds to thousands of biochemical activities on a single chip. In toxicology, these arrays can be used to screen for adverse protein–drug interactions, to detect post-translational modifications leading to disease, and to identify biomarkers for drug targets and early disease detection.

A recent advancement is the coupling of MS with LCM for identification of tumor markers specific for cancer. Specific cells of pathological interest are selected with LCM under direct microscopic visualization, laser captured, and removed from the tissues. The extracted lysate from the cells is applied directly to spots on the substrate of a surface-enhanced laser desorption/ionization (SELDI) MS, ionized, and desorbed from the surface, and a time-of-flight (ToF) proteomic profile of the entire cellular system is observed. This method has been recently applied to toxicology.

Several efforts are attempting to improve proteomic technologies to map and measure proteomes and subproteomes. However, no single proteomic platform seems to ideally suit and quantify the broad range of protein expression in a given cell/tissue system. More than one proteomic platform may likely be needed to distinguish the multiple forms and post-translational modifications of proteins, to address the inadequate annotation of proteomes, or to accomplish integration of proteomic data with genomic and metabonomic data. Additionally, advances in genomics data through investigations of pathways and subcellular structures induced by toxicity may guide studies in proteomics.

Metabonomics in Toxicology

The term metabonomics was derived from early work in Dr. Jeremy Nicholson's laboratory. This term along with metabolomics has been used in several citations interchangeably. Attempts have been made to clarify the definition of each term. It seems that agreement has been reached where metabonomics is the broader encompassing term of metabolite profiling and metabolomics refers specifically to profiling in cells.

This technology uses combinations of NMR, MS, and chromatography to profile multiple components in biofluids, tissues, or cells. The main advantage of metabonomics is the serial sampling of a biofluid noninvasively. The earliest papers used high-resolution ^{1}H-NMR alone for profiling. The technique became more sophisticated when bioinformatics tools, such as pattern recognition and expert systems, were applied to the data. Today, the following combinations of techniques are used: liquid chromatography–nuclear magne tic resonance (LC–NMR), magic angle spinning–nuclear magnetic resonance (MAS–NMR), gas chromatography–mass spectroscopy (GC–MS), LC–MS, capillary electrophoresis–mass spectroscopy (CE–MS), and LC–NMR–MS. The first technique listed in the combinations above refers to the method used to separate the multiple components of the sample, and these components are identified using the second technique.

Two of the earliest papers using metabonomics in toxicology were studies by Nicholson et al., which investigated mercury and cadmium toxicity in the rat. Each of these papers used an experimental design that reiteratively sampled a biological system over either dose or time using high-resolution ^{1}H NMR. The changes in the urinary excretion patterns correlated with the expected histological changes. However, an interesting note was that in the case of cadmium, a urinary metabolite related to nephrotoxicity was found that was undetectable using traditional methods. A more extensive study that included a-naphthylisothiocyanate and 2-bromoethylamine showed changes in the metabolite profiles ahead of the time point where the clinical chemistry or microscopic changes would be detected.

As with the previously described OMICS technologies, one emphasis has been to profile groups of compounds using metabonomics. Each compound gave a unique metabonomic profile and was successfully classified using pattern recognition techniques. A second emphasis was to be able to monitor not only biofluids, such as urine or plasma, but also tissues and cells. Moka et al. performed the first study to classify carcinoma biopsy samples by MAS-NMR. Since then, two studies have used metabonomics to investigate toxicity using a wider approach where urine, plasma, and tissue samples are all analyzed.

To collaborate and share information, a proposal for a users group in metabonomics was put forth. Since then, the Consortium for Metabonomic Toxicology (COMET) was formed and the first report from this group was given in 2003. This report describes what methodologies have been assessed, the development of a curated database for metabonomic profiles, and computer-based experts systems for data analysis.

Pharmacogenomics in Toxicology

Pharmacogenomics and pharmacogenetics are two terms that have created confusion because they have been used interchangeably and defined differently by several authors. The most widely accepted term, pharmacogenetics, is the study of an individual's response to a drug as determined by their genetic makeup. Pharmacogenetics as a field of study has been around for several decades. Early studies focused on observations of patient variability in metabolizing various drugs such as primaquine, succinylcholine, and dibucaine. In this chapter, the term "*pharmacogenomics*" will be used to refer to the use of high-throughput screening techniques for the detection of the genetic variation of an individual and its role in toxicity, especially in causing adverse effects.

In toxicology, most pharmacogenomics studies have focused on variations within the drug metabolizing enzymes (DMEs). These DMEs catalyze the phase I and phase II metabolic reactions. Several examples have been cited for arylamine N-acetyltransferase (NAT1 and NAT2), thiopurine-S-methyltransferase (TPMT), glutathione-S-transferase (GST), as well as the various cytochrome P450 enzymes (e.g., CYP2A6, CYP2C8, CYP2C9, CYP2C19, CYP2D6, and CYP3A4). Early studies showed that individuals with these genetic variations can be classified as "poor," "extensive," and "ultrarapid" metabolizers.

From a toxicity standpoint, this variability is extremely important in that poor metabolizers could accumulate the drug within their tissues causing a toxic response, whereas in extensive metabolizers, the drug has an extremely short half-life and may not stay around the tissues long enough to exert its desired effect. For example, an individual with the gene variant CYP2D6*2, which represents an "*ultrarapid metabolizer*," can possess a much higher activity for cytochrome P450 isozyme 2D6, whereas an individual with the gene variant CYP2D6*10 possesses a defective enzyme and therefore is a "*poor metabolizer*". Individuals who have slow or fast metabolism rates have been observed in several mammalian species.

Early examples of polymorphisms being detected in a high-throughput manner are studies that used oligonucleotide microarrays containing perfect-match and mismatch sequences. These studies investigated polymorphic changes in breast cancer, HIV infection, and cystic fibrosis. A more recent study used a chip containing over 11,000 SNPs to detect genetic variabilities in over 100 DNA samples—a high-throughput variation on associ ation studies. Another array format blended nanotechnology by using multiplexed nanoparticle probes with printed oligonucleotides to distinguish genetic polymorphic variants.

System Biology

Systems biology is a recent term that encompasses looking at the entire biological system from the molecular, cellular, tissue, organism, population, and finally, ecosystem levels. As Witkamp describes it, "systems biology is a realization that organisms do not consist of isolated subsets of genes, proteins and metabolites". It is also the application of network biology or comprehensive computational methods to analyze the data produced by the combination of OMICS technologies. The ultimate goal of toxicogenomics is to predict compound–cell and cell–cell interactions *in silico*, and the application of systems biology brings this one step closer.

In attempts to obtain this goal, several studies have correlated datasets from combined genomics and proteomic studies and combined genomics and metabonomics studies. An early toxicogenomics study by Cunningham et al. combined the datasets from the rat toxicity study with three hepatotoxins evaluated by gene expression microarrays described earlier with a matched proteomics arm. In this study, a portion of the gene and protein expression profiles matched but the remaining did not. Four other studies also tried correlating gene and protein expression in evaluating the effects of zinc, carbon tetrachloride, lithium, and bromobenzene. The experimental design for these studies used only one or two time points with one dose, and in all three studies, only a portion of overlap between gene and protein expression was observed. Finally, Coen et al. attempted to correlate metabonomics with genomics. They observed some overlap between the two technologies and, hence, concluded that these technologies are complementary in providing a view into toxicity.

A fully integrated approach using genomics, proteomics, and metabonomics was attempted by two groups of investigators. Schnackenberg et al. studied the hepatotoxicity effects of valproic acid. Correlative changes in glucose metabolism were shown by both metabonomics and proteomics methods. However, no significant changes were observed with the gene expression method. Kleno et al. used genomics, proteomics, and metabonomics to investigate the hepatotoxicity of hydrazine. Disruption in both glucose and lipid metabolism were present in all three datasets, and therefore, once again, these three technologies were shown to be complementary.

Future Technologies in Toxicogenomics

The field of toxicogenomics continues to evolve and develop. For all the technologies listed above, research is continuing to develop more efficient, more high-throughput versions. The field of nanotechnology may aid in this effort. The various engineered nanomaterials may enable the current microarray format to be redeveloped on a nanoscale level and provide more rapid and possibly instaneous results. Some of these engineered nanomaterials, such as single-walled carbon nanotubes, are being developed for applications in the communications and information technologies field and may lead to increased capacity and advances in bioinformatics.

The entire field of biosensors is being redeveloped on the nanoscale to nanosensors—from microelectronic membranes (MEMs) to nanoelectronic membranes (NEMs). A preliminary study done by Cunningham et al. assesses the toxicity of these nanomaterials using genomics. In this study, the gene expression profiles of three known nanoscale materials were compared and two were found to be more similar with each other. This similarity correlated with the similarity in their chemical structures. As more and more engineered nanomaterials are being made, the applications for these materials in the life sciences will only grow. As a result, their safety will also need to be assessed.

Facing the future, other new technological fields are making their way to the forefront of research and could have pertinent applications for investigating toxicity. RNA interference (RNAi) is a burgeoning area. This field was first thought to include only investigations of naturally-occurring microRNA (miRNA) molecules and synthesized short-interfering RNA (siRNA) molecules. An early paper used siRNAs to the aryl hydrocarbon receptor (AhR) and the AhR nuclear translocator (ARNT) to look at gene silencing. Since this 2003 paper, many references have now reported using siRNA molecules as knockout molecules to investigate mechanisms of toxicity. miRNA molecules, on the other hand, have been sequenced and printed on macroarrays and microarrays.

These array tools may allow the expression of these molecules, and consequently, their function to be investigated. Recently, other types of short non-coding RNA molecules have been reported as well as naturally-occurring siRNAs. It will be interesting to see what roles, if any, each of these new classes of short RNA molecules play in toxicity.

Another technological field is the exciting area of stem cells. Although work has been ongoing with adult stem cells for many years, research involving embryonic stem cells continues to hold great promise. Cell lines for mouse and rat have been used in several research areas to develop new animal models and devise new therapies. The next front is human embryonic stem (HES) cells. Currently, this tool is in the midst of an ethics and morality debate. However, the same debate was waged when fetal tissue was first used in the laboratory setting over two decades ago. If an investigator could direct the differentiation pathway of HES to more mature tissue-specific cells, the need for primary human tissue, which is already difficult to get, would be lessened. This application would increase dramatically the capability of *in vitro* toxicity assays.

Toxicogenomics is a growing and ever-changing field within toxicology. All of these advances in research and development could completely change the safety assessment landscape within just a few years. As the regulatory assays become more predictable, the time from discovery of a pharmaceutical agent to its market release will be lessened.

8

DNA Probes for Identification of Microbes

In 1997 and the first quarter of 1998, what we hereafter refer to as DNA probes were used primarily by those performing genetic-related research. Today (mid-2000), oligonucleotide (DNA, RNA, and related) probes in several guises are a growth industry in biotechnology, and their applications are widespread. In 1995, Theta Reports (*Gene Therapy/DNA Probes/PCR Markets*) predicted a phenomenal growth in polymerase chain reaction (PCR), DNA probes, and the successful use of gene therapy—they were correct about the first two. In 1996, the Frost & Sullivan Market Intelligence indicated that the 1995 market for DNA probes had been over $145 million, and predicted that it would reach $1.4 billion by 2003. Also in 1996, Business Communications Co., Inc., made similar predictions. DNA probes are the fastest growing area of in vitro diagnostics, expanding at the rate of 25% per year.

The most important differences between the earlier and the current version of DNA probes relate to the following:

1. Literature and applications have boomed; cumulative citations listed by Medline for "DNA probes"are currently 79,270.
2. Applications—especially of PCR—now embrace most aspects of life sciences, including agriculture, food science, and non-microbial disease states, as well as areas relating to human diseases.
3. Use of oligo-on-a-chip (DNA- or RNA-based array, also referred to in some instances as microchip) has burgeoned in pharmaceutical/biotech R&D. This approach, if not yet predominant, is becoming so in many applications.
4. Antisense therapeutics, which had lost favor due to a well-publicized Phase-I human death in mid-2000, are already rebounding. Some forms of antisense show very high potential as antimicrobials.

To focus the current version of "*DNA probes*" on microbiological and related issues, some background material has been abbreviated. This author also recommends that the genomics tyro read one or more of the basic references, of which the article by Keller and Marak is the most germane.

Rapid growth areas of science, such as oligo probes, are referenced most rapidly on the Internet. Formal print publication may appear 1-3 years after completion of the work. Many, but not all, Internet publications are refereed in a manner similar to that for print publications. Therefore, many of the references herein are from the Internet.

Although we have cited a very small proportion of the patent, regulatory, and market literature herein, the reader should note that:

1. Many productive scientists choose to file for letters patent in lieu of, rather than in addition to, conventional publication.
2. Negative findings may not find their way into scientific literature for a long time, if ever.
3. For a new commercial venture, first-rate technology is often insufficient; good business practice and adequate financing are equally important. Therefore, many small operations disappear.

Follow-up on vanished companies and products is difficult, unless they are acquired. For example, Biotech Research Laboratories and their peptide nucleic acid oligos (PNAs) were acquired by Boston Biomedica, Inc. Tracking BRL and its specifically targeted PNAs to BBI is simplified by web-page links, which are easy to follow for the reader with a modest knowledge of computer use.

Definitions

cDNA: Copy DNA, as by PCR or RT-PCR.

DNA probe: An oligonucleotide sequence that complements a sequence (usually of a gene) in or from an organism. Here, DNA is used generically in the description of probes.

dsDNA: Double-stranded DNA, as in the double helix.

Endonuclease: An enzyme that hydrolyzes (breaks) an oligonucleotide chain between particular bases only; consequently, the pattern of pieces of DNA (oligos) generated by the action of endonuclease on DNA of a particular organism is reproducible.

Genome: The entire DNA complement [gene(s)] of an organism; this includes the genetic information in viruses.

Morpholino oligo: An oligo containing the morpholino analog of the conventional backbone.

Nucleoside: Molecule containing a purine or a pyrimidine base linked to a pentose sugar.

Nucleotide: A phosphorylated nucleoside.

Oligonucleotide (also *termed oligos*): Usually a sequence of DNA or RNA with a phosphate backbone, but may have a sulfate, peptide, or morpholino backbone in place of a phosphate one, to reduce or eliminate oligo degradation by nucleases.

Phosphorothioate oligo: An oligo (usually a probe) containing S in place of P.

PNA oligomer: Peptide nucleic acid oligo; manufacturers include Boston Probes; the Danish company; Pantheco, and Research Genetics. These, like morpholino analogs, resist nuclease digestion.

Polymerase chain reaction: The method for producing, in vitro and fairly rapidly, millions

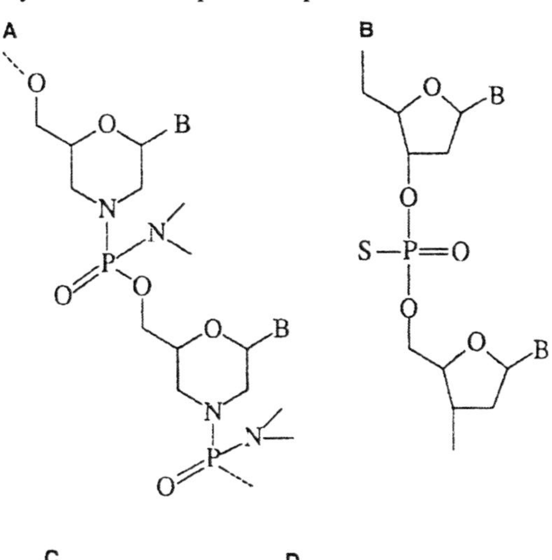

Fig. 8.1. Dinucleotide structures (as found in respective dinocleotides). A-morpholino analog; B-normal DNA or RNA; C-phosphorothioate analog of DNA; D-peptide nucleic acid.

of copies of a specific segment of DNA or RNA (amplification). The sequence of the ends of the portion to be copied must be known so that the primer can be annealed to the denatured oligo to be copied.

Primer: The segment of synthetic oligo that is added to one end of the DNA or RNA to be copied. The denatured oligo target is annealed with the primer, and DNA polymerase then adds complementary nucleic acids until the full copy is produced.

Reverse transcriptase (RT): The enzyme from RNA viruses that codes (cDNA) from RNA.

Sense strand: In dsDNA, the strand that codes for the protein that is generated from it. The other strand is complementary, and protects the sense strand.

ssDNA: Single-stranded DNA, as contrasted with dsDNA

Target of an oligonucleotide probe: Usually ribosomal RNA (rRNA), which (with uridine in place of thymine) is the complement to the sense strand of the dsDNA in the double helix.

Triplet code: Although the coding for the amino acid sequence of proteins is by sets of three nucleotides in the DNA, the actual blueprint for protein sythesis is in RNA transcribed from the DNA. For example, in the RNA copied from a gene, UAU (uracil–adenine–uracil) or UAC (C is cytidine in the second uracil) are triplet codes for tyrosine.

Abbreviated Background

Every characteristic of an organism (single-celled or multi-celled) is dictated by its genome. For example, all metabolic processes are determined by enzymes that are encoded in the genome (some enzymes are imported and/or exported from a microbial cell in plasmids, which are small closed DNA loops of genes separate from the microbial chromosome). In some viruses, the genome is ssDNAor RNA, but in the majority of organisms, including microbes, it is dsDNA. The double helix of dsDNA contains a sense strand, which carries the sequence of the nucleotide triplet codes that characterize the amino acid sequence of the protein they code for. The other nucleotide strand in dsDNA is complementary to the sense strand and stabilizes it.

Although some segments of the DNA in a microbial cell provide information that can identify the cell to species, there is only a single copy of DNA per cell. There may be 10^4 or more copies of the 16S rRNA per cell involved in the production of various proteins (usually enzymes) for use by the cell. The rRNA of molecular weight 16S (designated as Svedberg units in the ultracentrifuge) provides regions that are suitable for identification of the microbe to species.

A

B

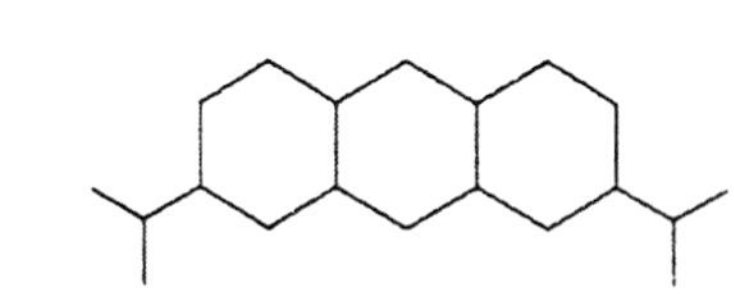

Fig. 8.2. Schematic of base pair in dsDNA (A) and acridine orange (AO) (B). The AO intercalates between sequential base pairs, extending the phosphate backbone.

Therefore, if the 16S rRNA of an organism can be made available to oligo probes, usually by opening the organism in some way, it is possible to see whether the rRNA of the microbe anneals (forms a duplex) with the labeled synthetic oligo probe of known sequence and identity. There are several ways of doing this. However, in my view, unless the genus of the organism is known with reasonably good probability, this method is inordinately expensive in the use of labeled probes.

Appropriate Use of Oligo Probes

In my view, before labeled probes are put to use for the identification of an unknown, the organism should be tentatively identified. Conventional (but effective) hand methods derived from *Bergey's Manual* can be painfully slow. The fatty acid methyl ester (FAME). technique are usually quite accurate and sufficiently rapid if the patient is not in extremis. Also, it is wise to remember that conventional bench methods (e.g., Bergey's) are dendritic, and for microbiologists lacking considerable experience, an error in any of the sequential steps may result in error in the identification. The earlier a mistake is made in a dendritic pattern, the greater the error in identification (i.e., if a bird's nest is near the end of a limb on the north side of the tree and one chooses to climb on a limb on the south side of the tree in search of the nest, one will be right about the nest being above ground, but remote from the objective).

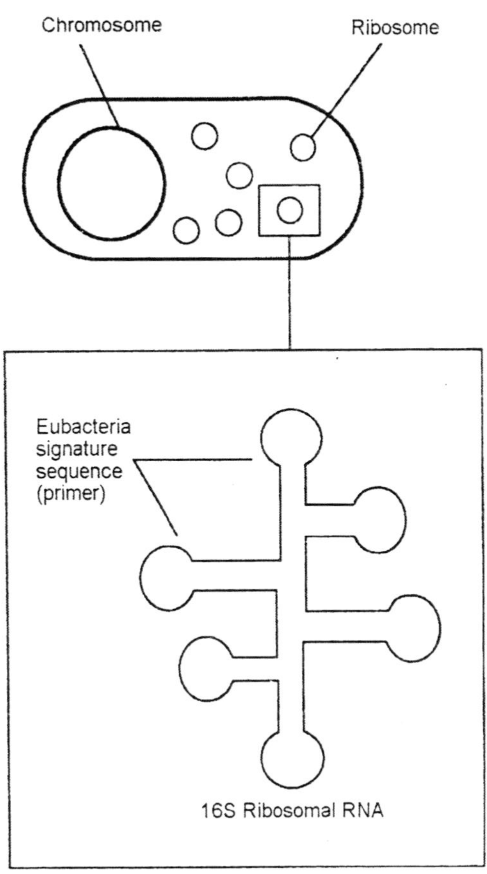

Fig. 8.3. Extrachromosomal ribosomes in a bacterium or fungus that contain 16S rRNA.

If preliminary information is available (e.g., indicators of pathogenicity), the most cost-effective and reliable approach may be to go directly to probes. Also, probes make best sense in widespread screening for specific diseases such as tuberculosis. In disease states, whether in humans, animals, or plants, symptoms may indicate the presence of one or a few pathogens. In such instances, the use of probes directly is sensible and economical. Machine identifications, based not on genomic but on chemical analyses, become confirming and often unnecessary.

Probes, depending on the oligo target in the organism, are for practical and definitive purposes. Errors with non-genomic machines (e.g., FAME profile by GC, or mass spectrometry/fuzzy logic profile, etc.) are because the organism sought is not in the machine library, or the concentration of key chemicals (almost always oligonucleotides, oligosaccharides, and/or FAME from the organism) is too low (insufficient cells or incomplete extraction).

For some very slow-growing organisms such as *Mycobacterium tuberculosis* and *M. leprae*, sufficient organisms may be present for analysis by probe in the sample fluid or tissue, in which case the use of penetrant aids such as DMSO facilitates the exposure of chemiluminescent-labeled oligo probes to the genome of the organism. The DNA of the organism then fluoresces under ultraviolet epi-illumination. The method with fluorescent-labeled probes when applied for the detection of cancers or genetic effects, to human or animal genes in tissue, is called fluorescent in situ hybridization (FISH).

Defined Oligo on Magnetic Beads

A very rapid technique employs specific oligos immobilized on Dynal magnetic beads. The special advantage is that the beads, covalently coupled to particular oligo sequences (or antigens, antibodies, or other binding entities), can be mixed in a nonmetallic container (e.g., test tube) with a solution or suspension so as to react even with very dilute targets (organisms, especially viruses). The beads are then concentrated simply by placing a magnet against the side of the container. The original solution, less the bead-reacted targets, is then removed and the beads rinsed in situ. The recovery of mRNA (terminal polyA sequence) is with poly dT beads.

The basic magnetic-bead patent appears to be the property of Dynal, but Clemente Associates produces Ni-bearing magnetic particles of 3- to 5-μm diameter for performing what they refer to as "*magnetic chromatography*," of cells, proteins, or both. Qiagen markets histidine-labeled Ni-containing agarose magnetic beads. Bangs Laboratories also produces 2 μm diameter beads with surface caboxyl groups for the coupling of binding ligands. Seradyn uses beads for DNA isolation. All of these can bear oligo probes. CPG, Inc. offers streptavidin magnetic porous glass for the binding of biotinylated molecules for a variety of oligo-probe-related purifications of cells, noncellular particles, and macromolecules, including DNAs and RNAs. Non-magnetic beads of a variety of matrices, ready for coupling by various chemistries to oligos, antibodies, antigens, or what-have-you, are available for column or suspension applications from Polymer Laboratories.

Polymerase Chain Reaction (PCR) and the Detection of Microbes

If a dozen copies of a pathogenic DNA virus are present per milliliter or gram in body fluid or beef tissue intended for sale, inoculation of the suspect source material into cell culture or in a test animal for analytical testing is a very lengthy, expensive process. It is unrealistic for use in the food industry or in a hospital, as are many other tests. If we seek particular viruses (e.g., rabies), the most rapid, practical, and effective means of detecting the virions is the PCR.

The primer used is an oligo specific to the organism to be detected. Commencing with the DNA recovered from one or several organisms, the multiplication of genomic material can be 10^7- to 10^8-fold in 35–90 min. By comparison, growing the virions in cell culture to equivalent numbers (to allow monoclonal antibody type analyses) usually requires 48 h or more. In cases where life hangs in the balance of an accurate analysis, those hours may be critical. Even with bacterial or fungal pathogens, the time required to generate sufficient genomic material for analysis by PCR is 35–45 min but 24–48 h in conventional culture on an appropriate nutfrient medium.

Reverse transcriptase PCR, (RT-PCR), runs the normal RNA to DNA sequence backward. Reverse transcriptase is an enzyme found in RNA viruses and, when added to a solution of RNA, deoxynucleotides, reverse transcriptase, etc., allows one to produce the DNA equivalent to the RNA recovered from an organism. The cDNA (DNA produced from RNA) recovered in sufficient amounts can then can be "clipped" using a well-characterized endonuclease and a cDNA "fingerprint" generated for comparison with the fingerprints of known RNA sources.

Immobilized Oligos or Genes in Analytical Arrays

Immobilized oligos in arrays (e.g., in the wells of microtiter plates or on glass slides) are used in the detection of cancer and precursor stages (e.g., mutations), in addition to drug screening of the interactions of candidate drugs (free) with human or animal gene sequences (immobilized). One possible approach involves the extraction of the gene of each of hundreds of bacterial species, grown as axenic (pure) cultures. In each of the wells of microtiter plates molded from polyethylene-co-acrylic acid, segments of the gene of a single bacterial species (prepared when the DNA from the cells of a particular colony are "clipped" with a known endonuclease) are added and immobilized to the bottom of the plate via the 3′-OH. A good immobilization system is the triazine method for coupling linear microbial DNA strands. To each of these plates, bearing (for example) ca. 100 wells and the genomes of 100 human microbial pathogens, is added one of the many varieties of possible synthetic oligos intended for test as potential drugs (limited mixtures, each unpurified but reproducible), each with a low toxicity label, preferably chemiluminescent rather than radioactive.

The drugs (e.g., PNAs) and immobilized microbial genomes are allowed a reaction time, rinsed, and then examined (automatically or by eye,) for retention of the synthetic candidate drugs by segments of the genomes of the various pathogens. In this way, it is possible to screen candidate oligos for

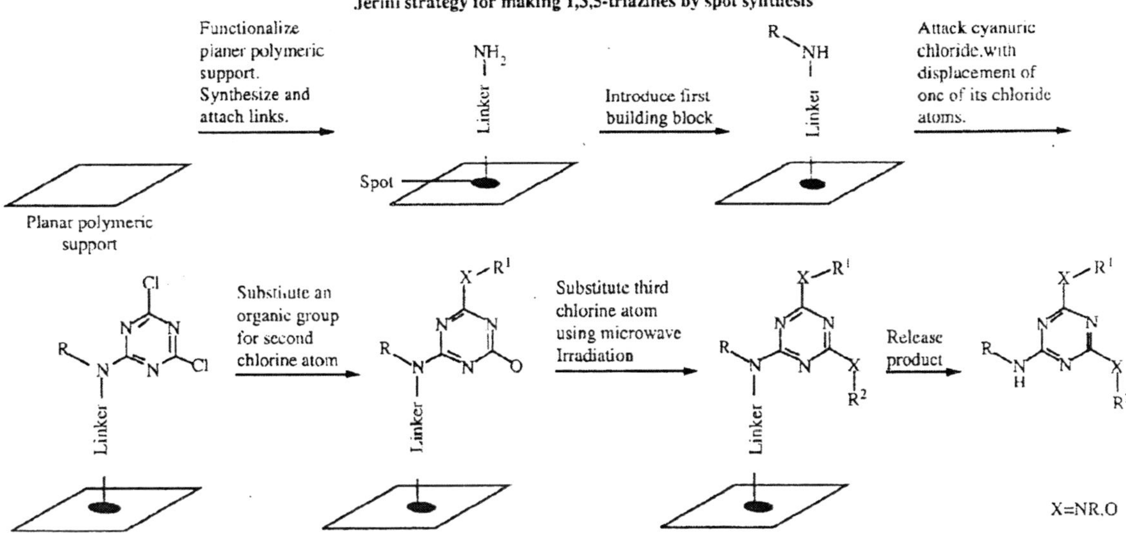

Fig. 8.4. Coupling microbial ssDNA or RNA or analogs via triazine to wells in a microtiter plate.

specific binding to immobilized genomes of known organisms, even if gene sequences of the pathogens are unknown, and the precise sequence that binds to a given pathogen's genome is known only with modest accuracy. In cases where this combinatorial-type approach to new product development appears promising, it can be automated, all or in part. Such systems are in widespread use in a variety of applications in the pharmaceutical industry. The example given is a variation of the method known as combinatorial chemistry. A variation on this method has been proposed by the U.S. National Institute of Environmental Health Sciences to evaluate chemicals as potential human toxins. Human genes, immobilized on microtiter-type plates, are exposed to known and unknown toxicants, with a view to seeking similarities in gene-binding patterns.

Specific Oligo Probes as Antimicrobials

The DNA of a cell must be copied if the cell is to reproduce. Also, certain enzymes are required for a cell to metabolize and function (as contrasted with the dormant state), and these are usually made in the cell as needed. Therefore, an antisense probe that reacts with, for example, a critical RNA in the cell, may effectively render the cell dormant. One can envision this in vitro and in vivo. But oligonucleotides are subject to degradation by nucleases which, depending on their specificity, clip a nucleotide at certain base sequences, usually rendering the oligo less functional or non-functional.

If a species-specific antisense oligo probe can be made resistant to enzymic degradation, and if it can readily enter a microbe, the probe not only identifies the organism, but also may shut down the metabolic potential of the cell. Antisense PNA oligos appear to meet these requirements and bind to sense with a lower dissociation constant (Kd) than does the phosphate-backbone antisense. PNA antisenses have the potential for use as very specific, low-toxicity microbicides for in vivo applications. The peptide analogs of DNA probes are protected by appropriate patents.

Antisense Probes as Therapeutics

The primary target of antisense probe studies is the ongoing cell proliferation in all cancers. Cancerous cells are not functional in, for example, gas transport in the lung. Like viruses, their anthropomorphized raison d'etre is only to reproduce, not to perform a service for the organism of which they are a part. On the other hand, normal cells have a finite lifetime and must occasionally be replaced.

The toxicants used in conventional chemotherapy and radiation not only kill a substantial proportion of the cells that are reproducing rapidly but also tend to destroy stem cells in the bone marrow and circulating plasma, which gives rise to the panoply of red cells, white cells, and platelets that are essential to a survival free of dialysis machines and other elaborate supports. For this reason, patient-sourced (autologous) stem cells ($CD34^+$), hopefully cancer-free, are recovered from the patient prior to radiation treatment or chemotherapy (or both) as "heroic" cancer therapy. The recipient of massive "chemotherapy," or radiation (or both), dies unless those healthy stem cells (removed from the patient prior to treatment) are injected intravenously (they find their way to the marrow) and replace the essential cells that chemotherapy or radiation has destroyed. In addition, although chemotherapy and radiation may "cure" a patient, the once-healthy cells that are not killed may be mutated in critical portions of the genome. It is fairly common that patients receiving "heroic" therapy develop new tumor sets 20 years downstream of the initial therapy. Ultimately, the exposure to these unselective toxicants that saved the patient may eventually kill the patient.

In theory, the beauty of antisense is that an anti-sense oligo probe does not damage all types of cells at random, and does not induce mutations. Antisense shuts down the propagation of some cells, and not others. Antisense therapy is distinct from gene therapy, in which a missing or malfunctioning gene (e.g., human clotting factor VIII gene in most hemophiliacs) is placed in autologous cells and returned to the patient. Professor Eric Wickstrom has done some excellent work in mouse models on antisense and Burkitt's lymphoma, rabies virus, and the human cMYC oncogene, to name a few systems. His group employs phosphorothioates, PNAs, and other variations on antisense. His patents on the synthesis and introduction of antisense into cells are germane.

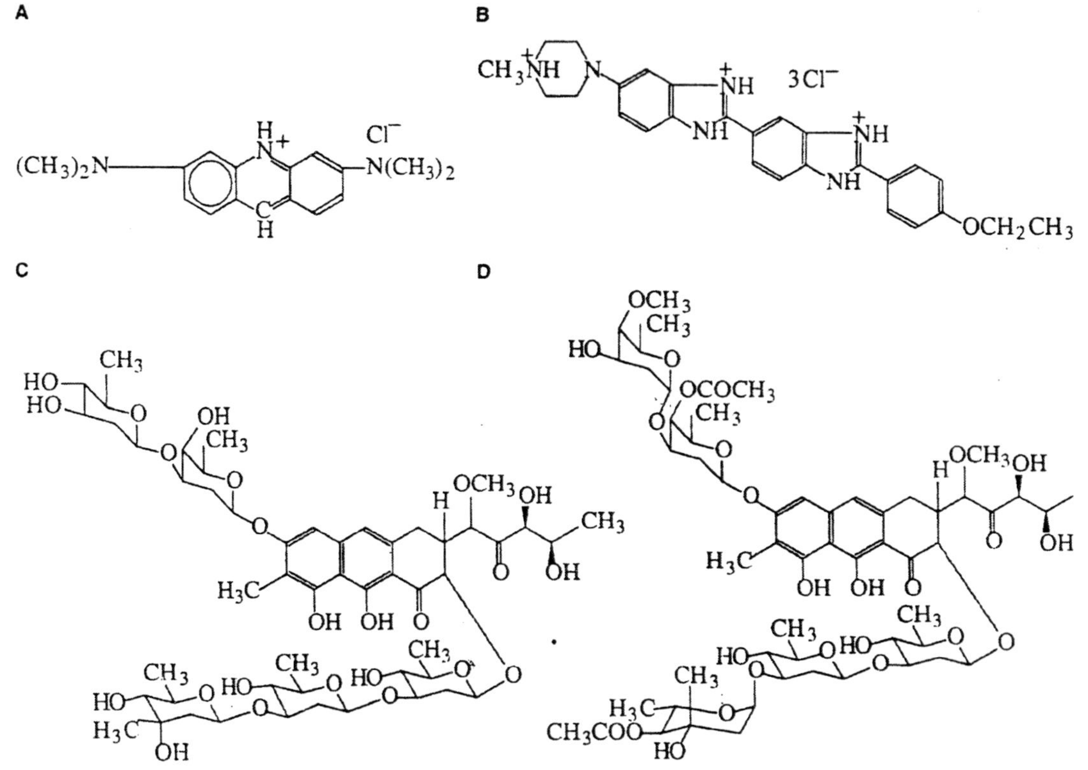

Fig. 8.5. Small organic molecules that interact with DNA and/or RNA and when excited with one wavelength of light, fluoresce in another. (A) acridine orange; (B) Hoechst 33,342; (C) mithramycin; (D) chromamycin A3.

Small, Non-specific Organic Probes that Locate Intact DNA

Some organic molecules have a high affinity (low K_d) for DNA and are stoichiometric but not specific in the manner of a complementary oligonucleotide. For example, acridine orange, is planar and intercalates between the paired sets of H-bonded base pairs (A–T, G–C) in dsDNA. Where AO penetrates into a cell and "reacts "with the dsDNA, the cell emits green light when excited with blue. AO also reacts with ssDNA or RNA by stacking on the charged phosphate of the backbone; ssDNA fluoresces in the red. Benzamides such as Hoechst 33342 bind to A–T-rich regions in the small groove of dsDNA. When sufficient dye is excited with blue light, light emission is red. The antibiotics mithramycin and chromamycin A3 bind to G–C regions of DNA. These small molecule probes of DNA (ds and ss) and RNA do not identify organisms, but indicate probable viability because the genome is intact. When cells in suspension or on a slide are stained and examined under a UV-epi-illuminated microscope or in a flow cytometer, with or without cell sorting, then viability can be estimated with fairly high precision and accuracy.

9

Single Nucleotide Polymorphism

To undertake partial, or complete, genome screens by association-based methodology for quantitative trait loci, multiple individuals have to be screened for large numbers of genetic markers. Consequently, much recent interest has focused on methods enabling accurate allele quantification in pooled deoxyribonucleic acid (DNA) samples. Microsatellites were the favored markers in initial studies, but the extraordinary wealth of data concerning single-nucleotide polymorphisms (SNPs) has turned attention to the quantification of SNP alleles in pools. All such approaches require accurate estimation of DNA concentrations, followed by the preparation of replicate pools, their validation, and application of procedures for determining allele frequencies. This chapter describes the important steps in preparing pools and surveys a variety of techniques that have been proposed for SNP detection. Finally, we describe the application of a generic approach using pooled DNA for detection of allele frequency differences between case and control populations based on primer extension protocols and outline a strategy for estimating SNP allele frequencies employing microarrays.

Historical Overview

The last decade has seen extraordinary success in the use of human linkage maps for identifying the genetic variants responsible for Mendelian, single- gene disorders. The virtues of linkage analysis are that it can be adapted to examine the co-segregation of a marker and a disease-conferring locus under a variety of proposed models that incorporate different inheritance patterns, penetrance values, and so on. A particular advantage is that linkage uses relatively few markers to scan the entire genome, typically using approx 400 evenly spaced microsatellites. Its range can extend over long genetic distances (up to 20 c*M*). For these reasons, linkage analysis is ideally suited for a systematic screen of the genome for disease-predisposing loci. Linkage analysis, however, has relatively low power to detect genes of small effect, and for this reason it has been relatively unsuccessful in applications to identify genes implicated in common disorders. Here, the expectation is that manifestation of the phenotype will depend on an underlying quantitative distribution of factors, both genetic and environmental. Many genes may each contribute only slightly to the overall predisposition and for this reason are referred to as quantitative trait loci (QTLs). Indeed, the challenge is to be able to detect QTLs that contribute as little as 1% to the genetic variance. Detection of such loci is essentially beyond the power of linkage analysis.

Association studies, in contrast, have the potential to detect genes of small effect. The sacrifice made to achieve this, however, is that markers must be the risk variant itself, or very tightly linked to the risk variant. For this reason, association analysis has until recently been used mainly for the study of polymorphisms within, or around, candidate genes that are involved in one of the pathways hypothesised to be relevant to disease aetiology. The possibility of using association analysis in a systematic screen of the entire genome was raised by Risch and Merikangas, who showed that, even if all the functional variants in the genome were examined and an appropriate Bonferroni correction were made for all these tests, association analysis would still have far greater power than linkage for detecting genes of minor effect.

The number of markers required for such an endeavour is likely to be large, possibly even up to hundreds of thousands, because successful detection of an association requires that the marker and QTL must be in linkage disequilibrium (LD) and this rapidly declines as a function of increasing genetic distance. Patterns of LD across the genome are highly variable, and to achieve reasonable coverage, intermarker distances of the order of 10 kb are thought to be necessary.

Thus, it seems likely that genome-wide association studies will require genotyping tens of thousands of markers. Furthermore, it is generally accepted that complex traits are influenced by many genes of varying, but small, effect size. Power to detect QTLs of 1% effect size will require thousands of individuals. There is, therefore, an urgent need to develop efficient high-throughput methodologies for detecting such markers. One way to reduce costs dramatically is to perform genotyping not on individual deoxyribonucleic acid (DNA) samples, but on pools made up of DNA from multiple individuals. For example, the allele frequencies in a sample of 500 cases and 500 controls can be measured from two pooled samples, rather than 1000 individual samples, reducing the genotyping costs by a factor of 500. Developments of this nature, coupled with high-throughput SNP genotyping methodologies, suggest that genome-wide association studies may soon become a feasible proposition.

Unfortunately, life is not so simple. There are problems in the use of pooled DNA for association analysis. For quantitative traits, pooling will result in loss of information concerning the variation among individuals of the same pool and in particular, it is difficult to examine multilocus haplotype effects or interactions, although some useful information can be extracted. Furthermore, allele frequency estimation from pooled DNA is subject to both bias and random measurement errors; however, careful attention to experimental design can minimize such difficulties. Nevertheless, little doubt exists that for laboratories equipped with conventional apparatus and resources, pooling provides the only feasible approach to large-scale, genome-wide association studies. In this chapter, we describe methodology that is designed to minimize problems of pool construction and provide sample protocols for two approaches designed to estimate SNP allele frequencies in pools.

SNP Detection and Allele Frequency Determination

SNPs generally reflect the existence of two alleles at appreciable frequency at a given nucleotide site. Although it is theoretically possible to have more than two alleles in the population, the following discussion assumes a simple biallelic system. The concept behind pooling subassumes that the constructed pool will represent the molecular equal equivalents of DNA from all members contributing to the pool. This requires two conditions to be met. Firstly, the DNA sampling and quantitation techniques are sufficiently sensitive and accurate to enable equimolar amounts of DNA from each individual to be combined. Second, the SNP genotyping assay works equally efficiently on each individual sample, so that each contributes proportionately to the final allele balance. At the technical level, the former is easier to achieve and monitor than the latter.

The latter depends upon the DNA samples being of equivalent integrity with regard to fragmentation and/or presence of interfering contaminants. One way to determine the equivalent integrity of the DNA samples is to employ TaqMan, or similar real-time polymerase chain reaction (PCR) approaches, to assess the amplification efficiency and, on the basis of the results, adjustments made so that each individual provides a similar number of template equivalents. Finally, because the detection efficiency may differ for the two alleles of a SNP, the application of a correction factor may be necessary to generate better estimates of the "true" frequencies. This factor generally referred to as "*K*," can be derived by examining the relative signal intensities obtained for the two alleles in known heterozygotes. Historically, restriction enzyme cleavage was the first technology applied to the detection of SNPs (i.e., restriction fragment length polymorphisms) and it has been applied to DNA pools; however, the problem of partial digestion and the relatively restricted number of potential target sites severely limits its applicability. There are now, however, a variety of technologies that have been developed for the estimation of SNP allele frequencies, many of which have been adapted for profiling of pooled DNA.

In many approaches, laser excitation of the fluorescently tagged products results in peaks representing the two alleles, whose heights in pooled samples are proportional to the allele frequencies. For some procedures, it is claimed that frequency estimates approaching the level of individual genotyping errors (i.e., 1–2%) can be achieved. Other strategies, such as Pyrosequencing, and those based on denaturing high-performance liquid chromatography, also can be modified for pooling analysis. Even higher throughput for SNP genotyping can be achieved by microarray and/or mass spectrometry technologies and, again, these techniques are being adapted for estimation of allele frequencies in pools.

Given the wide variety of approaches now available, further practical considerations in this chapter will be confined to SNP detection using microsequencing and to novel microarray-based technologies. Microsequencing has proved to be a robust technology, and kits are commercially available for ABI, Applied Biosystems sequencers, MegaBACE, and some other systems. Incorporation of different fluorescently tagged bases by primer extension at the SNP site enables allele products to be distinguished through both their mass and emission spectra. Tests on artificial pools indicate it to be a sensitive approach. Most recently, interest in employing commercially available microarrays, originally designed for multiple SNP detection on single individuals, for analysis of pooled DNA has led to exciting preliminary conclusions. We have investigated its applicability employing the Affymetrix GeneChip Human Mapping 10K Array Xba 131, a technology designed to genotype more than 10,000 SNPs using 250 ng genomic DNA. In addition to genotyping individual DNAs, we have shown that the Affymetrix GeneChip Human Mapping 10K Array Xba 131 can be employed accurately to estimate allele frequencies of DNA pools using the quantitative Relative Allele Signal (RAS) scores generated from the signal intensities on the microarray. It is highly probable that a very similar protocol will enable the interrogation of the next generation of microarrays displaying 120K SNPs spaced at roughly 20-kb intervals and hence a scan by association for the entire genome. For this approach using the 10K GeneChip, pooled genomic DNA is first digested using *Xba*I restriction enzyme. Adaptors, containing generic sequences, are then ligated onto the digested products. Next, a single PCR primer—optimized for short fragments—attaches to the ligated adaptors and amplifies all the DNA fragments. The PCR products are then purified, fragmented, end-labelled, and hybridized to the microarray ready for scanning employing an Affymetrix SNP array.

DNA Extraction

DNA can be prepared by standard SDS/poteinase K digestion and phenol extraction, or by application of generic spin column methods. All these can provide material that meets the general requirements for pooling and SNP detection. Our experience in SNP studies on pooled DNA is confined to DNA extracted from mouth swabs following exactly the procedures outlined by Freeman et al. This approach provides access to material sent by post and is a cheap and efficient procedure now tested for longer than 5 yr with no contraindications.

Pool Construction

Irrespective of the type of marker to be used, the first step in pool construction is the superficially simple one of collecting and combining equal quantities of DNA from case and control samples.

Depending on the method used for purification, quantification of DNA content by ultraviolet spectroscopy can lead to overestimation of the concentration and methods based on fluorimetry with a DNA-specific dye are to be preferred for their specificity. Because several dilutions may have to be undertaken, additional problems can be encountered through the pipetting of small volumes from viscous solutions. Repeated estimations of the samples are recommended. Finally, the fragment sizes of the DNA molecules are dependent on the extraction protocol, which may affect the efficiency of the PCR. It is worthwhile to check at least a subset of samples using a "real-time" PCR approach for the estimation of DNA template concentration. This measures template concentration by determining the number of PCR cycles required to reach a predetermined threshold level of product, which depends on the starting concentration of templates.

Validation of the Pooled DNA

To ensure that the allele frequencies estimated from the pooled DNA accurately reflect the allele frequencies of the individuals comprising the pool, it is recommended that the SNP genotype profile for the DNA pool should be obtained for 10 SNPs using whichever of the SNP genotyping methodologies

is appropriate. The allele frequencies estimated from pooled DNA can then be compared with the known SNP frequencies established by individual genotyping. For this purpose it is important that the pooled allele estimates should be corrected for preferential amplification of either allele.

Materials

SNaPshot to Assess SNP Frequencies in Pooled DNA

The following list of requirements and subsequent protocol is based on the analysis of a single pooled sample of DNA.

Amplification of genomic DNA

1. Pooled DNA sample @10 ng/μL
2. Taq polymerase. AmpliTaq or equivalent.
3. 40 m*M* deoxynucleotides triphosphates (dATP, dCTP, dGTP, dTTP).
4. 25 m*M* $MgCl_2$.
5. Deionized water.
6. Buffer (10X PCR reaction buffer.
7. PCR oligonucleotide primers (10 μM).
8. MJ Research thermal cycler (GRI or equivalent).
9. PCR Plates or strip tubes.

PCR purification

1. Shrimp alkaline phosphatase (SAP) 1 U/μL.
2. MJ Research thermal cycler.

SNaPshot reaction

1. SNaPshot multiplex ready reaction mix contained in the ABI PrismSNaPshot multiplex kit.
2. SNaPshot oligonucleotide primer @ 0.5 μM.
3. Deionized water.
4. MJ Research thermal cycler.

Postextension clean up

1. ExoSAP-IT (USB corporation).
2. MJ Research thermal cycler.

Electrophoresis on the 3100 genetic analyzer

1. ABI Prism 3100 genetic Analyzer with POP-4 and 36-cm array.
2. Matrix standard Set DS-02 [dR1 10, dRGG, dTAMRA, dROX, LIZ].
3. GeneScan-120 LIZ size standard (ABI).
4. Formamide Ultra.
5. ABI Prism Genotyper 3.7 NT software (ABI).

Microarray Estimation of SNP Frequencies in Pooled DNA Samples

As the protocols employed for labeling and hybridization to the Affymetrix microarrays do not differ significantly from those outlined in the manufacturer's handbook, it would be redundant to reproduce them here. We have found, however, that there are sections of the protocol that are particularly important to follow. In addition, for one step, we have found that an alternative protocol has worked better in our hands. A major modification in genotyping pools is the requirement to estimate allele frequency, rather than simply call homozygotes and heterozygotes.

Laboratory set-up

As noted in the manufacturer's protocol, correct laboratory set-up has been shown to be critical in the success of the Affymetrix GeneChip Mapping Assay. It is recommended that a single direction of workflow be employed to reduce the risk of contamination, particularly with PCR products. There are three principle "areas" that should be prepared before commencing the assay.

The most important area is a "pre-PCR Clean Room" in which restriction digest and ligation stages should be conducted. This room should be free of PCR products (amplicons) and the only DNA present should be that to be used in the assay. In addition to the usual precautions of wearing gowns and gloves, use of hairnets and safety masks are strongly encouraged. Individuals should not move from areas containing high amounts of PCR amplicons into the pre-PCR Clean Room directly without taking precautions to eliminate possible contaminants. A change of clothes and a shower is recommended for this purpose.

The second area is a "*PCR Staging Room*" in which the products from the ligation stage are prepped ready for the PCR reaction. The area should be essentially amplicon-free. It is acceptable to have the pre-PCR Clean Room and PCR-Staging room as one area, providing the workflow is unidirectional. This room (or area) should also contain any necessary reagents to set up the PCR but thermo-cycling amplification steps MUST be undertaken elsewhere (e.g., in the "Main Lab").

The "main lab" is where all subsequent reactions and steps of the procedure should take place. This area may have airborne PCR amplicons and DNA templates. To accommodate this laboratory setup, the GeneChip Mapping 10K Xba Assay kit is conveniently divided into three boxes, one for each area.

METHODS

SNaPshot to Assess SNP Frequencies in Pooled DNA

Pool construction

Genomic DNA purification and pool construction as described (**Subheadings 1.3.** and **1.4.**).

3.1.2. Primer Design

PCR oligonucleotide primers flanking the SNP region of interest can be designed using the web-based tool, Primer3, and should have predicted annealing temperatures (in 50 m*M* salt) of 58°C ± 1°C. The SNaPshot oligonucleotide primer must anneal to the complementary DNA strand directly adjacent to the SNP being interrogated. The optimal design is for a 20-mer with no extendable hairpin structures and to have annealing temperatures between 50 and 60°C. Primers can also be designed to be complementary to the anti-sense DNA strand, if it is problematic to design a primer for the sense strand.

Amplification of genomic DNA

1. Prepare the following reagents on ice to the following final concentrations with a final reaction volume of 10 μL in 1X PCR reaction buffer (add deionized water as necessary):

   2.5 m*M* $MgCl_2$
   0.8 m*M* dNTPs
   0.3 μ*M* forward PCR oligonucleotide primer
   0.3 μ*M* reverse PCR oligonucleotide primer
   1.6 U *Taq* polymerase
   Add 20 ng pooled genomic DNA (2 μL @10 ng/μL).

2. Perform amplification using a thermal cycler with the following standard conditions:

   96°C for 5 min;
   96°C for 45 s;
   62°C for 45 s; and
   72°C for 45 s;
   Decrease by 0.4 per cycle, 35 cycles
   72°C for 5 min.
   Store at 4°C if not proceeding directly to the next step.

PCR purification

The PCR template has to be purified to remove unincorporated PCR components, which otherwise would interfere in the subsequent SNaPshot thermal cycling reaction.

1. Vortex the ExoSAP-IT briefly to mix.
2. Mix 5 μL of PCR product with 2 μL of ExoSAP-IT.
3. Using a thermal cycler incubate for 15 min at 37°C and follow with an enzyme inactivation step of 80°C for 15 min.

   At this stage, samples can be stored at 4°C for short periods or 20°C for long-term storage.

SNaPshot reaction

This follows the protocol as described in the ABI Prism SNaPshot manual, with minor modifications:

1. Combine the following reagents on ice, to a final volume of 10 μL:

   2μL of ABI Prism SNaPshot ddNTP Ready Reaction Mix
   2 μL of purified PCR sample,
   0.25 μ*M* of SNaPshot extension primer (0.5 μL @ 0.5 μ*M*)
   5.5 μL of deionized water.

2. Mix, and then spin briefly.
3. Perform thermal cycling according to SNaPshot protocol:

   Thermal ramp (2°C/s) to 96°C;
   96°C for 10 s;
   Thermal ramp (2°C/s) to 50°C;
   50°C for 5 s;

Thermal ramp (2°C/s) to 60°C; and

60°C for 30 s.

Repeat for 25 cycles.

Maintain at 4°C if you cannot proceed directly to the next stage.

Postextension clean up

This step removes the 5' phosphoryl group of excess ddNTPs that would otherwise co-migrate with the SNP fragment of interest.

1. Add 1.0 U of SAP (1 U/μL) straight into the SNaPshot reaction mix.
2. Incubate on a thermal cycler for 37°C for 1 h followed by an enzyme inactivation step of 72°C for 15 min.

Electrophoresis on the 3100 genetic analyzer

1. Combine the following:
   0.5 μL of SAP cleaned samples.
   9.0 μL of Hi Di formamide.
   0.5 μL of GeneScan-120 LIZ size standard (ABI).
2. Load samples onto ABI Prism 3100 genetic analyser with POP-4 and 36-cm array, with the following run parameters:

Dye set:	E5
Run Module:	SNP36_pop4 default
Analysis module:	GS120analysisgsp.

Data analysis

Analyse data with GeneScan Analysis Software visualized in ABI Prism Genotyper 3.7 NT software.

Estimation of allele frequencies in the DNA pool

The allele frequencies are reflected in the relative peak heights displayed in the electropherogram trace. If the efficiency of detection is identical for each of the individual alleles, the relative peak heights (e.g., for allele A, this is calculated as the peak height of allele A divided by the sum of the peaks heights of alleles A and B; viz. A/[A+B]) provide a direct measure of allele frequency. In practice, the efficiencies of detection for the two alleles of a SNP may differ. This could be a result of unequal amplification of heterozygotes, differential efficiencies in the incorporation of the ddNTPS and unequal emission energies for the different florescent dyes.

Examining the deviation from 50:50 for known single individual heterozygotes can assess this and a correction can be applied to estimate the true allele frequency. Given signal strengths of H_A and H_B of a pooled sample, the corrected allele frequencies (f) for alleles A and B are $f_A = H_A/(H_A + KH_B)$ and $f_B = 1 - f_A$, where K = ratio of the signal for the allele which is less well amplified (A) to that of allele B (the better amplified). Sham et al. for a more in- depth discussion of pool design, replication issues, application of correction functions, and other aspects of experimental design that will help to reduce technical and sampling errors.

For many purposes, estimation and application of a correction coefficient, K, may be unnecessary if allele frequencies are being compared between groups, such as in case/control comparisons as it is the differences, rather than the absolute values, that are important. This particularly applies where allele frequencies are not in the extremes of their range as is likely to be the situation for significant QTLs for multi-factorial traits.

Microarray Estimation of SNP Frequencies in Pooled DNA Samples

Adjustment of pooled DNA preparations

The optimum concentration of pooled genomic DNA for use in the Affymetrix GeneChip Mapping Assay is 50 ng/μL. It is preferable that samples are diluted in reduced ethylene diamine tetraacetic acid (EDTA) TE buffer (0.1 m*M* EDTA; 10 m*M* Tris-HCL, pH 8.0) as the elevated EDTA concentration in regular TE (1.0 m*M* EDTA; 10 m*M* Tris-HCl; pH 8.0) may interfere with the assay's enzymatic reactions although use of standard TE has not proved to be a problem in our experience. A total of 250 ng DNA in a maximum volume of 15.5 μL is required for each assay; therefore, the minimum concentration of genomic DNA is approximately 16.1 ng/μL. As for individual DNA genotyping, all pooled samples must be free from contamination. Although contamination of individual genomic DNAs contributing to the pool is unlikely to affect the estimation of overall allele frequency, good practice indicates that contamination of any samples should be avoided. Until complete familiarity with the system and protocols is obtained we have found it best to work with small batches—adjustment of the starting material and reagents appropriate for 8 assays has proved optimal.

Ligation

Perform as per manufacturer's protocol.

PCR setup

Perform as manufacturer's protocol.

PCR product purification

To assess the quality of the amplified products obtained from the digested and ligated DNA, the following steps are important:

1. Run 3 μL of each PCR product mixed with 3 L of loading dye on a 2% TBE gel at 120 V for 1 h. Three distinct bands at approx 400, 710, and 875 bp should be observed against a background of other fragments.
2. Proceed to below; however, if this cannot be performed directly, the sample should be stored at -20°C.

PCR purification

The alternative protocol employing QIAGEN MinElute PCR Purification Kit was found to perform better as follows (*Note:* all buffers should be stored at 20–25°C):

1. Combine the four PCRs and aliquot five equal volumes to five 1.5-mL collection tubes.
2. Mix five volumes PB buffer to 1 vol PCR.
3. For each PCR, place a MinElute column in a 2-mL collection tube and stand in a suitable rack.
4. Add each PB buffer/PCR mix to center of a MinElute column and centrifuge at maximum for 1 min to bind DNA to membrane of MinElute column.
5. Discard through-flow and place each column back in the used collection tube then add 750 μL of PE buffer to each MinElute column.
6. Centrifuge at maximum for 1 min to wash DNA bound to column.
7. Discard through-flow and place the column back in its used collection tube.
8. Centrifuge at maximum for an additional minute, then discard through-flow and collection tubes. (*Note:* the additional centrifigation has been shown to be essential for recovering required yields of DNA).
9. Place MinElute Columns in clean 1.5-mL collection tubes and add 10 μL of EB Buffer to the center of each MinElute column, let each column stand for 1 min, and then centrifuge at maximum

for 1 min. (*Note:* here, it is essential that EB Buffer be added to the center of the MinElute column.)

10. Collect the purified PCR products from the five tubes representing each sample and combine so each sample is now contained in a single 1.5-mL collection tube
11. Dilute 4 μL of each purified PCR sample in 156 μL of Molecular Biology Grade Water (1 in 40 dilution).
12. Quantify each purified sample applying the convention that 1 absorbance unit at 260 nm equals 50 μg/mL for dsDNA. The expected concentration should be around 11 ng/μL. At least 20 μg of purified PCR product in 45 μL is required for fragmentation. If fragmentation cannot be performed after PCR purification, the sample should be stored at -20°C.

Fragmentation

Perform as per manufacturer's protocol.

Labeling

Perform as per manufacturer's protocol.

Hybridization

Perform as per manufacturer's protocol.

Washing and staining

Perform as per manufacturer's protocol.

Scanning

Perform as per manufacturer's protocol.

Estimation of allele frequencies

Allele frequency estimates are derived from RAS scores, for sense (RAS 1) and antisense (RAS2) strands using GDAS software. We have routinely found that the average of RAS 1 and RAS2 (RAS_{av}) provides the best estimate of allele frequency for any particular DNA pool. RAS scores should vary between 0 (for a BB homozygote) and 1.0 (for an AA homozygote), and heterozygotes should generate a relative allele signal of approx 0.5. Depending on the efficiency of detection of the two alleles for any SNP, the RAS scores for an individual heterozygote may vary from this and a correction can be introduced to compensate for this.

Notes

1. Experimental errors that are unique to pooling can inflate the test statistic and so potentially contribute to an increase in false-positive associations (type 1 errors) if they are ignored. There are three main sources of variance unique to pools: (i) sampling errors (which depends on the N of the pools and the allele frequency), can be addressed by making randomly selected independent DNA pools; (ii) random experimental variance in pool formation due to quantitation and pipetting errors can be addressed by making independent replicate DNA pools of the same individuals; (iii) finally, measurement error in the determination of the allele frequencies in the DNA pool can be addressed by repeated measurements of the same DNA pool. By incorporating such steps into the experimental design, these variances can be determined and accounted for in the test statistic.
2. To balance type I and type II errors, we recommend using a multistage replication design. For example, comparing DNA pools of extreme cases (bottom 15- 25%, assuming the trait under investigation is continuously distributed) against DNA pools of extreme controls (top 15-25%). This could be followed by a within-family study that will protect against hidden population stratification, for example comparing lower versus higher DNA pools of co-twins in discordant sibling pairs. Finally, individual genotyping should be used to confirm the results.

3. It is likely that the PCR product produces a faint image. To visualize the bands it is therefore recommended that the sensitivity of the visualization software is maximized.
4. During generation of RAS scores in GDAS, the default parameters for signal detection can be lowered to increase signal detection, and thus the number of non-redundant RAS scores. As RAS scores are incorporated into an algorithm that is used to call the genotypes of individuals, it is not recommended to lower these defaults by too much. For pooled DNA however, we have found that increasing signal detection by reducing the default parameters by 25 to 50%, still yield reliable RAS scores used to estimate allele frequency. It is worth noting that RAS scores generated using default parameters are not altered when the defaults are lowered and thus remain the most accurate of the RAS scores generated.

Analysis of Single Nucleotide Polymorphisms

From the preceding chapters, it is evident that there is a critical need to better understand the instances where pharmacogenomics will be of value for the pre-market development or the post-market prescribing of individualized medicines. In order to enable both the experimental assessment of the utility of pharmacogenomics and ultimately its reduction to routine clinical practice where appropriate, there is an ongoing need for improved assay methods for the analysis of single nucleotide polymorphisms (SNPs), the most abundant type of genetic variant in the human genome. The purpose of the present chapter is to provide a general discussion of strategic and experimental issues related to the choice of suitable genotyping methodologies for various research and clinical settings. The reader is referred to other chapters in this monograph that provide further technical details of many of the emerging SNP genotyping technologies that will be briefly summarized here.

SNP Analysis Technologies

When comparing currently available and newly emerging technologies for their suitability in SNP genotyping assays, it is important to consider both the needs and the resources of potential end users. In this regard, study design and/or sample number can determine, and be limited by the availability of, a suitable genotyping technology. Assay cost is an important consideration for the choice of a method, and can place significant practical constraints on study design. On one hand, in clinical diagnostic settings where relatively small numbers of patient samples might require analysis for a validated genetic variant over a given time period, assay accuracy may be more important than cost per assay. On the other hand, both low assay cost and capability for high assay throughput (speed and volume of sample processing) will be important for early-stage novel drug target discovery studies that will require the analysis of large numbers of genome-wide or candidate-gene SNP markers in large numbers of clinical DNA specimens.

The ideal genotyping technology is thus likely to be one with sufficient flexibility to adapt to a variety of different study designs or SNP throughputs—in terms of both the number of SNPs that require analysis per DNA sample and the number of patient DNA samples that require analysis. Such flexibility requires the ability to adapt the assay technology to different throughputs, which in turn may require a variety of detection methods and instrumentation platforms to cover the spectrum of cost, throughput, and convenience in a robust and optimally accurate fashion.

In this regard, it is useful to distinguish between the analytical biochemistries that form the basis of different SNP genotyping assays, and the variety of novel platforms and methods of detection, or readout, of the genotyping results. Although genotyping readout and genotyping platform (which includes devices for automation, miniaturization, and multiplexing) will strongly influence the throughput and cost components of a given assay technology, the fundamental nature of the underlying biochemistry primarily determines the potential accuracy and robustness of the method. With this in mind, the next section focuses on a discussion of some assay biochemistries, the particular features of which will determine the degree to which they may be ported to various detection, automation, and multiplexing platforms.

Assay Biochemistries

As mentioned above, the central core component of a genotyping technology is contained within the assay biochemistry. In this regard, a general distinction may be made between those methods that rely primarily upon differential hybridization stringency for their specificity, and those that derive specificity primarily from the ability to detect a product of an enzymatic reaction. A number of methods also use combinations of hybridization and enzyme reactions, with varying degrees of contribution to specificity from each of the two components.

Hybridization-Based Approaches

The specificity of hybridization-based approaches in SNP genotyping relies on the fact that the melting temperatures of DNA–DNA or DNA–RNA hybrids that perfectly match are higher than those that do not. Thus experimental conditions may be found where differential rates or equilibrium levels of hybridization may be distinguished, even for single-base mismatches such as would occur in the presence of a SNP. Original hybridization-based approaches that employed the hybridization of radioactively labeled oligonucleotides on Southern blots of human genomic DNA suffered from all of the practical disadvantages of classical restriction fragment length polymorphism (RFLP) analysis, including use of large quantities of starting genomic DNA and the use of tedious and hazardous hybridization methods. The use of PCR reaction products and substitution of nonradioactive labels improved the assays, but the requirement for gel electrophoresis made high-throughput problematic. More recent methods that utilize the monitoring of the kinetics of probe hybridization to target DNA with changes in hybridization temperature, termed dynamic allele-specific hybridization (DASH) can now allow for greater specificity and higher throughput in a solely hybridization-based discrimination method.

Enzyme-Based Approaches

Because of the high inherent catalytic specificity of enzymes for their substrates, enzyme-based approaches to SNP genotyping generally possess a higher degree of assay fidelity than those primarily dependent on hybridization for their specificity. Historically, the standard method for genotyping of SNPs and of other types of genetic variants, RFLP analysis, is an enzymatic approach that relies upon the exquisite selectivity of bacterial restriction endonucleases for short stretches of defined DNA sequence that act as recognition sites for DNA strand cleavage. Thus in instances where a SNP changes a restriction enzyme recognition sequence, differential digestion of normal and variant sequences can be observed. First iterations of this approach required the digestion of large quantities of genomic DNA, electrophoretic separation of digested fragments, transfer of fragments to nitrocellulose or nylon membranes and detection of fragment size differences by hybridization with a radiolabeled probe complementary to the fragments. Advancements in the method, most notably prior PCR amplification of defined DNA segments containing SNP sites and PCR-mediated introduction of novel restriction sites, have improved the conservation of starting material, the ability to detect fragments visually in gels without the need for labeled probe hybridization and the applicability to a broader range of SNP variant sites in the genome. However, the major drawback to such methods is still the requirement for electrophoretic separation of digested products, which severely limits the throughput and automatability of the method and increases reagent and labor costs.

Dideoxy DNA sequencing represents another example of an enzymatic approach to genotyping, which uses the specificity of DNA polymerase to incorporate appropriate nucleotide bases opposite a primed single-stranded DNA template, followed by size separation of terminated polymerase-extended reaction products by gel electrophoresis to detect the identity of nucleotide variants at defined sites. DNA sequencing remains the gold standard to which other genotyping methods are compared, and is also the method of choice for discovering new SNPs among DNA samples from populations or for confirming and localizing those discovered using scanning methods such as single-strand conformation polymorphism (SSCP) analysis or denaturing HPLC. With respect to the genotyping of pre-existing SNPs, major disadvantages of DNA sequencing include the ongoing requirement for electrophoretic separation of extended DNA fragments (which restricts the platform and hampers throughput), potential technical difficulties in detecting heterozygosity at a particular SNP locus when genotyping from uncloned PCR products, and the higher cost of reagents associated with the requirement to extend reactions by many more nucleotide bases than the polymorphic site under investigation.

An alternative method of DNA sequencing, called *Pyrosequencing* uses a series of enzymatic reactions to enable the continuous readout of short stretches of DNA sequence without the requirement for electrophoretic fragment separation. The method may be useful for low-throughput research and clinical diagnostic applications, but is unlikely to be applied to high-throughput applications.

Another variation of DNA sequencing is called single-base primer extension, or minisequencing. Primer extension in its original form involves the annealing of an oligonucleotide primer to a single-stranded PCR product (analogous to the primer annealing step in DNA sequencing reactions) at a location which lies immediately adjacent to, but not including, the polymorphic SNP site, followed by the addition of DNA polymerase and subsequent enzymatic extension of the primer in the presence of only chain-terminating dideoxynucleotides, which may be labeled in a variety of ways to facilitate subsequent detection of the identity of the single incorporated nucleotide. As with DNA sequencing, an important distinguishing feature of primer extension is that specificity arises not from primer hybridization but rather from the catalytic activity of the DNA polymerase. An additional advantage of primer extension over classical sequencing is that electrophoretic separation is not required to detect the extended product, but rather any one of a number of simple methods to detect the label attached to the incorporated dideoxynucleotide. Finally, the simplicity of the biochemistry allows reactions to be performed either in solution or on primers attached to solid supports, providing flexibility with regard to platforms and capacity for reaction multiplexing.

Combined Hybridization/Enzymatic Approaches

One of the most commonly used small-scale genotyping methods is allele- specific PCR amplification, which combines allele-selective PCR primer hybridization with a subsequent PCR reaction. Conditions are optimized so that hybridization and subsequent amplification occur only when the PCR priming oligonucleotide is perfectly matched with the target site (usually with the polymorphic site at the 3′ end of the oligonucleotide). The result of the test is therefore determined electrophoretically as either the presence or absence of a PCR product. Again, a major drawback of this method for high-throughput applications is the requirement for gel electrophoresis and visualization of product, a process that is not amenable to automation. It is also important to note that in this assay accuracy is still dependent solely on differential hybridization specificity, which must be carefully optimized for each polymorphic site to be analyzed and is therefore difficult to multiplex. A number of newer assays have been designed to introduce an enzymatic step in order to improve the specificity, and therefore the overall accuracy, of hybridization-based assays.

Oligonucleotide ligation assays (OLA) are an example of this approach, where addition of a DNA ligase to a hybridization reaction results in the attachment of an oligonucleotide to an immobilized capture DNA only when the fragments are perfectly matched. The Invader assay utilizes a sequence specific cleavage enzyme called a cleavase to release a quenched fluorescent dye label when hybridization of a perfectly complementary oligonucleotide produces a unique structure that is recognized by the enzyme. Although a potential significant advantage of this assay is the elimination of the requirement for prior PCR amplification of target sequence, the method currently requires the use of a relatively large quantity of input genomic DNA, which can often be a scarce and valuable commodity. The TaqMan assay uses the exonuclease activity of Taq DNA polymerase to liberate a fluorescent signal from a quenched probe oligonucleotide when the sequence is perfectly complementary to a target, but not when the sequence differs.

Detection Methods

As mentioned above, most classical genotyping methods have typically relied upon the electrophoretic separation of DNA fragments in order to visually detect differences in size or fragmentation patterns between allelic variants. Although the advent of capillary electrophoresis in DNA sequencing has enabled the throughput of these detection methods to be improved considerably, such systems require a significant capital outlay and there are still limitations to the scale of genotyping studies that can be performed. For this reason, a number of detection methods that do not require electrophoretic fragment separation have been developed. Mass spectrometry may be used to simultaneously identify oligonucleotide fragments that differ by as little as a single nucleotide. This method has been applied to a variation of the primer extension genotyping assay, whereby fragments differing in size by one or a few nucleotides are generated in primer extension reactions, and detected by their mass differences.

Other detection methods used in conjunction with the primer extension biochemistry include the use of an enzyme-linked immunochemical assay that produces different color reactions corresponding to the allelic variants in micotiter plate wells, and fluorescently labeled dideoxynucleotides that can be detected on microarrays of immobilized extended oligonucleotides. Fluorescence polarization (FP) has been used as an effective detection marker for primer extension, Invader and TaqMan assays, and is based on the observation that the degree of emitted FP of a labeled molecule is proportional to its molecular mass. Thus by monitoring the FP of a fluorescent dye during an enzyme reaction, changes in the molecular mass can be detected without sample purification or electrophoresis. Other approaches using fluorescence to monitor the course of enzyme reactions in SNP genotyping make use of the ability of an adjacent molecule to quench the fluorescence of a fluorophore. Reactions that result in the removal of the quencher or its movement away from the fluorophore will result in termination of the quenching and emission of a fluorescent signal. A variation of this theme is the recent development of molecular beacons, which are single oligonucleotide-based molecules containing both a fluorophore and a quencher, such that hybridization of the molecule produces a conformational change that releases the quenching and produces a fluorescent signal.

Platforms

In order to produce integrated genotyping systems that meet the practical needs of a broad range of experimental uses, a variety of system embodiments have been developed. These are designed so as to optimize assay convenience, reliability, sample usage, cost-effectiveness, and throughput, as required for the application. For many future genomic applications, the requirement for cost-effective, large-scale genotyping of large numbers of SNPs will be required. Three of the most popular means by which to achieve cost-effective high-throughput genotyping include miniaturization, process automation, and reaction multiplexing. Automation, which involves robotic sample handling and reagent delivery to assays, will not be discussed further here. Miniaturization and multiplexing are of considerable value in dramatically reducing reagent usage, assay time, and overall genotyping cost. One of the most effective ways of achieving this is through the use of a variety of novel microarray technologies. Microarrays may in fact be considered as miniaturized multiplexing devices, enabling the simultaneous reaction and detection of multiple samples. Classical microarrays are two-dimensional immobilized spotted arrays of DNA or oligonucleotides on glass slides, with the locations of specific sequences being pre-defined. Traditional expression microarrays use immobilized DNA to hybridize with cDNA, which has been synthesized from isolated tissue mRNA, in order to obtain semi-quantitative measures of transcript levels in the tissues.

Microarrays may also be used very effectively for primer extension based SNP genotyping, whereby oligonucleotide primers specific for the interrogation of particular SNPs are immobilized in defined locations on arrays, incubated with pooled target PCR products and extended with fluorescently labeled dideoxynucleotides. The presence and identity of the extended fluorescent labels can then be detected by automated fluorescence imaging of the microarrays. Alternatively, a variation on this approach is the use of the so-called *universal arrays*, where the primer extension oligonucleotide is synthesized with a further generic "tag" sequence attached, that is complementary to a sequence immobilized on a microarray. In this embodiment, multiplexed primer extension reactions can be performed in solution, followed by incubation of the extended products with the microarray in order to capture the extended products for detection on the microarray. Another microarraying technique involves the use of labeled micro- spheres as the attachment matrix instead of glass slides. In this case, the array is a three-dimensional solution array rather than a two-dimensional glass array, and the identity and fluorescence of the attached products can be measured by flow cytometry of the microspheres.

A recent innovation for the labeling of microspheres involves the use of fluorescent semiconductor nanocrystals, or quantum dots, which create a spectral bar code for microsphere identification. The method allows for a high level of genotyping reaction multiplexing, due to the ability to create a large number of unique identifying signatures. From the above discussion, it is clear that there are a large number of methods now available for the genotyping of SNPs in pharmacogenomic studies. No single combination of biochemistry, detection method, and platform will be able to meet the needs of every genotyping "customer."Thus the potential user of genotyping assays must therefore carefully assess the needs of one's own genotyping laboratory, and determine the relative importance of throughput, cost-effectiveness, speed of analysis, accuracy, and availability of existing and projected equipment and infrastructure capabilities in making choices of one or more appropriate embodiments to meet those needs.

10

Cell-based Therapeutics

Throughout the 1980s and early 1990s, the term 'biopharmaceutical' had become virtually synonymous with 'proteins of therapeutic use'. Nucleic-acid-based biopharmaceuticals, too, harbour great potential. Current developments in nucleic-acid-based therapeutics centre around gene therapy, as well as antisense technology (including RNAi) and aptamer technology, all of which are discussed later in this chapter. These technologies have the potential to revolutionize medical practice. Despite all the hype, however, it is important to note that by early 2007 at least, only three nucleic-acid-based products had gained approval worldwide: one antisense-based product (tradename Vitravene), one aptamer (tradename Macugen) and one gene therapy product (tradename Gendicine, approved only in China). In contrast, some 165 protein-based biopharmaceuticals had been approved by early 2007. The full benefit of nucleic-acid-based medicines will accrue only after the satisfactory resolution of several technical difficulties currently impeding their routine medical application. Cell-based medicines also harbour tremendous potential. Although a small number of such products have gained approval, none is a stem-cell-derived product.

Gene Therapy

The fundamental principle underpinning gene therapy is theoretically straightforward, but difficult to achieve in practice satisfactorily. The principle entails the stable introduction of a gene into the genetic complement of a cell, such that subsequent expression of the gene achieves a therapeutic goal. The potential of gene therapy as a curative approach for inborn errors of metabolism and other conditions induced by the presence of a defective copy of a specific gene (or genes) is obvious.

Table 10.1 Some diseases for which gene-based therapeutic approaches are currently being appraised in clinical trials

Cancer, various forms	AIDS
Cystic fibrosis	Haemophilia
Familial hyper-cholesterolaemia	Severe combined immunodeficiency diseases (SCID)
Gaucher's disease	α_1-antitrypsin deficiency
Purine nucleoside phosphorylase deficiency	CGD
Rheumatoid arthritis	Peripheral vascular disease

An increased understanding of the molecular basis of various other diseases, including cancer, some infectious diseases (e.g. AIDS) and some neurological conditions, also suggests a role for gene therapy in combating these. Indeed two-thirds of all gene therapy trials conducted to date aim to treat cancer. The first such trial was initiated in the USA in 1989. Thus far, some 1200 different clinical studies have/are being undertaken worldwide. The majority (estimated at 67 per cent) have/are being undertaken in the USA, with most of the remaining trials being undertaken in Europe (mainly in the UK and in Germany). The majority of trials (62 per cent) are in early stage (phase I) and only some 2.2 per cent of all trials have reached phase III. Despite the initial enthusiasm, only a handful of such studies have revealed a therapeutic benefit to the patient.

Moreover, gene therapy, like all other medical interventions, is not without associated risk. A US patient died in 1999 as a result of participating in one such trial. Even more disturbingly, the ensuing FDA investigation unearthed allegations that at least six other deaths attributed to clinical trial treatments had gone unreported to the regulatory agency; and further, that only a fraction of serious adverse effects had been reported. As a result, regulatory regulation and monitoring of gene therapy trials has been increased. Further serious adverse effects, including some fatalities, have been reported subsequently, as discussed later. Such disappointing results do not reflect any flaw in the concept of gene therapy. They instead reflect the need to develop more effective technical means of accomplishing gene therapy in practice. These initial studies have highlighted the technical innovations required to achieve successful gene transfer and expression. These, in turn, should render future ('*second-generation*') gene therapy protocols more successful.

Basic Approach to Gene Therapy

The desired gene must usually be packaged into a vector system capable of delivering it safely inside the intended recipient cells. A variety of vectors can be used to effect gene transfer. These include both viruses (particularly retroviruses and adenoviruses) and non-viral carriers, such as plasmid-containing liposomes/ lipoplexes. Each such vector has its own unique set of advantages and disadvantages, as discussed subsequently in this chapter.

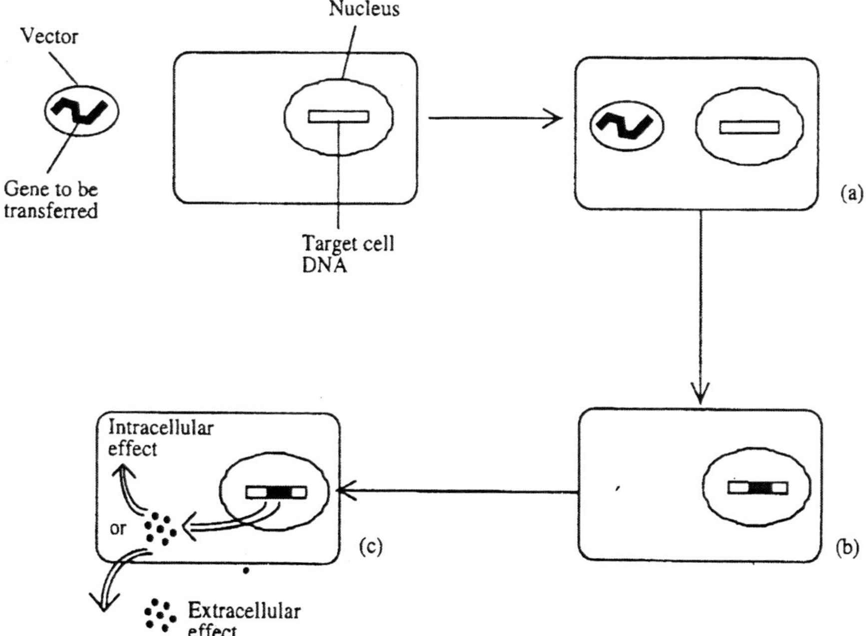

Fig. 10.1. Simplified schematic representation of the basis of gene therapy. (a) Entry of the therapeutic nucleic acid; (b) Transfer of the nucleic acid into the nucleus of the recipient cell. (c) The foreign gene is expressed, resulting in the synthesis of the desired protein product.

Table 10.2 Vector systems used to deliver genes into mammalian cells

Viral-based vector systems	*Non-viral-based vector systems*
Retroviruses	Nucleic-acid-containing liposomes
Adenoviruses	Molecular conjugates
Adeno-associated virus	Direct injection of naked DNA
Herpes virus	CaPO4 precipitation
Polio virus	Electroporation
Vaccinia virus	Particle acceleration

Once assimilated by the cell, the exogenous nucleic acid must now travel/be delivered to the nucleus. In some cases, the mechanism by which this transfer occurs is understood, at least in part (e.g. in the case of retroviral vectors). In other cases (e.g. use of liposome vectors or naked DNA), this process is less well understood. At a practical level, gene therapy protocols may entail one of three different strategies.

The *in vitro* approach entails initial removal of the target cells from the body. These are then cultured *in vitro* and incubated with vector containing the nucleic acid to be delivered. The genetically altered cells are then reintroduced into the patient's body. This approach represents the most commonly adopted protocol to date. In order to be successful, however, the target cells must be relatively easy to remove from the body, and reintroduce into the body. Such *in vitro* approaches have successfully been undertaken utilizing various body cell types, including blood cells, stem cells, epithelial cells, muscle cells and hepatocytes.

A second approach involves direct injection/administration of the nucleic-acid-containing vector to the target cell, *in situ* in the body. Examples of this approach have included the direct injection of vectors into a tumour mass, as well as aerosol administration of vectors (e.g. containing the cystic fibrosis gene) to respiratory tract epithelial cells.

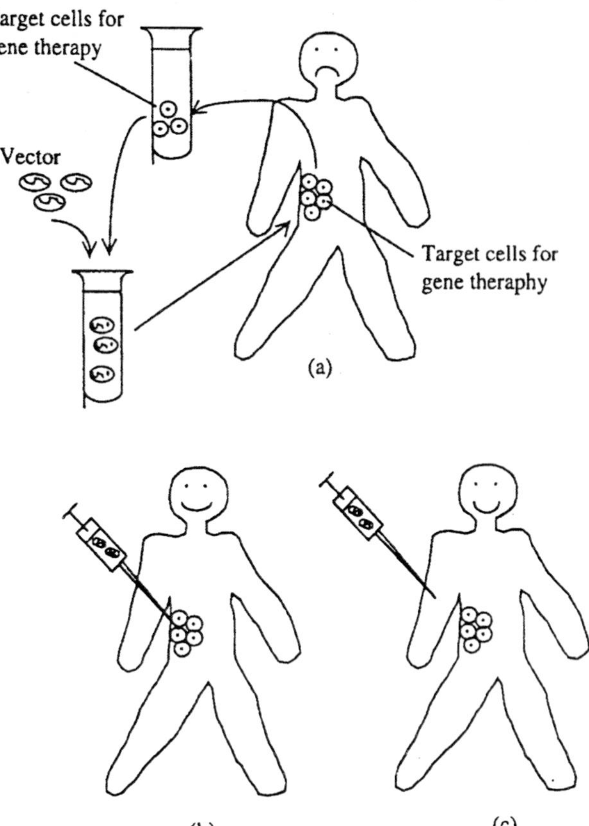

Fig. 10.2. The various practical approaches that may be pursued when undertaking gene therapy.

Although less complicated than the *in vitro* approach, direct *in situ* injection of vector into the immediate vicinity of target cells is not always feasible. This would be true, for example, if the target cells are not localized to one specific area of the body (e.g. blood cells). An alternative (*in vivo*) approach entails the development of vectors capable of recognizing and binding only to specific, predefined cell types. Such vectors could then be administered easily by, for example, i.v. injection. Through appropriate biospecific interactions, they would only deliver their nucleic acid payload to the specified target cells. The simplicity and specificity of this approach renders it the method of choice.

However, thus far, no such vector systems have been developed for routine therapeutic use. Intensive efforts to develop these are underway, and a number of different strategies are being pursued. For example, the inclusion of an antibody on the vector surface, which specifically binds a surface-antigen uniquely associated with the target cell, would allow selective delivery. Another approach entails engineering the vector to display a specific hormone that would bind only to cells displaying the hormone receptor. The feasibility of this approach has been demonstrated using retroviral vectors engineered to display EPO on their surface.

Some Additional Questions

The choice of vector, target cell and protocol used will depend upon a number of considerations. The major consideration is obviously what the ultimate goal of the gene therapy treatment is in any given case. For example, in some instances it may be to correct an inherited genetic defect, whereas in other instances it may be to confer a novel function upon the recipient cell. An example of the former would be the introduction of the cystic fibrosis transmembrane conductance regulator (CFTR) gene (the cystic fibrosis gene) into the airway epithelial cells of cystic fibrosis sufferers. An example of the latter would be the introduction of a novel gene into white blood cells whose protein product is capable of in some way interfering with HIV replication. Such an approach might prove an effective therapeutic strategy for the treatment of AIDS.

An additional consideration that may influence the protocol used is the desired duration of subsequent expression of the gene product. In most cases of genetic disease, long-term expression of the inserted gene would be required. In other instances (e.g. some forms of cancer therapy or the use of gene therapy to deliver a DNA-based vaccine), short-term expression of the gene introduced would be sufficient/desirable. For most applications of gene therapy, straightforward expression of the gene product itself will suffice. However, in some instances, regulation of expression of the transferred gene would be required (e.g. if gene therapy combating insulin-dependent diabetes mellitus was to be considered). Achieving such expressional control over transferred genes is a pursuit that is only in the early stages of development.

The choice of target cells is another point worthy of discussion. In some instances, this choice is predetermined, e.g. treatment of the genetic condition, familial hypercholesterolaemia, would require insertion of the gene coding for the low-density lipoprotein receptor specifically in hepatocytes.

In other cases, however, some scope may be available to choose a target cell population. Even in the case of redressing some genetic diseases, it may not be necessary to correct genetically the exact population of cells affected. For example, a hallmark of several of the best characterized genetic diseases is the exceedingly low production of a circulatory gene product. Examples include clotting factors VIII and IX, a lack of which leads to haemophilia. It may be possible to correct such defects by introducing the appropriate gene into any recipient cell capable of exporting the gene product into the blood. Is such cases, choosing a target cell could be made upon practical considerations, such as their ease of isolation and culture, their capacity to express (and excrete) the protein product, and their half lives *in vivo*. Several cell types, including keratinocytes, myoblasts and fibroblasts, have been studied in this regard. It has been shown, for example, that myoblasts, into which the factor IX gene and the growth hormone gene have been introduced, could express their protein products and secrete them into the circulation.

Vectors Used in Gene Therapy

A list of the various vectors capable of introducing genes into recipient cells has been provided in Table 10.2. These vectors are conveniently categorized as being viral-based or non-viral-based systems. The main vector systems developed, thus far, are discussed in somewhat more detail below.

Retroviral Vectors

Some 24 per cent of all gene therapy clinical trials undertaken to date have employed retroviral vectors as gene delivery systems. Retroviruses are enveloped viruses. Their genome consists of ssRNA of approximately 5–8 kb. Upon entry into sensitive cells, the viral RNA is reverse transcribed and eventually yields double-stranded DNA. This subsequently integrates into the host cell genome. The basic retroviral genome contains a minimum of three structural genes: *gag* (codes for core viral protein), *pol* (codes for reverse transcriptase) and *env* (codes for the viral envelope proteins). At either end of the viral genome are the long terminal repeats (LTRs), which harbour powerful promoter and enhancer regions and sequences required to promote integration into the host DNA. Also present, immediately adjacent to the 5′ LTR, is the packing sequence (ψ). This is required to promote viral RNA packaging.

The ability of such retroviruses to (a) effectively enter various cell types and (b) integrate their genome into the host cell genome in a stable, long-term fashion, made them obvious potential vectors for gene therapy.

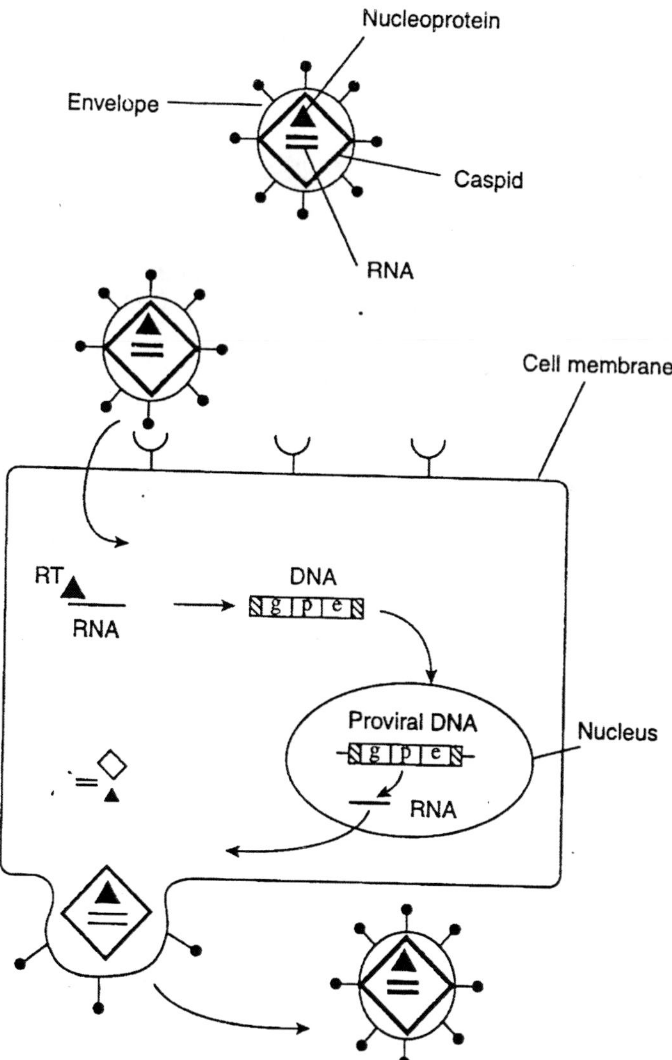

Fig. 10.3. The retroviral life cycle.

The construction of retroviruses to function as gene vectors entails replacing the endogenous viral genes, required for normal viral replication, with the exogenous gene of interest. Removal of the viral structural genes means that the resulting vector cannot itself replicate. In order to generate mature virion particles harbouring the vector nucleic acid, this genetic material must be introduced into a *'packing cell'*. These are recombinant cells that have previously been engineered to contain the *gag*, *pol* and *env* structural genes. In this way, packing cells are capable of producing mature, but replication-deficient, viral particles, harbouring the gene to be transferred. These viral particles function as so-called one-time, single-hit gene transfer systems.

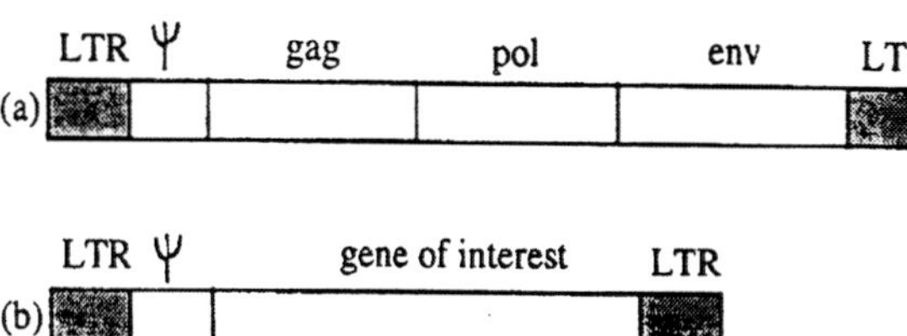

Fig. 10.4. Schematic representation of (a) the proviral genome of a basic retrovirus and (b) the genome of a basic engineered retroviral vector carrying the gene of interest.

More recently, various modifications have been introduced to this basic retroviral system. The inclusion of the 5′ end of the *gag* gene is shown to enhance levels of vector production by up to 200-fold. Additionally, specific promoters have been introduced in order to attempt to control expression of the inserted gene. Most work has focused upon the use of tissue-specific promoters in an effort to limit expression of the desired gene to a specific tissue type.

The most commonly employed (recombinant deficient) retrovirus used in this regard has been derived from the Maloney murine leukaemia virus (MoMuLV).

Retroviruses display a number of properties/characteristics that influence their potential as vectors in gene therapy protocols. These may be summarized as follows:

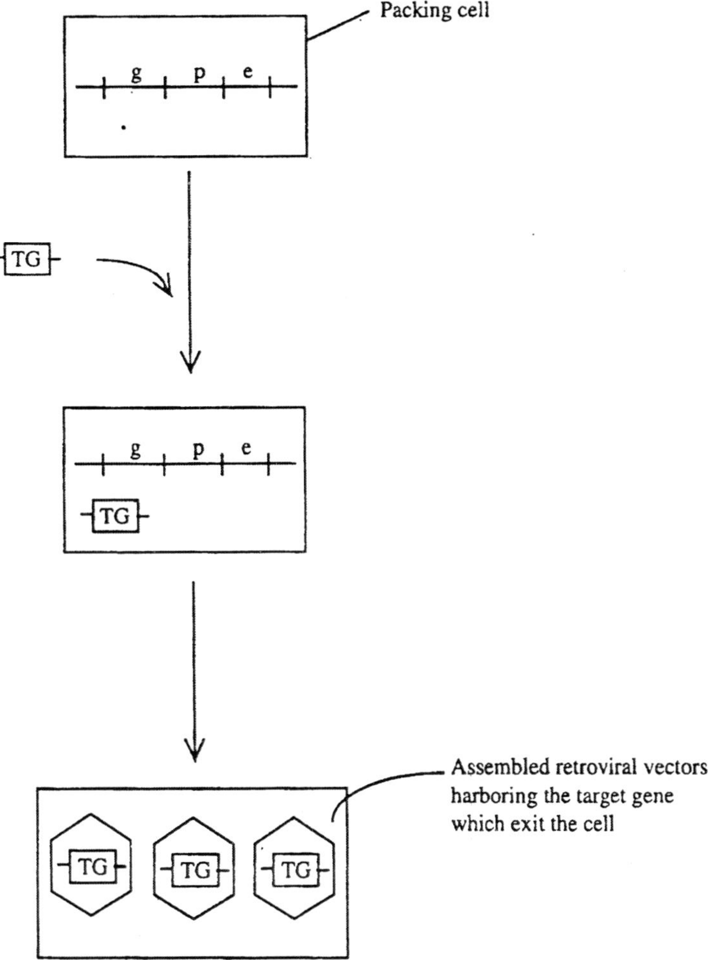

Fig. 10.5. The use of packing cells to generate replication-deficient retroviral vectors. The packaging cell is an engineered animal cell into which the retroviral gag (g), pol (p) and env (e) genes have been introduced.

1. Retroviruses as a group have been studied in detail and their biochemistry and molecular biology are well understood;
2. Most retroviruses can integrate their proviral DNA only into actively replicating cells;
3. The efficiency of gene transfer to most sensitive cell types is very high, often approaching 100 per cent;
4. Integrated DNA can be subject to long-term, relatively high-level expression;
5. Proviral DNA integrates randomly into the host chromosomes;
6. Retroviruses are promiscuous, in that they infect a variety of dividing cell types;
7. Complete copies of the proviral DNA are passed on to daughter cells if the original recipient cell divides;
8. Good, high-level, titre stocks of replication-incompetent retroviral particles can be produced;
9. Safety studies using retroviral vectors have already been carried out on various animal species.

The fact that they have been well studied, display almost 100 per cent transduction efficacy in sensitive cells and that the transferred genes are usually subject to long-term, fairly high-level expression renders retroviruses powerful potential vectors. These advantages form the basis of their widespread use in this regard. However, many of their other characteristics serve to curtail the application of retroviruses as gene therapy vectors. From a practical standpoint, retroviral vectors are relatively labile.

Thus, although retroviruses are relatively easy to propagate, they are often damaged by subsequent purification and concentration, which are steps essential for their clinical use. In most instances, their ability to infect only dividing cells clearly restricts their use. Their lack of selectivity in terms of the dividing cell types they infect is also a disadvantage. They will not infect all dividing cell types: the entry of any specific retrovirus is dependent upon the existence of an appropriate viral receptor on the surface of a target cell. As the identity of most retroviral receptors remains unknown, it remains difficult to predict the entire range of cell types any retrovirus is likely to infect during a gene therapy protocol. Integration and expression of the exogenous gene in cells other than target cells could result in physiological complications.

An additional drawback with regard to retroviral-based vectors is the propensity of the transferred gene to integrate randomly into the chromosomes of the recipient cells. Integration of the transferred DNA in the middle of a gene whose product plays a critical role in the cell could irrevocably damage cellular function. For example, disruption of a central metabolic enzyme could cause cell death, and disruption of a tumour suppresser gene could give rise to cellular transformation. In addition, integration of the proviral nucleic acid to sites adjacent to quiescent cellular proto-oncogenes could result in their activation.

The theoretical complications posed by random chromosomal integration became a medical reality in 2002, when two children who had received retroviral-based gene therapy 2 years previously developed a leukaemic-like condition. The initial clinical trial aimed to treat X-linked severe combined immunodeficiency (SCID-X1), a hereditary disorder in which T-lymphocytes and NK cells in particular do not develop, due to a mutation in the gene coding for the ãc cytokine receptor subunit. The clinical consequence is near abolition of a functional immune system.

The trial entailed retroviral-mediated *ex vivo* transduction of haematopoietic stem cells from 10 young SCID-X1 sufferers, with subsequent re-infusion of the treated cells. A marked and prolonged clinical response in which the condition was essentially reversed was observed in 9 out of the 10 patients. The prolonged response was likely due to the transduction of pluripotent progenitor cells with self-renewal capacity. However, the two youngest patients (1 and 3 months old at the time of treatment) developed uncontrolled proliferation of mature T-lymphocytes 30 months and 34 months after gene therapy respectively.

It has subsequently been shown that this leukaemia-like condition was triggered by proviral integration at a site near the LM02 proto-oncogene promoter, leading to gene activation. This development resulted in an initial ban on further retroviral-based gene therapy trials in some world regions, and the proportion of trials undertaken subsequently using retroviral-based systems has dropped significantly.

Adenoviral and Additional Viral-based Vectors

A number of additional viral types may also prove useful as vectors in the practice of gene therapy. Chief amongst these are the adenoviruses. Adeno-associated virus, the herpes virus, and a number of other viruses, are also being considered.

Adenoviruses are relatively large, non-enveloped structures, housing double-stranded DNA as their genetic material. Their genome is much larger (approximately 35 kb) and more complex than those of retroviruses. In most instances, only a small fraction of this genome is removed when constructing an adenovirus-based vector. Upon cellular infection, adenoviral DNA becomes localized in the nucleus, but does not integrate into the host cell DNA. Usually, infection by wild-type adenoviruses is associated with, at worst, mild clinical symptoms in humans. As potential vectors for gene therapy, adenoviruses display a number of both advantages and disadvantages, and they have been used in over 300 gene therapy trials to date. Their major advantage relates to their ability to infect non-dividing cells efficiently and the usually observed expression of large quantities of the desired gene products. However, the failure of the adenoviral-based DNA to integrate into the host cell generally means that its survival and, hence, the duration of gene expression, is limited. Adenovirus-based vectors, carrying various marker genes (i.e. a gene whose expression product is easily detected), have been administered to animals. Marker gene expression has been subsequently noted in various tissues, including heart, liver, muscle, bone marrow, central nervous system and endothelial cells. Duration of marker gene expression ranged from 2–3 weeks to several months.

Table 10.3 Some characteristic advantages and disadvantages of adenoviruses as potential vectors for gene therapy. Refer to text for further details

Advantages	*Disadvantages*
Adenoviruses are capable of gene transfer to non-dividing cells	Adenoviruses are highly immunogenic in man
They are easy to propagate in large quantities	The duration of expression of transferred genes can vary, and is usually transient
High levels of gene expression are usually recorded	Infection of permissive cells with wild-type adenovirus usually results in cell lysis
They are relatively stable viruses	Adenoviruses display a broad selectivity in the cell types they can infect

Whereas short-term, high-level gene expression may be appropriate for some gene therapy applications, it would be of less use for the treatment of, for example, genetic diseases, where long-term gene expression would be required. This could be achieved, in theory, by repeat administration of the adenoviral vector. However, adenoviruses prompt a strong immune response, which limits the efficacy of repeat administration. Indeed, the gene therapy trial death in 1999, as mentioned previously, was apparently caused by a severe and unexpected inflammatory reaction to the adenoviral vector used. Additional viruses that may prove of some use as future viral vectors include adeno-associated virus and herpes virus. Adeno-associated virus is a very small, single-stranded DNA virus: its genome consists of only two genes. It does not have the ability to replicate autonomously and can do so only in the presence of a co-infecting adenovirus (or other selected viruses).

Although it is found in the human population, it does not appear to be associated with any known diseases. Not surprisingly, only relatively small genes can be introduced into adeno-associated viral vector systems. Such systems, however, do provide a mechanism of gene transfer into non- dividing cells. It also seems to facilitate long-term expression of the transferred genetic material. In contrast to adenoviruses, nucleic acid transferred by adeno-associated viruses appears to be integrated into the recipient cell genome.

The herpes simplex virus represents another potential vector system that is receiving increased attention. Because herpes simplex virus is a neurotrophic virus, it may prove to be particularly useful in delivering genes to neurons of the peripheral and central nervous system. Upon infection, herpes simplex virus usually remains latent in non-dividing neurons, with its genome remaining in an unintegrated form. Thus far, it has proven difficult to generate a replication-incompetent, but yet viable, herpes simplex particle. Moreover, some of the replication-incompetent viruses generated still retain an ability to damage/destroy the cells they infect. Although herpes-based vector systems one day may prove useful in gene therapy, suitable and safe vector variants of herpes simplex virus must first be generated and tested. An additional virus that has more recently gained some attention as a possible vector is that of the sindbis virus. A member of the alphavirus family, this ssRNA virus can infect a broad range of both insect and vertebrate cells. The mature virion particles consist of the RNA genome complexed with a capsid protein C. This, in turn, is enveloped by a lipid bilayer in which two additional viral proteins (El and E2) are embedded. The E2 polypeptide appears to mediate viral binding to the surface receptors of susceptible cells. The major mammalian cell surface receptor it targets appears to be the highly conserved, widely distributed laminin receptor. The sindbis virus is simple, robust, capable of infecting non-dividing cells and generally supports high levels of gene expression. However, it does display a broad host range and, hence, lacks the inherent targeting specificity characteristic of an idealized viral vector.

Recently, a novel recombinant sindbis virus, displaying altered host cell specificity, has been generated. Scientists inserted a nucleotide sequence coding for the IgG binding domain of *Staphyloccus aureus* into the E2 viral gene. Disruption of the E2 gene renders its protein product incapable of binding laminin (hence, destroying the natural viral tropism). However, the protein A domain allows the chimaeric E2 product to bind monoclonal antibodies. This altered virus may prove to be a useful generic or 'null' vector, potentially capable of being specifically targeted to any desired cell type. This would simply necessitate pre-incubation of the virus with monoclonal antibodies raised against a surface antigen unique to the proposed target cell population. Binding of the monoclonal antibody to the protein A domain would ensue and the immobilized monoclonal antibody would dictate the cell type targeted.

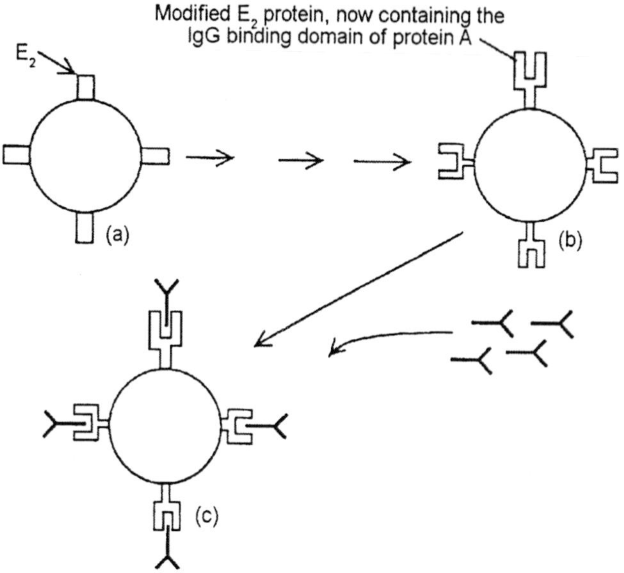

Fig. 10.6. Generation of engineered sindbis virus capable of being targeted to bind specific cell types.

Initial studies using this system have proved encouraging. The altered virus (without associated monoclonal antibody) failed to infect a wide variety of human cell lines. By initially incubating with monoclonal antibody of the appropriate specificity, however, the viral particles were capable of efficiently transducing cells expressing surface receptors such as CD4, CD33 and human leukocyte antigen.

A number of other issues must now be addressed including determining if the IgG–protein A affinity is sufficiently high to keep the antibody associated with the virus *in vivo*. The full potential of this approach will also require more detailed characterization of surface markers uniquely associated with different cell types. However, the approach exemplifies the types of technical innovation now being introduced that will make second-generation vectors more suited to their role in gene therapy.

Manufacture of Viral Vectors

Viral vector manufacture for therapeutic purposes involves initial viral propagation in appropriate animal cell lines, viral recovery, concentration, purification and formulation. The manufacture of alternative viral vectors likely follows a substantially similar approach. Master and working banks of both the viral vector and the animal cell line will have been constructed during the drug development process. Manufacture of a batch of vector, therefore, will be initiated by the culture of packing cells in suitable animal cell bioreactors. To date, bioreactor size of 100 l or less have been used, which are sufficient to satisfy clinical trial demand. The packing cells are then seeded with the replication-deficient virus, allowing vector propagation. After a fixed time the viral-infected cells are collected (harvested) by microfiltration or centrifugation and the cells are then homogenized in order to release the viral vector. Traditionally, adenoviral vectors (and indeed many other animal cell viruses) were purified from such a crude mixture by caesium chloride density-gradient centrifugation. While appropriate to laboratory-scale operations, this method is unsuitable for large-scale viral recovery due to scale-up issues and cost.

Alternative purification methods based upon column chromatography are thus employed on an industrial scale. Major '*contaminants*' present in this crude viral vector preparation include some intact animal cells, cellular debris, and intracellular molecules, most notably animal cell protein and nucleic acid. Intact cells/ cellular debris is removed by filtration. The release of large amounts of cellular DNA increases the solution viscosity and complicates downstream processing. The purification protocol, therefore, usually entails the physical degradation of DNA by addition of a nuclease enzyme. A solvent/detergent treatment step is then undertaken as a safety step in order to inactivate any enveloped contaminant viruses that might also be present. High-resolution purification is usually achieved by a combination of ion-exchange and gel-filtration chromatography, with product concentrations steps being undertaken by ultrafiltration if necessary. The final product is then filter sterilized and filled into glass vials. The purified vectors generally may be stored either refrigerated or frozen, and they display useful shelf lives of 2 years or more.

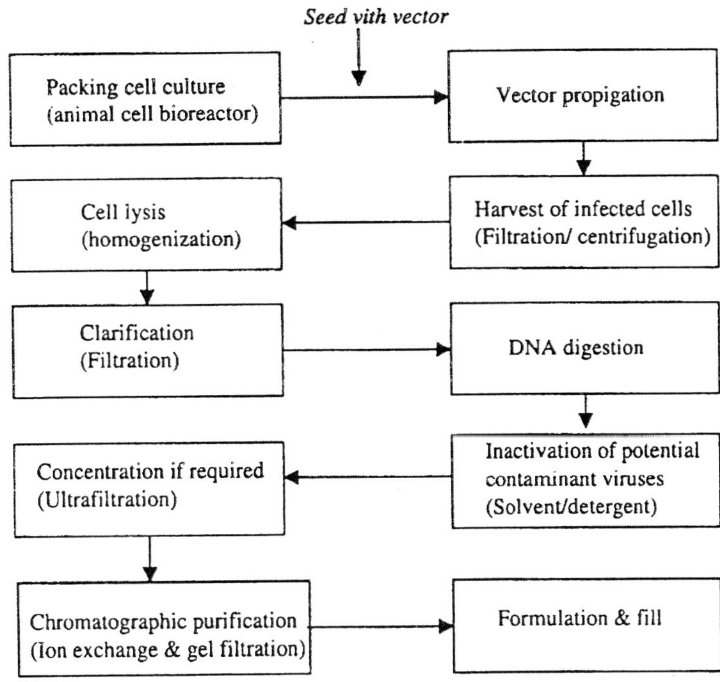

Fig. 10.7. Large-scale manufacture of adenoviral vectors for usefor gene-therapy-based clinical protocols.

Non-viral Vectors

Although viral-mediated gene delivery systems currently predominate, a substantial number of current clinical trials use non-viral-based methods of gene delivery. General advantages quoted with respect to non-viral delivery systems include:

1. Their low/non-immunogenicity;
2. Non-occurrence of integration of the therapeutic gene into the host chromosome (this eliminates the potential to disrupt essential host genes or to activate host oncogenes).

The initial approach adopted entailed administration of 'naked' plasmid DNA housing the gene of interest. This avenue of research was first opened in 1990, when it was shown that naked plasmid DNA was expressed in mice muscle cells subsequent to its i.m. injection. The plasmid DNA concerned housed the β-galactosidase gene as a reporter. Subsequent expression of β-galactosidase activity could persist for anything from a few months to the remainder of the animal's life. The transfection rate recorded was low (1–2 per cent of muscle fibres assimilated the DNA), and the DNA was not integrated into the host cell's chromosomes.

Up until this point, it was assumed that naked DNA injected into animals would not be spontaneously taken up and expressed in host cells. This finding vindicated the cautious approach taken by the FDA and other regulatory authorities with regard to the presence of free DNA in biopharmaceutical products.

Scientists have also since demonstrated that DNA (coated on microscopic gold beads) propelled into the epidermis of test animals with a '*gene gun*', is expressed in the animal's skin cells. Furthermore, the introduction in this fashion of DNA coding for human influenza viral antigens resulted in effective immunization of the animal against influenza. Similar results, using other pathogen models, have also now been generated. It is assumed that expressed antigen is secreted by the cell and, in this way, is exposed to immune surveillance. Further research has illustrated that systematic administration via i.v. injection rarely achieves meaningful cell transfection. This is most likely due to the high nuclease levels present in serum. In contrast, free nuclease activity in muscle tissue is extremely low.

Modern non-viral-based systems generally entail complexing/packaging the gene of interest (present, along with appropriate promoters, etc., in a circular plasmid) with additional molecules, particularly

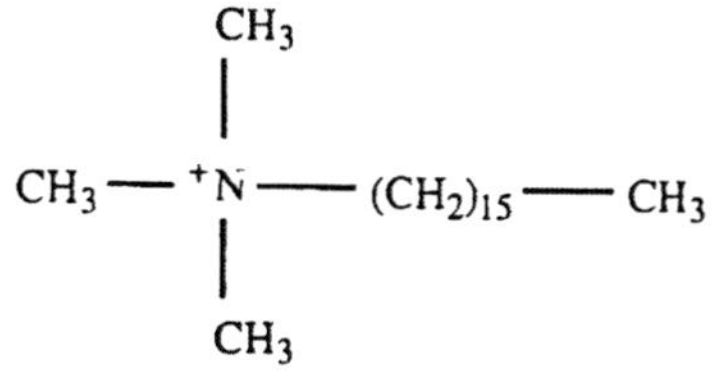

$CH_3-{}^{+}N(CH_3)_2-(CH_2)_{15}-CH_3$

CTAB

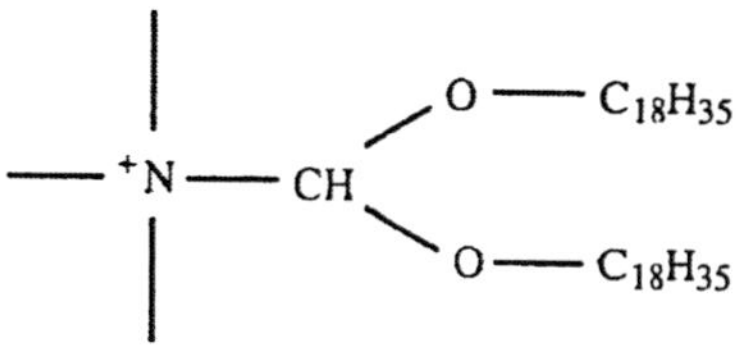

$-{}^{+}N-CH(O-C_{18}H_{35})(O-C_{18}H_{35})$

DOTMA

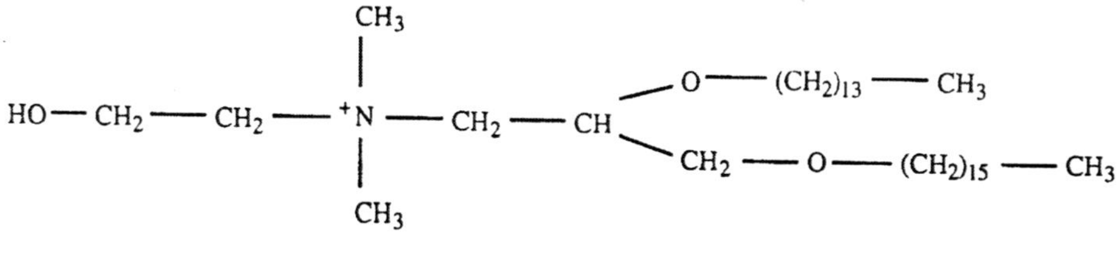

$HO-CH_2-CH_2-{}^{+}N(CH_3)_2-CH_2-CH(O-(CH_2)_{13}-CH_3)(CH_2-O-(CH_2)_{15}-CH_3)$

DMRI

$^{+}NH_3-[CH((CH_2)_4{}^{+}NH_3)-C(=O)-NH]_n-CH((CH_2)_4{}^{+}NH_3)-COO^-$

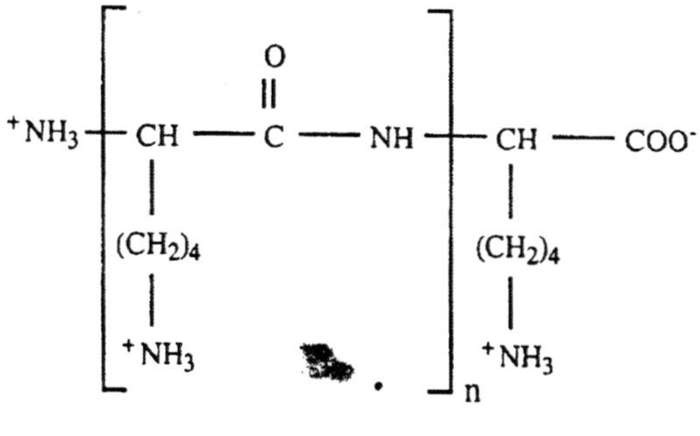

Polylysine

Fig. 10.8. Structure of some cationic lipids and polylysine.

various lipids or some polypeptides. These generally display a positive charge and, hence, interact with the negatively charged DNA molecules. The function of such carrier molecules is to stabilize the DNA, protect it from, for example, serum nucleases and ideally to modulate interaction with the biological system (e.g. help target the DNA to particular cell types, or away from other cell types).

The most commonly used polymers are the cationic lipids and polylysine chains. Cationic lipids can aggregate in aqueous-based systems to form vesicles/liposomes, which in turn will interact spontaneously with DNA. Initially, the negatively charged plasmid DNA probably acts as a bridge between adjacent vesicles. Further DNA/vesicle interactions quickly generate a complex three-dimensional lattice-like system composed of flattened vesicles (some of which probably rupture) interspersed with plasmid DNA. The lipid component of such '*lipoplexes*' should, therefore, provide a measure of physical protection to the therapeutic gene.

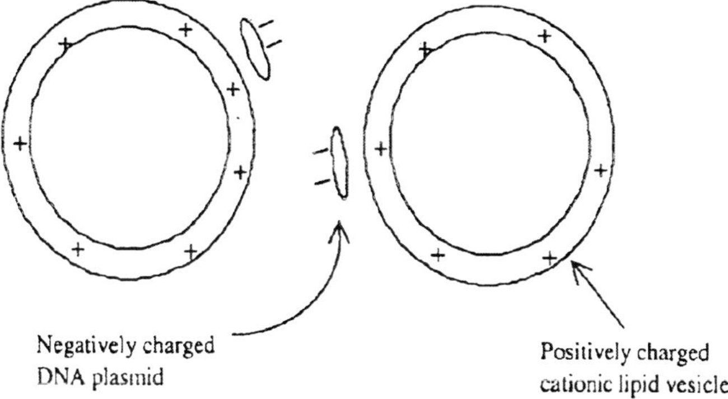

Fig. 10.9. Initial interaction of plasmid DNA with cationic vesicles.

Gene therapy results to date using this approach have been mixed. The process of lipoplex formation is not easily controlled; hence, different batches made under seemingly identical conditions may not be structurally identical. Furthermore, *in vitro* test results using such lipoplexes can correlate very poorly with subsequent *in vivo* performance. Clearly, more research is required to underpin the rational use of lipoplexes for gene therapy purposes. The same is true for other polymer-based synthetic gene delivery systems, the most significant of which is the polylysine-based system. Polylysine molecules, due to their positive charge, can also form electrostatic complexes with DNA. However, the stability of such '*polyplexes*' in biological fluids can be problematic. Furthermore, polyplexes tend to be rapidly removed from circulation, prompting a low plasma half-life. These difficulties can be alleviated in part by the attachment of PEG molecules. PEG attachment is also used to increase the serum half-life of various therapeutic proteins, such as some interferons.

No matter what their composition, such synthetic gene delivery systems also meet various biological barriers to efficient cellular gene delivery. Viral vector-based systems are far less prone to such problems, as the viral carrier has evolved in nature to overcome such obstacles. Obstacles relate to:

1. Blood-related issues;
2. Biodistribution profile;
3. Cellular targeting;
4. Cellular entry and nuclear delivery.

Whereas lipoplexes/polyplexes generally protect the plasmid from serum nucleases, the overall positive charge characteristic of these structures leads to their non-specific interactions with cells (both blood cells and vascular endothelial cells) and serum proteins. Also, following i.v. injection, such DNA complexes in practice tend to accumulate in the lung and liver. Targeting of DNA complexes to specific cell types also poses a considerable (largely unmet) technical challenge. Approaches, such as the incorporation of antibodies directed against specific cell surface antigens may provide a future avenue of achieving such cell-selective targeting. However, it is currently believed that ionic interactions constitute a predominant binding force between the positively charged lipoplexes/polyplexes and the negatively charged eukaryotic cell surface. Such electrostatic interactions may even override more biospecific interactions characteristic of antibody- or receptor-based systems. Currently, probably the most effective means of delivering such vectors to target tissue/cells is to inject them into/beside the target area.

However targeted to the appropriate cell surface, if it is to be clinically effective, the therapeutic plasmid must enter the cell and reach the nucleus intact. Cellular entry is generally achieved via endocytosis. A proportion of endocytosed plasmid DNA escapes from the endosome by entering the cytoplasm, thereby escaping liposomal destruction. The molecular mechanism by which escape is accomplished is, at best, only partially understood. Anionic lipid constituents of lipoplexes, for example, may fuse directly with the endosomal membranes, facilitating direct expulsion of at least a portion of the plasmid DNA into the cytoplasm. Generally, the DNA is released in free form (i.e. uncomplexed to any lipid). Some attempts have been made to rationally increase the efficiency of endosomal escape. One such avenue entails the incorporation of selected hydrophobic (viral) peptides into the gene delivery systems. Many viruses naturally enter animal cells via receptor-mediated endocytosis. These viruses have evolved efficient means of endosomal escape, usually relying upon membrane- disrupting peptides derived from the viral coat proteins.

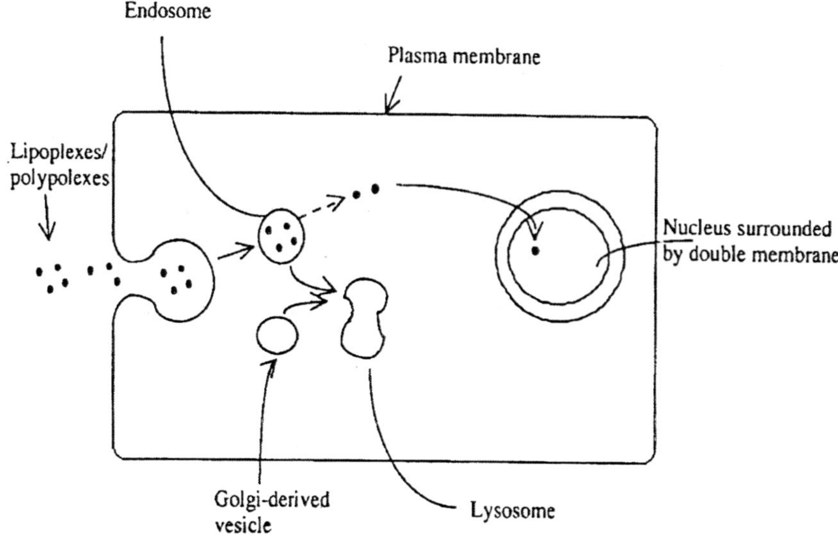

Fig. 10.10. Overview of cellular entry of (non-viral) gene delivery systems, with subsequent plasmid relocation to the nucleus.

Once in the cytoplasm, a proportion of plasmid molecules are likely degraded by cytoplasmic nucleases, effectively further reducing transfection efficiencies. There are two potential routes by which plasmid DNA could reach the nucleus:

1. Direct nuclear entry as a consequence of nuclear membrane breakdown associated with mitosis;
2. Transport through nuclear pores, which may occur via passive diffusion or specific energy-requiring transport processes.

Overall, it is estimated that only one in 10^4–10^5 plasmids taken up by endocytosis will enter the nucleus intact and be successfully expressed.

Manufacture of Plasmid DNA

Prior to its manufacture, researchers would have constructed an appropriate vector housing the therapeutic gene and introduced it into a producer microorganism, usually *E. coli*. Routine large-scale plasmid manufacture then entails culture of a batch of producer microorganisms by fermentation, followed by plasmid extraction and purification. In this regard, the overall approach used resembles the approaches taken in the large-scale manufacture of recombinant therapeutic proteins. Fermentation promotes microbial cell replication and, thus, the biosynthesis of large quantities of plasmid. Subsequent to fermentation, the microbial cells are harvested (collected) by either centrifugation or microfiltration. Following resuspension in a low volume of buffer, the cells must be disrupted in order to release the plasmids therein. This appears to be most commonly achieved by the addition of a lysis reagent consisting of NaOH and SDS. The combination of high pH and detergent action disrupts the microbial cell wall/membranes with consequent release of the intracellular contents. In addition to the desired plasmid DNA, this crude mixture will also contain various impurities, which must be removed by subsequent downstream processing steps. Notable impurities include:

1. Cell wall debris and some intact cells;
2. Proteins;
3. Genomic DNA;
4. RNA;
5. Low molecular mass metabolites;
6. Endotoxin.

After lysis is complete, the next step can entail the addition of a high-salt neutralization solution, such as potassium acetate. This promotes formation of aggregates of genomic DNA and SDS–protein complexes, which can subsequently be removed by centrifugation or filtration. The plasmids can then themselves be precipitated from the resultant solution by the addition of appropriate solvent (usually either isopropanol or ethanol). Upon resuspension, the plasmid preparation can then be subjected to chromatographic purification. The major contaminants likely still present include RNA, genomic DNA fragments, nicked or other plasmid variants, and endotoxins. Gel-filtration chromatography can effectively remove contaminants that differ substantially in shape/size from the desired plasmid. These can include most genomic DNA fragments, RNA and (most) endotoxins. It can also achieve partial removal of plasmid variants, such as open circular plasmids from the main (supercoiled) plasmid preparation. Ion exchange can remove many protein contaminants, as well as RNA. However, genomic DNA and endotoxins generally co-purify with the plasmid DNA. Additional chromatographic approaches based upon reverse-phase and affinity systems have been developed at laboratory scale at least. A significant feature of plasmid purification employing capture chromatography (i.e. involving plasmids binding to the chromatographic beads) is the low plasmid-binding capacities observed. The pore size of commercially available capture chromatographic media is insufficiently large to allow entry of plasmids, restricting binding to the bead surface. Binding capacities can, therefore, be 100-fold or more lower than those observed when the same media are used to purify (much smaller) therapeutic proteins.

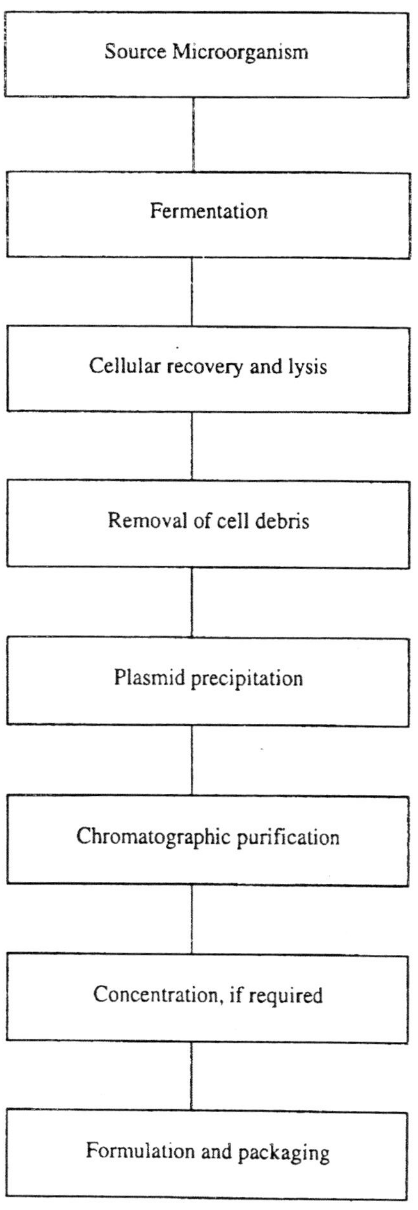

Fig. 10.11. Overview of the manufacturing process for the large-scale production of plasmid DNA.

Purified plasmids may then be analysed using various analytical techniques. Freedom from contaminating nucleic acid/proteins can be assessed electrophoretically. Endotoxin and sterility tests would also be routinely undertaken. The purified plasmid DNA must next be formulated to yield the final non-viral delivery system. Formulation studies relating to such systems remain an area requiring further investigation. Most work reported to date relates to formulating/stabilizing lipoplex-based gene delivery systems. Aqueous suspensions of these (and other) non-viral-based systems tend to aggregate quickly (in a matter of minutes to hours). In order to circumvent this problem, the final delivery systems were often actually formulated at the patient bedside in earlier clinical trials.

Research aimed at identifying appropriate stabilizing excipients/formulation formats is ongoing. Simple freezing is an option, particularly as frozen formulations would be immune to agitation-induced aggregation. However, the process of freezing, particularly slow freezing, in itself induces aggregation. This can be minimized by flash freezing (e.g. by immersion in liquid nitrogen), although this approach may not prove practicable at an industrial scale. The addition of cryoprotectants may help minimize this problem, and initial studies indicate that various sugars (e.g. glucose, sucrose and trehalose) show some potential in this regard. Another avenue under investigation relates to the generation of a final freeze-dried product. Again, issues such as the (relatively) slow freezing process characteristic of industrial-scale freeze-driers complicate attaining this goal in practice.

Gene Therapy and Genetic Disease

Well over 4000 genetic diseases have been characterized to date. Many of these are caused by lack of production of a single gene product or are due to the production of a mutated gene product incapable of carrying out its natural function. Gene therapy represents a seemingly straightforward therapeutic option that could correct such genetic-based diseases. This would be achieved simply by facilitating insertion of a 'healthy' copy of the gene in question into appropriate cells of the sufferer.

Although simple in concept, the application of gene therapy to treat/cure genetic diseases has, thus far, made little impact in practice. The slow progress in this regard is likely due to a number of factors. These include:

1. The number of genetic diseases for which the actual gene responsible has been identified and studied are relatively modest, although completion of the human genome project should rapidly accelerate identification of such genes.
2. As discussed previously, none of the first-generation gene-delivering vectors have proven fully satisfactory.
3. Some genetic diseases are quite complex, with several organs/cell types being affected. In most instances, it has proven difficult in practice to introduce the required gene into all the affected cell types.
4. Regulation of expression levels of the genes transferred has proven problematic.
5. Drug companies often display greater interest in applying gene therapy to more prevalent diseases, such as cancer. The patient population suffering from many genetic diseases is relatively modest. In some instances, a limited patient population may not be sufficient to allow the developing company to recoup the cost of drug development.

Many of the initial attempts to utilize gene therapy in practice focused upon haemoglobinopathies (e.g. sickle cell anaemia and thalassaemias). These conditions were amongst the first genetic disorders to be characterized at a molecular level, with the defect centring around the haemoglobin α- or β-chain genes. Furthermore, the target cells in the bone marrow could be removed and subsequently replaced with relative ease. However, these conditions proved to be a difficult initial choice for the gene therapist. The production of the appropriate quantities of functional haemoglobin is dependent not only upon the presence of α- and β-globin genes of the correct sequence, but also upon detailed regulation of gene expression. Such tight regulation of expression of transferred genes is beyond the capability of gene therapy technology as it currently stands.

Table 10.4. Some examples of genetic diseases for which the defective gene responsible has been identified

Disease	*Defective genes protein product*
Haemophilia A	Factor VIII
Haemophilia B	Factor IX
Thalassemia	β-globin
Sickle cell anaemia	β-globin
Familial hypercholesterolaemia	Low-density protein receptor
Severe combined immunodeficiency	Adenosine deaminase
Severe combined immunodeficiency	Purine nucleoside phosphorylase
Niemann-Pick disease	Sphingomylinase
Gaucher's disease	Glucocerebrosidase
Cystic fibrosis	Cystic fibrosis transmembrane regulator
Emphysema	α_1-Antitrypsin
Leukocyte adhesion deficiency	CD18
Hyperammonaemia	Ornithine transcarbamylase
Citrullinaemia	Arginosuccinate synthetase
Phenylketonuria	Phenylalanine hydroxylase
Maple syrup disease	Branched chain α-ketoacid dehydrogenase
Tyrosinaemia type 1	Fumarylacetoacetate hydrolase
Glycogen storage deficiency type 1A	Glucose-6-phosphatase
Fucosidosis	α-L-Fucosidase
Mucopolysaccharidosis type VII	β-Glucuronidase
Mucopolysaccharidosis type I	α-L-Iduronidase
Galactosaemia	Galactose-1-phosphate uridyl transferase

Another early genetic disease for correction by gene therapy was SCID. One form of this disease is caused by a lack of adenosine deaminase (ADA) activity. ADA is an enzyme that plays a central role in the degradation of purine nucleosides (it catalyses the removal of ammonia from adenosine, forming inosine, which, in turn, is usually eventually converted to uric acid). This leads to T- and B-lymphocyte dysfunction. Lack of an effective immune system means that SCID sufferers must be kept in an essentially sterile environment.

When compared with treating diseases such as thalassaemia, regulation of the level of expression of a corrected ADA gene was believed to be less important for a successful therapeutic outcome. (In most, though not all, metabolic diseases caused by an enzyme deficiency, it appears that expression of even a fraction of normal enzyme levels is sufficient to ameliorate the disease symptoms.)

Gene therapy trials aimed at counteracting ADA deficiency were initiated in 1990. The first recipient was a 4-year-old SCID sufferer. The protocol used entailed the isolation of the child's peripheral lymphocytes, followed by the *in vitro* introduction of the human ADA gene into these cells, using a retroviral vector. After a period of expansion (by culture *in vitro*), these treated cells were re-injected into the patient. As the lymphocytes (and, by extension, the corrective gene) had a finite life span, the therapy was repeated every 6–8 weeks. This approach appeared successful, in that it has resulted in a marked and sustained improvement in the recipient's immune function. Critically, however, interpretation of this outcome was made more difficult owing to the later revelation that the patient also initiated more conventional SCID therapy just prior to the gene therapy treatment. A second retroviral-based trial aiming to treat a different form of SCID has also been discussed earlier in this chapter.

Haematopoietic (and intdeed other) stem cells are attractive potential gene therapy recipient cells because they are immortal. Successful introduction of the target gene into these cells should facilitate ongoing production of the gene product in mature blood cells, which are continually derived from the stem cell population. This would likely remove the requirement for repeat gene transfers to the affected individual.

The routine transduction of haematopoietic stem cells has, thus far, proven technically difficult. They are found only in low quantities in the bone marrow, and there is a lack of a suitable assay for stem cells. However, recent progress has been made in this regard, and routine transduction of such cells will likely be achievable within the next few years.

Additional genetic diseases for which a gene therapy approach is currently being evaluated include familial hypercholesterolaemia and cystic fibrosis. Familial hypercholesterolaemia is caused by the absence (or presence of a defective form of) low-density lipoprotein receptors on the surface of liver cells. This results in highly elevated serum cholesterol levels, normally accompanied by early onset of serious vascular disease. The gene therapy approaches that have been attempted thus far to counteract this condition have entailed the initial removal of a relatively large portion of the liver. Hepatocytes derived from the liver are then cultured *in vitro*, with gene transfer being undertaken using retroviral vectors. The corrected hepatocytes are then usually infused back into the liver via a catheter. Although studies in animals have been partially successful, transduction of only a small proportion of the hepatocytes is normally observed. Subsequent expression of the corrective gene can also be variable. *In vivo* approaches to hepatic gene correction, using both viral and non-viral approaches, are also currently being assessed.

The cystic fibrosis (*cf*) gene was first identified in 1989. It codes for CFTR, a 170 kDa protein that serves as a chloride channel in epithelial cells. Inheritance of a mutant *cftr* gene from both parents results in the cystic fibrosis phenotype. While various organs are affected, the most severely affected are the respiratory epithelial cells. These cells have, unsurprisingly, become the focus of attempts at corrective gene therapy. Cystic fibrosis is the most common inherited mono- genetic disease in Europe and the USA, and sufferers have a typical life expectancy of less than 40 years. Over a third of the 100 or so gene therapy trials thus far undertaken to treat inherited disorders have specifically targeted cystic fibrosis.

Several vectors have been used in an attempt to deliver the cystic fibrosis gene to the airway epithelial cells of sufferers. The most notable systems include adenoviruses and cationic liposomes. Vector delivery to the target cells can be achieved directly by aerosol technology. Delivery of CFTR cDNA to airway epithelial cells (and subsequent gene expression) has been demonstrated with the use of both vector types. However, in order to be of therapeutic benefit, it is essential that 5–10 per cent of the target cell population receive and express the CFTR gene. This level of integration has not been achieved so far; and, furthermore, gene expression has often been transient.

Gene Therapy and Cancer

To date, the majority of gene therapy trials undertaken aim to cure not inherited genetic defects, but cancer. The average annual incidence of cancer reported in the USA alone stands at approximately 1.4 million cases. Survival rates attained by pursuit of conventional therapeutic strategies (surgery, chemo/radiotherapy) stand at about 50 per cent. Initial gene therapy trials aimed at treating/curing cancer began in 1991. Various strategic approaches have since been developed in this regard. Numerous trials aimed at assessing the application of gene therapy for the treatment of a wide variety of cancer types are now underway.

Table 10.5 Some therapeutic strategies being pursued in an attempt to treat cancer using a gene therapy approach.

Modifying lymphocytes in order to enhance their anti-tumour activity
Modifying tumour cells to enhance their immunogenicity
Inserting tumour suppressor genes into tumour cells
Inserting toxin genes in tumour cells in order to promote tumour cell destruction
Inserting suicide genes into tumour cells
Inserting genes, such as a multiple drug resistance (*mrd*) gene, into stem cells to protect them from chemotherapy induced damaged
Counteracting the expression of oncogenes in tumour cells by inserting an appropriate antisense gene

Although many of the results generated to date provide hope for the future, gene therapy thus far has failed to provide a definitive cure for cancer. The lack of success is likely due to a number of factors, including:

1. A requirement for improved, more target-specific vector systems.
2. A requirement for a better understanding of how cancer cells evade the normal immune response.
3. For ethical reasons, most patients treated to date were suffering from advanced and widespread terminal cancer (i.e. little/no hope of survival if treated using conventional therapies). Cancers at earlier stages of development will probably prove to be more responsive to gene therapy.

Table 10.6 Some specific cancer types for which human gene therapy trials have been initiated

Breast cancer	Colorectal cancer
Malignant melanoma	Tumours of the central nervous system
Ovarian cancer	Renal cell carcinoma
Small-cell lung cancer	Non-small-cell lung cancer

One of the earliest cancer gene therapy trials attempted involved the introduction of the TNF gene into TILs. The rationale was that if, as expected, TIL cells reintroduced into the body could infiltrate the tumour, TNF synthesis would occur at the tumour site (where it is required). This approach has since been broadened, by introducing genes coding for a range of immunostimulatory cytokines (e.g. IL-2, IL-4, IFN-γ and GM-CSF) into TILs. A variation of this approach involves the introduction of such cytokine genes directly into tumour cells themselves. It is hoped that reintroduction of such cytokine-producing cells into the body will result in a swift and effective immune response, i.e. killing the tumour cells and vaccinating the patient against recurrent episodes. In most instances so far, this strategy has been carried out in practice by removal of target cells from the body, culture *in vitro*, introduction of the desired gene (mainly using retroviral vectors), followed by reintroduction of the altered cells into the body.

An alternative anti-cancer strategy entails insertion of a copy of a tumour suppresser gene into cancer cells. For example, a deficiency in one such gene product, p53, has been directly implicated in the development of various human cancers. It has been shown *in vitro* that insertion of a p53 gene in some p53-deficient tumour cell lines induces the death of such cells. A potential weakness of such an approach, however, is that 100 per cent of the transformed cells would have to be successfully treated to fully cure the cancer. Tumour suppressor-based gene therapy in combination with conventional approaches (chemotherapy or radiotherapy) may, therefore, prove most efficacious, and the sole gene-therapy-based medicine approved to date (in China only) is based upon this approach.

Yet another strategy that may prove useful is the introduction into tumour cells of a 'sensitivity' gene. This concept dictates that the gene product should harbour the ability to convert a non-toxic pro-drug into a toxic substance within the cells• - thus leading to their selective destruction. The model system most used to appraise such an approach entails the use of the thymidine kinase gene of the herpes simplex virus.

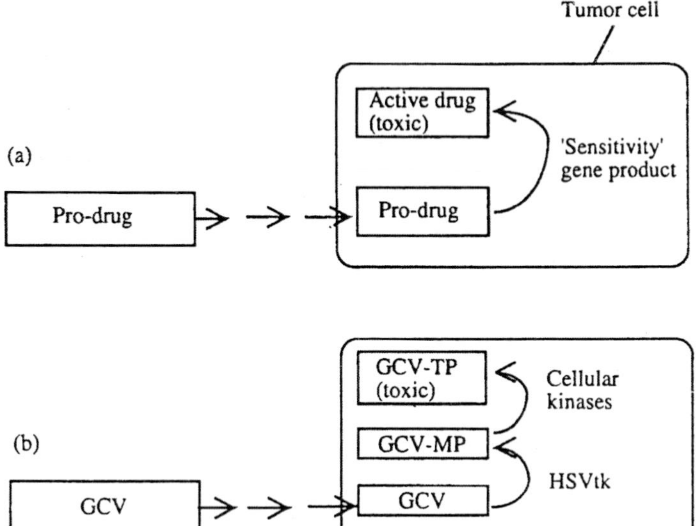

Fig. 10.12. Schematic representation of the therapeutic retionale underpinning the introduction of a 'sensitivity' gene into tumour cells in order to promote their selective destruction.

A different gene therapy-based approach to cancer entails introduction of a gene into haematopoietic stem cells in order to protect these cells from the toxic effects of chemotherapy. Most cancer drugs display toxic side effects which usually limits the upper dosage levels that can be safely administered. One common toxic side-effect is the destruction of stem cells. If these cells could be protected or made resistant to the chemotherapeutic agent, it might be possible to administer higher concentrations of the drug to the patient. In practice, such a protective effect could be conferred by the multiple drug resistance (type 1; MDR-1) gene product. This is often expressed by cancer cells resistant to chemotherapy. It functions to pump a range of chemotherapeutic drugs (e.g. daunorubicin, taxol, vinblastine, vincristine, etc.) out of the cell. Animal studies have confirmed that introduction of the MDR-1 gene into stem cells protects these cells subsequently from large doses of taxol. This approach is now being appraised in patients receiving high-dose chemotherapy for a range of cancer types, including breast and ovarian cancer and brain tumours.

Gene Therapy and AIDS

It is likely that gene therapy will prove useful in treating a far broader range of medical conditions than simply those of inherited genetic disease and cancer. A prominent additional disease target are those diseases caused by infectious agents, particularly intracellular pathogens such as HIV. The main strategic approach adopted entails introducing a gene into pathogen-susceptible cells whose product will interfere with pathogen survival/replication within that cell. Such a strategy is sometimes termed '*intracellular immunization*'.

One such anti-AIDS strategy being pursued is the introduction into viral-sensitive cells of a gene coding for an altered (dysfunctional) HIV protein, such as *gag*, *tat* or *env*. The presence of such mutant forms of *gag*, in particular, was shown to be capable of inhibiting viral replication. This is probably due to interference by the mutated *gag* product with correct assembly of the viral core. An additional approach entails the transfer to sensitive cells of a gene coding for antibody fragments capable of binding to the HIV envelope proteins. This may also interfere with viral assembly in infected cells.

Scientists have also generated recombinant cells capable of synthesizing and secreting soluble forms of the HIV cell surface receptor, i.e. the CD4 antigen. It has been suggested that release of such soluble viral receptors into the blood would bind circulating virions, hence blocking their ability to 'dock' at sensitive cells. Although this proved to be the case *in vitro*, early *in vivo* studies have not proved as encouraging. Yet additional therapeutic approaches to AIDS, based upon antisense technology, will be discussed later in this chapter.

Gene-based Vaccines

An additional gene-therapy-based approach to vaccination is also now under investigation. The approach entails the administration of a DNA vector housing the gene coding for a surface antigen protein from the target pathogen. In this way, the body itself would produce the pathogen-associated protein. Theoretically, virtually any body cell could be targeted, the only requirement being that target cells export the resultant antigenic protein such that it is encountered by the immune system. Additionally, gene expression need only be transient, i.e. just sufficiently long to facilitate the induction of an immune response. Target conditions for gene-based vaccines thus far having entered clinical trials include malaria, hepatitis B and AIDS.

Some Additional Considerations

In addition to some technical difficulties outlined earlier, a number of non-technical issues must be satisfactorily addressed before its practice becomes widespread. Chief amongst these issues are the questions of public perception, ethics and costs.

Gene therapy is not, and will not be, an inexpensive therapeutic tool. The cost of such treatments will likely be broadly similar to the cost of present-day biopharmaceuticals. However, if proven successful in treating many currently incurable conditions, the cost:benefit ratio will almost certainly greatly favour its medical use.

Public perception and ethical considerations are, in some ways, interlinked. The ability to so readily modify our genetic complement holds great therapeutic promise. However, strict regulations overseeing the use of this technology are required (and are currently being enforced). Without proper controls, the danger exists that gene therapy could eventually be used to 'improve' human characteristics. The technical know-how to underpin a new era of eugenics is now almost a reality. The most important safeguard aimed at preventing eugenic-type developments is already in place. Currently, gene therapy is restricted to somatic cells; the genetic manipulation of human germ cells is banned. Any genetic alterations achieved thus will not be transmitted to future generations. Like many other technologies, there is no 'going back' in relation to gene therapy. The challenge is to ensure that human genetic manipulation is used only for purposes that clearly represent the 'common good'.

Antisense Technology

Various disease states are associated with the inappropriate production/overproduction of gene products. Examples include:

1. The expression of oncogenes, leading to the transformed state;
2. The overexpression of cytokines during some disease states with associated worsening of disease symptoms;
3. The overproduction of angiotensinogen, - which ultimately results in hypertension.

An additional example includes the intracellular transcription and translation of virally encoded genes during intracellular viral replication. In all such instances, the medical consequences of such inappropriate gene (over)expression could be ameliorated/prevented if this expression could be down-regulated. A nucleic-acid-based approach to achieve just this is termed '*antisense technology*'.

The antisense approach is based upon the generation of short, single-stranded stretches of nucleic acids (which can be DNA- or RNA-based) displaying a specific nucleotide sequence. These are generally termed '*antisense oligonucleotides*'. These oligonucleotides are capable of binding to DNA (at specific gene sites) or, more commonly, to mRNA derived from specific genes. This binding, in most cases, occurs via Watson–Crick-based nucleotide base pair complementarity. Binding prevents expression of the gene product by preventing either the transcription or translation process.

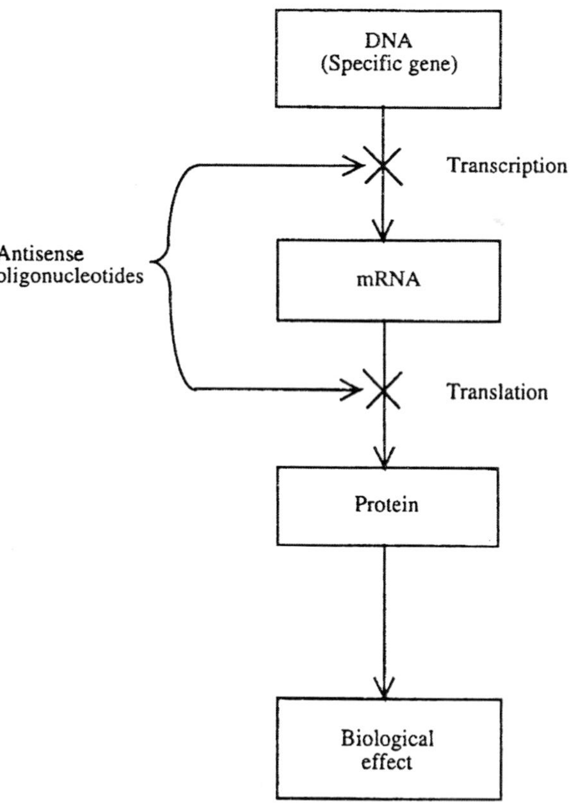

Fig. 10.13. Overview of the concept of the antisense approach: the end goal is the prevention of expression of a particular gene product by either blocking the transcription or translation of that gene.

Antisense Oligonucleotides and Their Mode of Action

The nucleotide sequence of an mRNA molecule contains the encoded blueprint that dictates the amino acid sequence of a protein. Because of this, the mRNA sequence is said to make '*sense*'. (This mRNA, therefore, is complementary to an '*antisense*' DNA strand, i.e. it is the antisense strand of DNA in a given gene that serves as template for the mRNA synthesis.) As long as at least part of the nucleotide sequences of any mRNA is known, it becomes potentially possible to synthesize chemically an oligonucleotide, either a ribo- or deoxyribonucleotide, whose base sequence is complementary to at least a section of the mRNA sequence. As long as such an 'antisense' oligonucleotide can enter the cell, the complementarity of sequences can promote hybridization between the mRNA and the antisense oligonucleotide.

Successful binding, however, does not depend alone upon Watson–Crick base complementary. It is also influenced by higher-order secondary and tertiary structures adopted by the RNA. Intramolecular complementary base pairing can occur (particularly within transfer and ribosomal RNA, but also messenger RNA), resulting in the formation of short duplex sequences, separated by stems and loops. Such higher-order structure seems to be functionally important, conferring recognition motifs for proteins and additional nucleic acids, as well as helping to stabilize the RNA. Regions engaged in intramolecular base pairing are obviously poor targets for antisense oligos. It is thus desirable to synthesize a nucleotide whose sequence is complementary to an accessible sequence along the mRNA backbone. Various approaches are taken to identify such suitable sequences (remember, the entire sequence of the mRNA will be known). The 'blind' or 'shotgun' approach entails synthesizing large numbers of oligos targeted to various (often overlapping) regions of the mRNA. The ability of each oligo to block translation of the mRNA is then directly assessed in an *in vitro* assay system using cell-free extracts. The second design approach entails the use of various computer programs to interrogate the mRNA sequence in an attempt to predict its higher-order structure (and hence identify accessible sequences). This approach remains to be optimized. The translation initiation sites of mRNAs are often popular targets because

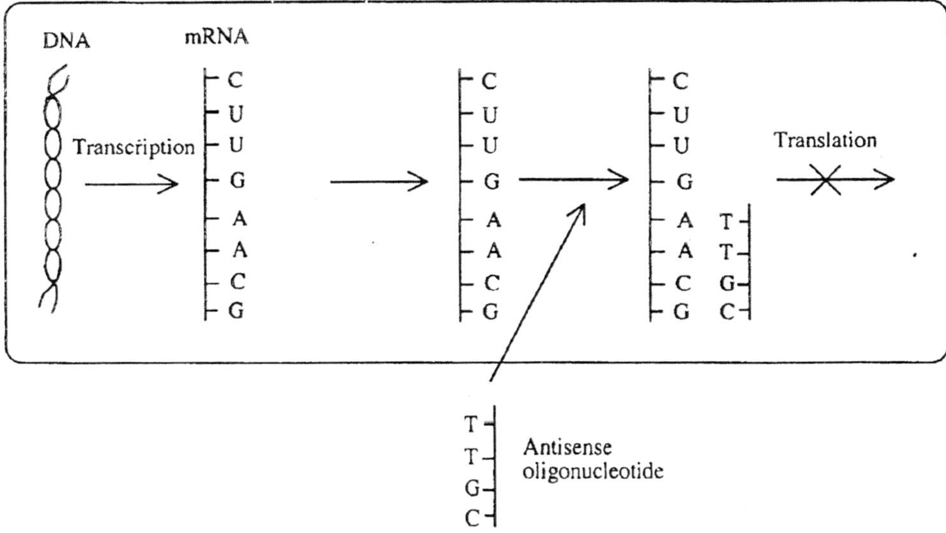

Fig. 10.14. Outline of how an antisense oligonucleotide can prevent synthesis of a gene product by blocking translation. In practice, antisense oligos are 12-18 nucleotides in length.

they are essential to translation and they are generally free from secondary structure. However, sequence homologies can exist within these sequences in unrelated genes. This reduces the specificity of the blocking effect and could lead to clinically significant side effects.

Binding results in the blocking of translation of the mRNA and, hence, prevents synthesis of the mature gene's protein product. The prevention of mRNA translation by duplex formation with antisense oligonucleotides appears to be underpinned by various mechanisms, including: (a) the oligonucleotides act as steric blockers, i.e. prevent proteins involved in translation, or other aspects of mRNA processing, from binding to appropriate sequences in the mRNA; (b) the generation of duplexes also likely allows targeting by intracellular RNases such as RNaseH. This enzyme is capable of binding to RNA–DNA duplexes and degrading the RNA portion of the duplex (most synthetic antisense oligonucleotides are DNA based).

Uses, Advantages and Disadvantages of 'Oligos'

Antisense oligonucleotides (oligos) are being assessed in preclinical and clinical studies as therapeutic agents in the treatment of cancer, as well as a variety of viral diseases (e.g. HIV, hepatitis B, herpes and papillomavirus infections). They also have potential application in treating other disease states for which blocking of gene expression would likely have a beneficial effect. Such medical conditions include restenosis, rheumatoid arthritis and allergic disorders. Cancer, however, remains the most common target indication. The favoured approach is to target genes whose expression/up-regulation triggers or fuels tumorigenesis. These include products of the BCL-2, survivin and clusterin genes. The BCL-2 oncogene products drive neoplastic progression by enhancing cell survival via inhibition of apoptosis. Survivin is generally not expressed in healthy tissue, but expressed at high levels in a range of common cancer types, including lung, colon, breast and prostate cancers. It plays an important role in both promoting cell division and inhibiting apoptosis. The clusterin gene codes for a cytoprotective '*chaperone*' protein whose up-regulation is associated with various human cancers.

As potential drugs, antisense oligos display a number of desirable characteristics, the most significant of which is their likely specificity. Statistical analysis reveals that any specific base sequence of 17 or more bases is extremely unlikely to occur more than once in a human cell's nucleic acid complement.

It thus follows that an oligonucleotide of 17 or more nucleotide units in length, which is designed to duplex successfully with a specific mRNA species, is unlikely to form a duplex with any other (unintended) mRNA species. Most synthetic oligos, therefore, are in the region of 17 nucleotide units long. These will display virtually an absolute specificity for the target sequence. Additional advantages of the oligonucleotide antisense approach include:

1. *Relatively low toxicity*: thus far, most trials report relatively few significant side effects. This is likely due to the highly specific nature of oligo duplexing, and the fact that they are 'natural' biomolecules. Some toxicity may, however, by triggered by non-specific binding to proteins, and most antisense agents appear to promote pro-inflammatory effects at high dosage levels.
2. The requirement for only low levels of the oligo to be present inside the cell, as target mRNA is, itself, usually present only in nanomolar concentrations.
3. The ability to manufacture oligos of specified nucleotide sequence is relatively straightforward using automated synthesizers.

However, native antisense oligonucleotides also suffer from a number of disadvantages, which are ultimately responsible for numerous disappointing trial results, and the fact that, after almost two decades of clinical investigation, only a single product has gained approval to date. Disadvantages include:

(a) sensitivity to nucleases;

(b) very low serum half lives;

(c) poor rate of cellular uptake;

(d) orally inactive.

Some progress has been made to overcome such difficulties, and continued progress in the area is expected to render the next generation of oligos more therapeutically effective.

Native oligonucleotides display a 3′–5′ phosphodiester linkage in their backbone. These are sensitive to a range of nucleases naturally present in most extracellular fluids and intracellular compartments. The half-life of native oligonucleotides in serum is only of the order of 15 min, and oligoribonucleotides are less stable than oligodeoxynucleotides. Selective modification of the native phosphodiester bond can render the product resistant to nuclease degradation.

Modification usually entails replacement of one of the free (non-bridging) oxygen atoms of the phosphodiester linkage with an alternative atom or chemical group. Most commonly, the oxygen has been replaced with a sulfur atom and the resultant phosphorothioates display greatest clinical promise. Phosphorothioate-based oligos, 'S-oligos', display increased resistance to nuclease attack while remaining water-soluble. They are also easy to synthesize chemically and they display a biological half-life of several hours. Most antisense oligos currently assessed in clinical trials are S-oligos, as is the sole antisense agent approved for general medical use to date. Further modified oligos may well improve product pharmacokinetic and pharmacodynamic properties, as alluded to towards the end of the next section.

Oligonucleotide Pharmacokinetics and Delivery

Oligo administration during many clinical trials entails direct i.v. infusion, often over a course of several hours. S.c. and, in particular, intradermal administration is usually also associated with high bioavailability. Oligos bind various serum proteins, including serum albumin (as well as a range of heparin- binding and other proteins that commonly occur on many cell surfaces). Targeting of naked oligos to specific cell types, therefore, is not possible. Following administration, these oligos tend to distribute rapidly to many tissues, with the highest proportion accumulating in the liver, kidney, bone marrow, skeletal muscle and skin. They do not appear to cross the blood–brain barrier. Binding to serum proteins provides a repository for these drugs and prevents rapid renal excretion.

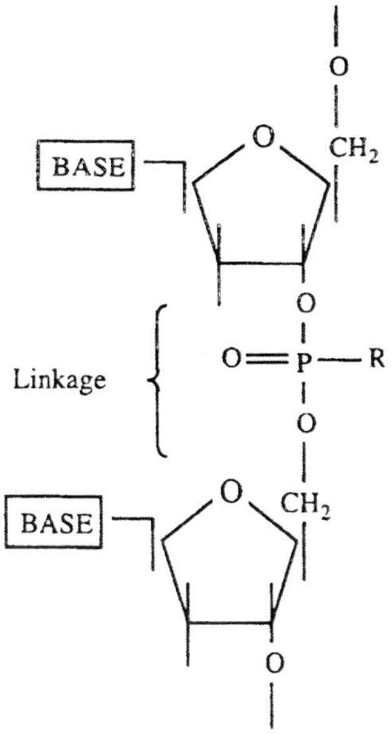

Linkage name	Substituent (R)
Phosphorothioate	$-S^-$
Methylphosphonate	$-CH_3$
Methylphosphotriester	$-O-CH_3$
Ethylphosphotriester	$-O-CH_2-CH_3$
Alkylphosphoramidate	$-NH-CH_3$

Fig. 10.15. Major types of modification potentially made to an oligo's phosphodiester linkage in order to increase their stability or enhance some other functional characteristics.

The precise mechanism(s) by which oligos enter cells is not fully understood. Most are charged molecules, sometimes displaying a molecular mass of up to 10–12 kDa. Receptor-mediated endocytosis appears to be the most common mechanism by which charged oligos, such as phosphorothioates, enter most cells. One putative phosphorothioate receptor appears to consist of an 80 kDa surface protein, associated with a smaller 34 kDa membrane protein. However, this in itself seems to be an inefficient process, with only a small proportion of the administered drug eventually being transferred across the plasma membrane.

Uncharged oligos appear to enter the cell by passive diffusion, as well as possibly by endocytosis. However, elimination of the charges renders the resultant oligos relatively hydrophobic, thus generating additional difficulties with their synthesis and delivery. Attempts to increase delivery of oligos into the cell mainly centre on the use of suitable carrier systems. Liposomes, as well as polymeric carriers (e.g. polylysine-based carriers), are gaining most attention in this regard.

An alternative system, which effectively results in the introduction of antisense oligonucleotides into the cell, entails application of gene therapy. In this case, a gene, which when transcribed yields (antisense) mRNA of appropriate nucleotide sequence, is introduced into the cell by a retroviral or other appropriate vector. This approach, as applied to the treatment of cancer and AIDS, is being appraised in a number of trials.

Oligos, including modified oligos, appear to be ultimately metabolized within the cell by the action of nucleases, particularly 3′-exonucleases. Breakdown metabolic products are then mainly excreted via the urinary route. Even phosphorothioate oligos display serum and tissue half-lives of less than a day. As a consequence, continuous or frequent i.v. infusions are required for product administration. Some progress has been reported in the development of second-generation phosphorothioate oligos with improved pharmacokinetic characteristics. The most promising development entails the modification of the ribose sugar found in the repeat nucleotide structure. Attachment (at the 2′ position) of methyl (-CH_3) or methoxy ethyl (-$CH_2CH_2OCH_3$) groups increases product stability, as well as product potency (by enhancing binding affinity for RNA). However, these changes also abrogate the product's ability to activate RNaseH, a primary mechanism of inducing its antisense effect. This, in turn, may be overcome by the more recent development of chimaeric phosphorothioate oligos; in which 2′-modified sugar nucleotides are placed only at the ends of the molecule, leaving a nuclease-compatible gap in the middle.

Manufacture of Oligos

In contrast to the biopharmaceuticals discussed thus far (recombinant proteins and gene therapy products), antisense oligonucleotides are manufactured by direct chemical synthesis. Organic synthetic pathways have been developed, optimized and commercialized for some time, as oligonucleotides are widely used reagents in molecular biology. They are required as primers, probes and for the purposes of site-directed mutagenesis. The nucleotides required (themselves either modified or unmodified as desired) are first reacted with a protecting chemical group. Each protected nucleotide is then coupled in turn to the growing end of the nucleotide chain, itself attached to a solid phase. After coupling, the original protecting group is removed and, when chain synthesis is complete, the bond anchoring the chemical to the solid phase is hydrolysed, releasing the free oligo. This may then be purified by HPLC. The most common synthetic method used is known as the phosphoramidite method, which uses a dimethoxytrityl protecting group and tetrazole as the coupling agent. Automated synthesizers that can quickly and inexpensively synthesize oligos of over 100 nucleotides are commercially available.

Additional Antigene Agents: RNA Interference and Ribozymes

RNAi and ribozymes represent two additional approaches to gene silencing/down-regulation with therapeutic potential. RNAi is an innate cellular process that achieves silencing of selected genes via an anti- sense mechanism. It shares many characteristics with the antisense-based approach described above, but also some important differences, e.g. in the exact mechanism by which the antisense effect is achieved. RNAi probably evolved initially in primitive organisms in order to protect their genomes from viruses, transposons and additional insertable genetic elements, and to regulate gene expression. The RNAi pathway was first discovered in plants, but it is now known to function in most, if not all, eukaryotes. RNAi represents a sequence-specific post-translational inhibition mechanism of gene expression, induced ultimately by dsRNA, be it produced naturally or synthesised *in vitro* and introduced into a cell. Entry of dsRNA triggers its cleavage into short (21–23 nucleotide long) sequences called short interfering RNAs (siRNAs). This cleavage is catalysed by a cellular nuclease enzyme called 'Dicer'. The siRNA is incorporated into a multi-subunit effector complex known as an RNA-induced silencing complex (RISC), which also contains several nucleic acid processing enzymes (a helicase, an endonuclease and an exonuclease). The double-stranded siRNA then unwinds (a process promoted by the helicase activity), and the 'sense' strand of the dsRNA is discarded. The remaining 'antisense' siRNA strand then facilitates RISC binding to a specific mRNA via Watson–Crick base complementarity, which is then degraded by RISC nuclease activity.

RNAi technology has obvious therapeutic potential as an antisense agent, and initial therapeutic targets of RNAi include viral infection, neurological diseases and cancer therapy. The synthesis of dsRNA displaying the desired nucleotide sequence is straightforward. However, as in the case of additional nucleic-acid-based therapeutic approaches, major technical hurdles remain to be overcome before RNAi becomes a therapeutic reality. Naked unmodified siRNAs for example display a serum half-life of less than 1 min, due to serum nuclease degradation. Approaches to improve the RNAi pharmacokinetic profile include chemical modification of the nucleotide backbone, to render it nuclease resistant, and the use of viral or non-viral vectors, to achieve safe product delivery to cells. As such, the jury remains out in terms of the development and approval of RNAi-based medicines, in the short to medium term at least.

Certain RNA sequences can function as catalysts. These so-called ribozymes function to catalyse cleavage at specific sequences in a specific mRNA substrate. Many ribozymes will cleave their target mRNA where there exists a particular triplet nucleotide sequence G–U–C. Statistically, it is likely that this triplet will occur at least once in most mRNAs. Ribozymes can be directed to a specific mRNA by introducing short flanking oligonucleotides that are complementary to the target mRNA. The resultant cleavage of the target obviously prevents translation. One potential advantage of ribozymes is that, as catalytic agents, a single molecule could likely destroy thousands of copies of the target mRNA. Such a drug should, therefore, be very potent. Again, however, ribozymes suffer from similar complications to antisense-based products in terms of their development as biopharmaceuticals, and no such product is likely to gain approval for some time to come.

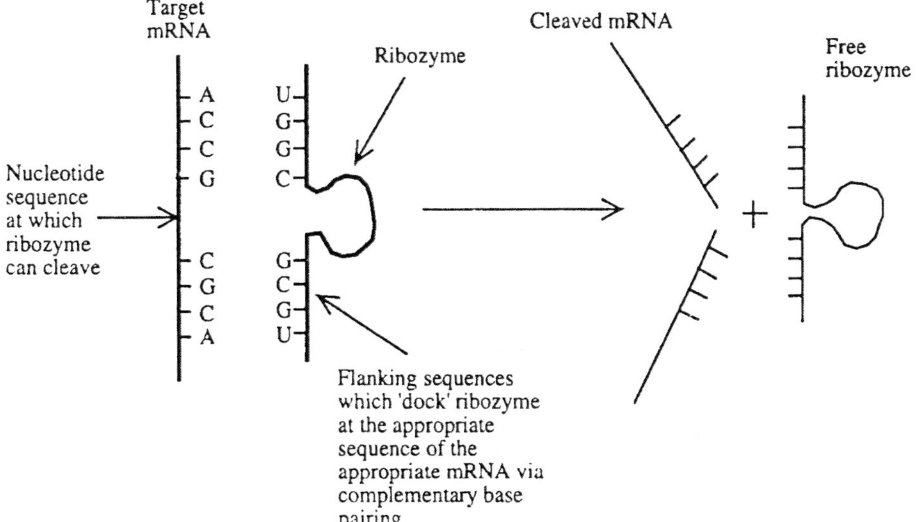

Fig. 10.16. Outline of how ribozyme technology could prevent translation of specific mRNA, thus preventing synthesis of a specific target protein.

Aptamers

Aptamers are single-stranded DNA or RNA-based sequences that fold up to adopt a unique three-dimensional structure, allowing them to bind a specific target molecule.

Binding displays high specificity, and aptamers capable of distinguishing between closely related isoforms or different conformational states of the same protein have been generated. Binding affinity is also high. It is in the low nanomolar to picomolar range, which is comparable to the binding affinity of an antibody for the antigen against which it was raised.

Aptamer technology was first developed in 1990. It entails the initial generation of a large aptamer library, with subsequent identification of individual aptamers binding a target ligand via an appropriate selection strategy. DNA aptamer libraries are usually generated via direct chemical synthesis and amplified by PCR. RNA libraries are usually generated by *in vitro* transcription of synthetic DNA libraries. Identification of specific aptamers binding the target molecule is most easily undertaken by an automated *in vitro* selection approach known as systematic evolution of ligands by exponential enrichment (SELEX).

Most libraries contain up to 10^{15} species. Because of their high binding specificity and affinity, aptamers (like antibodies) are/may prove useful for affinity-based purification, target validation and drug discovery, diagnostics and therapeutics. One such product has been approved for general medical use to date. A modest number of additional aptamers are in clinical trials, aimed at treating conditions including infectious diseases, cancer and haemophilia. Aptamers appear to display low immunogenicity; but, when administered systemically, they are quickly excreted via size-mediated renal clearance. In order to prevent renal removal, such aptamers are usually conjugated to PEG. PEG may also help further protect the aptamers from degradation by serum nucleases; native aptamers are prone to nuclease attack, but their half-lives can most effectively be extended via chemical modification, as discussed earlier in the context of antisense agents.

Cell-and Tissue-based Therapies

Recent progress relating to the identification, isolation and manipulation of stem cells has made this cell type a focus of enormous attention, both within the scientific and general communities. Although stem cells harbour great medical potential, their routine application to the treatment of medical conditions (so-called regenerative medicine) remains a distant prospect, as discussed below. In contrast, fully differentiated cells or groups of cells (organs and tissues) are currently in routine medical use. Such products include cells or tissues used for the purposes of transplantation, as well as a small number of engineered cell-based products.

Transplantation entails the transfer of living cells/tissue/organs from a donor to a recipient. In some cases (e.g. many skin grafting procedures) the donor and recipient are actually the same individual, and this is termed autologous transplantation. More usually, however, the donor and recipient are different individuals, and this is termed *allogeneic transplantation*.

Common forms of transplantation include whole blood transfusions, bone marrow transplantations, skin grafting and transplantation of a wide range of organs, including kidneys, liver, pancreas, lungs and heart. Improvements in surgical transplant techniques, along with the availability of effective immunosuppressive drugs (including some antibody-based drugs, render 1-year success rates for most organ transplants in the 75–95 per cent range.

Tissue/organs destined for transplant are rarely considered to be pharmaceutical products. The material for transplant is usually harvested directly by clinicians via surgical or other appropriate techniques, followed by direct transplantation without significant *in vitro* processing.

'Tissue- or cell-engineered' products represent a small but significant subgroup of cell-based products. Such products also consist of/contain fully differentiated cells but do undergo some modification or formulation *in vitro* prior to their medical use. Examples include Carticel and Apligraf, a skin substitute used in the treatment of certain ulcers, which is composed of keratinocytes and fibroblasts derived from human neonatal foreskin tissue and bovine collagen.

Stem Cells

The therapeutic application of stem cells has long been a dream of medical sciences, but recent discoveries and technical advances have brought this dream somewhat closer to being a reality. Stem cells are usually defined as undifferentiated cells capable of self-renewal that can differentiate into more than one specialized cell type.

Such cells are often classified on the basis of their original source as either embryonic or adult stem cells. As the name suggests, embryonic stem cells are derived from the early embryo, whereas adult stem cells are present in various tissues of the adult species. Much of the earlier work on embryonic stem cells was conducted using mouse embryos. Human embryonic stem cells were first isolated and cultured in the laboratory in 1998. Research on adult stem cells spans some four decades, with the discovery during the 1960s of haematopoietic stem cells in the bone marrow. However, the exact distribution profile, role and ability to manipulate adult stem cells (particularly those outside of the bone marrow) are subjects of intense current research, and for which more questions remain than are answered.

Embryonic stem cells are derived from pre-implant-stage human embryos, usually at the blastocyst stage (the blastocyst is a thin-walled hollow structure containing a cluster of cells, known as the inner cell mass, from which the embryo arises). These embryos are invariably ones initially generated as part of *in vitro* fertilization procedures but which are destined to be discarded, either due to poor quality or because they are in excess to requirement. There are an estimated 400 000 *in vitro* fertilization-produced embryos in frozen storage in the USA alone, of which some 2.8 per cent are likely to be discarded.

Culture of human embryonic stem cells starts with the recovery of the blastocyst's inner cell mass. One common recovery procedure is termed '*immunosurgery*'. The process entails the initial treatment of blastocysts with pronase (a cocktail of proteolytic enzymes), which effectively degrades the outer protective membrane known as the '*zona pellucida*'. The blastocysts are next treated with anti-human whole serum antibody and guinea pig complement, which triggers complement-mediated lysis of the blastocyst outer cell layers (the trophoblast), allowing recovery of the inner cell mass. The latter cells are then cultured under defined conditions in order to allow them to multiply while remaining undifferentiated.

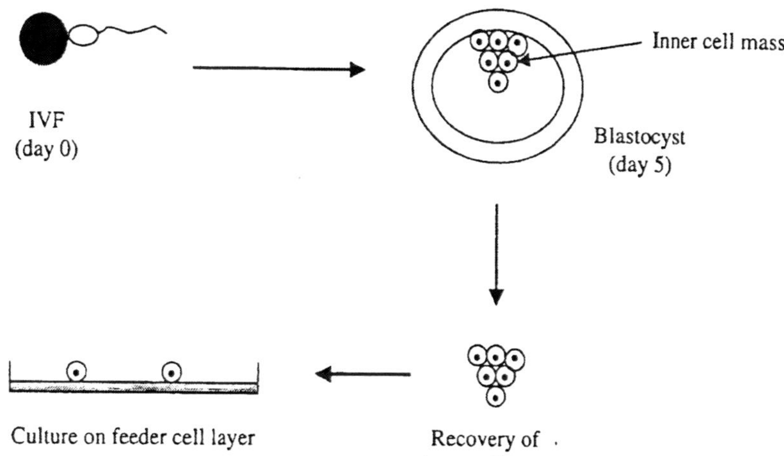

Fig. 10.17. Overview of the generation and culture of human embryonic stem cells.

In addition to cell culture media, the culture vessels often contain a layer of 'feeder' cells (e.g. mouse fibroblasts), irradiated in order to prevent their growth and division. These feeder cells can serve two functions: (a) to provide a suitable substratum with which the embryonic stem cells can interact, aiding in their growth and division; (b) feeder cells can release often ill-defined nutrients into the medium, which can again support stem cell growth. The presence of a feeder cell layer would represent a complication in the downstream processing of stem cells for therapeutic use, and could represent a potential source of pathogenic contaminants. More recently, culture systems have been developed in which the feeder cell layer is replaced by fibronectin (a glycoprotein found on the cell surface) or matrigel (a protein-rich membrane extract from a mouse sarcoma cell line).

Substantial research work remains ongoing in order to identify an optimal cell culture medium composition that will facilitate strong cell growth while remaining in an undifferentiated state. Basic animal cell culture media are often supplemented with serum as a nutrient source. It is known that the addition of the cytokine LIF can sustain mouse embryonic stem cells in the undifferentiated state, but LIF alone cannot achieve this in the context of human embryonic stem cells. Research, therefore, continues with a view to optimize culture media composition for such human cell lines. Whereas the culture of human embryonic stem cell lines requires the maintenance of cells in an undifferentiated state, the application of such cells in regenerative medicine requires the subsequent controlled differentiation of such cells to generate a specific desired cell type (e.g. a specific neuron type to treat a specific neurodegenerative disease, etc.). The process by which any stem cell differentiates naturally to form a specific cell is hugely complex and understood only in outline and only for a few cell types. Differentiation is dependent upon several concerted signals from effector molecules such as cytokines. A major challenge, therefore, is to gain a more complete understanding of how differentiation into specific cell types is driven and controlled. Only with such knowledge will come the ability to grow specific cells (and ultimately tissue/organ types) from stem cells for the purposes of regenerative medicine.

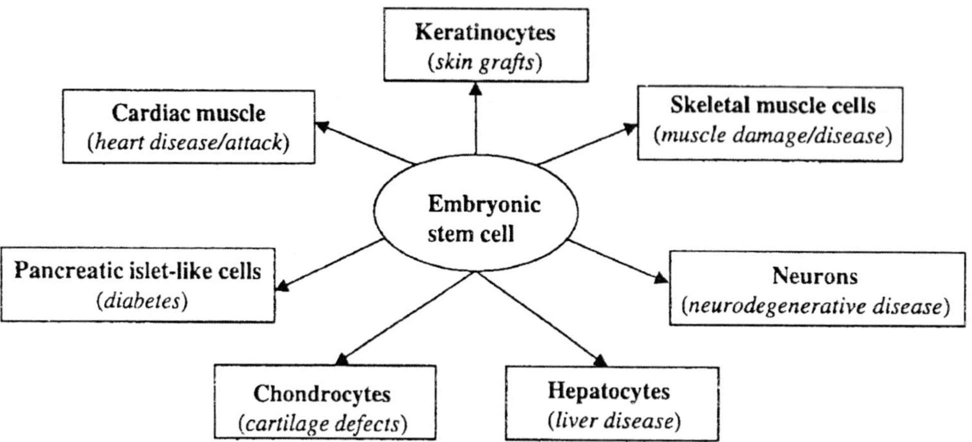

Fig. 10.18. Some cell types reported to have been produced via in vitro directed differentiation from either mouse or human embryonic stem cells.

Although only in its infancy, some progress has been reported in elucidating details of selected directed differentiation pathways, initially in the context of mouse embryonic stem cells, but latterly also in the context of human embryonic stem cells. This progress has largely been the result of empirical studies and is largely achieved in one or more of three ways: (a) manipulation of culture media composition; (b) alteration of the surface characteristics of the matrix on which the cells are grown (e.g. adhesive feeder cells or specific protein-based matrices); (c) via introduction of specific regulatory genes into the stem cells themselves. The ability to generate dopaminergic-like neurons represents a significant milestone in the attempt to apply regenerative medicine to the treatment of Parkinson's disease. This neurodegenerative condition, which effects some 2 per cent of adults over the age of 65, is triggered by the death of this cell type in the brain. Parkinson's disease, therefore, is likely to be one of the first clinical targets in the development of regenerative medicines.

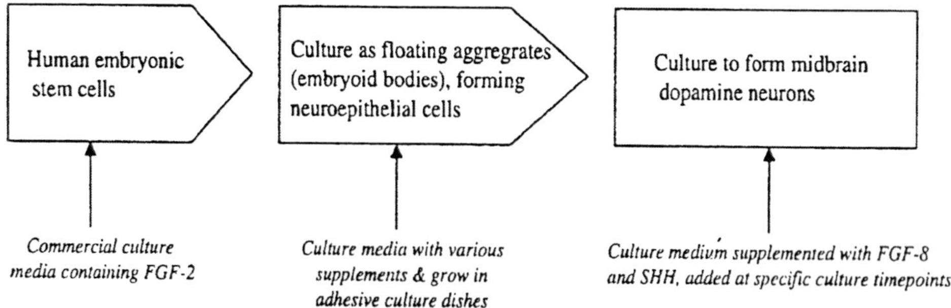

Fig. 10.19. Simplified schematic overview of the directed differentiation of human embryonic stem cells to form differentiated dopamine like neurons.

Adult Stem Cells

The main focus of stem cell research over the last few decades has been directed to embryonic stem cells. However, more recently, research upon and an understanding of various populations of adult stem cells has gathered pace. Adult stem cells are undifferentiated cells found amongst differentiated cells in a tissue or organ. These cells can renew themselves and can differentiate to yield the major cell types characteristic of the tissue in which they reside. The main physiological role of adult stem cells, therefore, appears to be to maintain and to repair (to a certain extent at least) the tissue in which they reside.

For many years it was believed that adult stem cell populations were present in a very limited number of tissue types, and that they could only differentiate into cells characteristic of the tissue in which they reside. Recent research challenges both of these assertions. Adult stem cells are being discovered in a growing number of tissues, including bone marrow, peripheral blood and blood vessels, the brain and spinal cord, skeletal muscle, skin, liver, pancreas, digestive system, cornea and retina. Identification and study of such cells can be made difficult by the low levels in which they are normally found, the presence of many additional cell types and the difficulties in culturing them. Much basic research is required to answer fundamental questions regarding adult stem cells, including: How many types exist and where are they located? What was their ultimate source? What level of plasticity do they exhibit? What factors stimulate their relocation and differentiation at a site of tissue damage?

The use of adult, as opposed to embryonic, stem cells in regenerative medicine would have a number of significant advantages. It would overcome moral/ethical difficulties associated with blastocyst destruction. It would also allow for autologous transplantation of cells, i.e. adult stem cells could be harvested from a patient, cultured and differentiated *in vitro* and then reintroduced back into the patient. This would overcome potential immunological complications and a requirement to use immunosuppressive drugs. Hurdles to this approach not only include the difficulties in isolating and successfully culturing these cells, but also ascertaining the level of plasticity exhibited by adult stem cells. This refers to the range of potential fully differentiated cell types that could be produced from adult stem cell populations, and such investigations represent a very active area of current stem cell research.

Future Direction

Every few decades a medical innovation is perfected that profoundly influences the practice of medicine. Widespread vaccination against common infectious agents and the discovery of antibiotics serve as two such examples. Many scientists now believe that the potential of nucleic-acid- and cell-based technologies rivals even the most significant medical advances achieved to date.

It is now just over a decade since the first nucleic-acid-based drugs began initial tests. Several such drugs will likely be in routine medical use in less than a decade more. The application of gene technology could also change utterly the profile of biopharmaceutical drugs currently on the market. Virtually all such products are proteins, currently administered to patients for short or prolonged periods, as appropriate. Gene therapy offers the possibility of equipping the patient's own body with the ability to synthesize these drugs itself, and over whatever time-scale is appropriate. Taken to its logical conclusion, gene therapy thus offers the potential to render obsolete most of the biopharmaceutical products currently on the market. Regenerative medicine, too, although still in its infancy, harbours enormous future medical potential. Of all the biopharmaceuticals discussed throughout this text, nucleic-acid- and cell-based drugs may well turn out to have the most profound influence on the future practice of molecular medicine.

11

NUCLEIC ACID-BASED THERAPIES

The ability to control the gene expression of a desired cellular population via the delivery of nucleic acids has inspired applications in clinical and basic science. In the past, nonviral gene delivery referred to the delivery of plasmid DNA (pDNA) whereby the expression of a target protein, which could restore normal biological function or aid during wound healing, would be increased. More recently, however, the term *gene delivery* has expanded to include the delivery of small interfering RNA (siRNA) and oligonucleotides (ON), which can be used to decrease or down-regulate the expression of a target protein. Ongoing clinical trials using gene delivery as a therapeutic agent include cancer, cystic fibrosis, adenosine deaminase deficiency, and infectious diseases such as acquired immunodeficiency syndrome (AIDS). Gene delivery employs both viral and nonviral vectors to deliver nucleic acids. Although viral delivery strategies are in general more efficient than their nonviral counterparts, an increasing concern about immune responses to viral vectors *in vivo*, which could pose additional risks for patients under going gene therapy, has motivated the development of nonviral delivery vectors that aim to synthetically mimic biologically produced viruses.

Nonviral delivery vectors have to be engineered to be able to package plasmid DNA to form particles that can (1) travel through biological fluids without losing activity, (2) target appropriate cells, (3) be internalized by the targeted cell population, and (4) finally trafficked to the intracellular site of action (e.g., nucleus and/or cytosol). Furthermore, the ideal delivery system would achieve the above-mentioned points while being non-immunogenic and nontoxic. Although there have been numerous approaches to the engineering of delivery vectors, this chapter will focus mainly on nonviral delivery vectors that show promising approaches to overcome the delivery limitations mentioned above or that have been tested *in vivo*. Strategies to administer nonviral delivery vectors *in vivo* can be divided into two main approaches: systemic delivery or direct injection of DNA nanoparticles and the implantation of a matrix that releases "naked" DNA or DNA nanoparticles. Systemic delivery aims at engineering delivery vectors that can be delivered non-invasively through a bodily fluid such as intravenously, transdermally, and orally, while targeting an appropriate tissue (e.g., tumor) or organ (e.g., lung). Local delivery, on the other hand, aims at bypassing the tissue-targeting step by delivering the nonviral vectors directly (or nearby) to the site of action, typically with the use of a polymeric matrix. The polymeric matrix can be designed to slowly release the DNA nanoparticles to the local environment where cells can internalize them or can be designed so that it can be infiltrated with local cells that can take up the DNA nanoparticles residing inside the matrix. Design parameters for targeted cellular internalization and intracellular trafficking are similar for systemic and local delivery approaches; however, the design of the vector physical properties such as surface coating and particle size must be tailored to the method of application.

Systematic and Direct Injection Delivery

In vivo production and secretion of therapeutic proteins by DNA delivery can be achieved through either systemic or local administration, each providing a unique opportunity for gene therapy. Systemic delivery allows noninvasive access to many target cells and tissue that are not accessible by direct administration. The most common approach involves the complexation of naked DNA with cationic lipids (lipoplexes) or cationic polymers (polyplexes) that package the DNA into nano-sized aggregates. The major factors limiting the *in vivo* effectiveness for systemically delivered lipoplexes and polyplexes is colloidal instability and ineffective targeting. For intravenous administration, complexes are rapidly eliminated from the blood stream (<30 minutes) and found mostly in the liver and to a lesser extent in organs with fine capillary beds like skin, muscle, and intestine. The interaction of biomolecules from the physiological fluid with the complexes induces aggregation and dissociation of the complexes, which limits bioavailability and internalization. The association of serum components (albumin, heparin, lipoprotein, or specific opsonins) with polyplexes and lipoplexes, which can target the complex for clearance by macrophages and is affected by the surface charge density and surface morphology of complexes. Cationic formulations (i.e., lipoplexes and polyplexes) can provide an enhanced stability against degradation and may allow for a more efficient interaction with the negatively charged endothelial cell; however, noncationic or less cationic formulations may be required to avoid accumulation in the reticuloendothelial system. Variations in the charge ratio may be used as part of a passive targeting strategy. For lipoplexes delivered intravenously, different formulations (e.g., charge ratio) can be used to target the lung, liver, blood cells, or tumors.

To avoid the difficulties of crossing the endothelium and nonspecific uptake by the liver, DNA can be delivered directly to the target tissue by injection of polyplexes, lipoplexes, or microspheres with encapsulated DNA. Injection of lipoplexes and polyplexes into the desired tissue can be used to achieve *in vivo* gene transfer. However, transfection depends on the physico-chemical properties of the complexes and the rate of clearance from the tissue, which varies from tissue to tissue and depends on factors such as the lymph supply. Nevertheless, polyplexes have been found to be sufficiently small and stable so as to diffuse throughout the brain ventricular spaces after a local injection injection.

Formulations

Unprotected plasmid DNA (naked DNA) is unstable under *in vivo* conditions, due to rapid degradation by serum nucleases. Therefore, carriers or vectors are necessary to protect DNA or RNA from degradation to facilitate uptake into specific cells, and to transfer the DNA or RNA their target location (e.g., nucleus or cytosol). Delivery vectors for systemic delivery are designed to increase gene transfer function by enhancing the stability of DNA, the efficiency of cellular uptake and intracellular trafficking, and the biodistribution of DNA. In this section, the formulations that have been developed to deliver nucleic acids such as plasmid DNA (pDNA), oligonucleotide (ON), or small interfering RNA (siRNA) will be reviewed.

Cationic polymers

Cationic polymers have been used since the late 1980s as formulations for nucleic acid delivery. Cationic polymers contain high densities of primary, secondary, or tertiary amines, some of which are protonated at neutral pH. This high density of positive charges allows the cationic polymers to form stable condensed structures with pDNA, termed polyplexes, which are capable of entering the cell. Furthermore, polyplexes protect the DNA from nucleases found in serum and other extracellular environments. The structure of frequently used cationic polymers, which have been used *in vivo* to deliver therapeutic genes, although many novel polymers are being developed, including polyallylamine, peptoids, poly(dimethyl aminoethyl methacrylate) poly(trime-thyl aminoethyl methacrylate), poly(β-amino ester), and poly(phosphoester). Cationic polymers vary widely in molecular architecture, ranging from linear to highly branched molecules, which influences their complexation with nucleic acids as well as their transfection efficiency. In addition to providing positive charges for DNA complexation, the primary amines also serve as functional groups to chemically modify the polymers with ligands and peptides that can enhance one or more of the steps in the transfection process. Furthermore, tertiary and some secondary amines are typically neutral at physiological pH and have been found to aid in intracellular trafficking by facilitating the release of the polyplexes from the endosome though endosomal buffering.

Interaction of cationic polymers with DNA

Cationic polymers form aggregates with DNA, termed polyplexes, via electrostatic interactions, which protect the nucleic acid from degradation. During the complexation of DNA with cationic polymers, the extended structure of DNA is changed to a more condensed configuration forming aggregates in the nanometer size range. Polyplexes typically give rise to particles with spherical, globular, or rod-like structures, which are 20 to 200 nm in diameter but can reach up to 1000 nm. Evidence that electrostatic interactions mediate the complexation of cationic polymers include Fourier transform infrared resonance (FTIR) data showing a reduction of the asymmetric phosphate stretching vibration of plasmid DNA after complexation with polyethyleneimine (PEI). Furthermore, microcalorimetric measurements have shown that complex formation between the graft copolymer poly(ethylene oxide)-PEI and a poly(dTA) result from the formation of ion pairs between ionized amino groups of PEI segments of the copolymer and the phosphate groups of DNA. An increase in salt concentration generally results in a decrease binding affinity between the cationic polymer and the DNA probably due to a charge shielding effect at the higher salt concentrations.

The complexation and condensation behavior depend on the polymer's physical properties, including molecular weight, density of charges, whether it is linear or branched, and the ratio of polymer to DNA. The molecular weight of the cationic polymer influences both the condensation behavior as well as the complex size. In general, for most cationic polymers, an increase in molecular weight results in a decrease of complex size until a condensation limit is achieved. For example, for PEI, it has been found that molecular weights higher than 25 kDa showed no further increase of complex size, whereas molecular weights of 2 kDa or lower result in a decreased ability to complex DNA to form small complexes. The stability and size of the polyplexes formed between cationic polymers and DNA have also been correlated to primary amine content. Low branched PEI (low density of primary amines) requires higher N/P rations to complete condensation compared with highly branched derivatives (high density of primary amines). Last, complex size tends to decrease with an increasing polymer-to-DNA ratio.

Polyplexes as cellular transfection agents

In addition to reducing the size of DNA and protecting the DNA from degradation by serum nucleases, binding of polycations to DNA typically results in polyplexes having a net positive charge. This positive charge has been found to be essential for efficient transfection. It is thought that the positively charged polyplexes electrostatically interact with the negatively charged proteoglycans of the cell membrane, resulting in nonspecific adsorptive endocytosis. The polyplexes, which are now trapped inside the endosomes, need to escape before endosome–lysosome fusion occurs, which would result in polyplex degradation inside the lysosomes. Cationic polymers such as PEI have the advantage over other cationic polymers [e.g., poly(amino acids)] in that they do not require an endosomal lysotropic agent to be added to achieve efficient transfection. Once released from the endosome the polyplexes need to transport the DNA to the nucleus where it can be transcribed or siRNA or ON to the cytosol, where they can mediate gene downregulation. The transition from the cytosol to the nucleus is not well understood, and it depends on the physical properties of the polymer and the cell cycle and degree of mitotic activity of the cells. To aid the transition from the cytosol to the nucleus cationic polymers have been modified with nuclear localization sequences typically derived from viruses. Full unpackaging or decomplexation of the siRNA and ON in the cytosol is critical for their action. Strategies to enhance decomplexation involve the introduction of environmentally sensitive bonds, reducing the affinity of the cationic polymer for the DNA and the delivery of enzymes that can degrade the cationic polymer. Although positively charged polyplexes promote efficient transfection *in vitro*, they lead to aggregation and low transfection *in vivo* with most polyplexes accumulated in the liver after systemic administration. The aggregation of polyplexes has been attributed to the presence of negatively charged proteins in serum, which can mediate bridging of multiple polyplexes together.

Poly(ethylenimine)

In recent years, poly(ethylenimine) has emerged as a widely used cationic polymer to mediate gene transfer *in vivo* and *in vitro*, resulting in two commercially available transfection products ExGene and jetPEI. PEI has a protonatable hydrogen every two carbons in its structure, making it the polycation with the highest density of protonable amines. Branched PEI is synthesized using the acid catalyzed ring opening polymerization of aziridine, resulting in a theoretical 1 : 2 : 1 ratio of primary to secondary to tertiary amines. However, C-13 nuclear resonance spectroscopy measurements have shown that the degree of branching is closer to 1 : 1 : 1 for most commercially available PEIs, which indicates a higher degree of branching. Linear PEI, on the other hand, is synthesized by ring opening polymerization of 2-ethyl-2-oxazoline followed by acid hydrolysis. Linear and branched PEI can be purchased in a wide variety of molecular weights ranging from less than 1000 Da to 1.6×10^3 kDa; however, the range most typically used for gene delivery is 5 to 25 kDa, mostly due to toxicity caused by higher molecular weight PEIs. PEI forms complexes with DNA ranging from 77 to 300 nm in size at N/P ratios ranging from 6 to 10. High-molecular-weight PEI forms smaller, more stable particles and achieves higher transfection efficiencies than low-molecular-weight PEI; however, it is more toxic. Similarly, highly branched PEI forms smaller particles that are more stable than low-branched PEI and achieves higher transfection efficiencies, but again, it is more toxic than low-branched PEI.

PEI has be used extensively *in vivo* to deliver DNA and siRNA locally to the brain cornea, tumors, and vasculature and systemically to the lung and tumors. The charge of the DNA/PEI complexes delivered *in vivo* have a profound effect on their organ targeting. Delivery of positively charged complexes in the tail vein in mice resulted in gene transfer primarily in the lungs, whereas surface shielding transferring-PEI–DNA complexes resulted in preferential gene delivery to distantly growing tumors.

Poly (amino acids)

Cationic poly(amino acids) are some of the most commonly used cationic polymers for gene delivery. Cationic peptides such as polylysine are commercially available in a variety of molecular weights. However, commercially available PLLs are highly polydisperse. To synthesize monodisperse peptides, solid phase synthesis is used that involves the immobilization of the growing peptide on a solid support and a series of protecting/deprotecting synthetic steps (e.g., Fmoc chemistry). The sequential addition of each amino acid provides peptides an absolute level of control over the sequence of the growing peptide, which allows for the specific attachment of targeting ligands or other desired modifications anywhere along the molecule.

PLL and its derivatives are the most commonly used cationic peptides for gene delivery, typically used at charge ratios (+/–) ranging from 3 : 1 to 6 : 1. As increasing amounts of PLL are added to DNA, the structure changes from circular to thick, flattened to compact, and finally to toroids and rods at a charge ratio of 6 : 1. The diameter and cross section of the toroids are approximately 140 nm and 44 nm, respectively. As with other cationic polymers, the ideal length of the PLL represents a balance between two competing effects: effective condensation and cytotoxicity. Relative to low molecular weight, the high-molecular-weight PLL forms tighter, smaller condensates that are more resistant to the effects of salt concentration and sonication. Cell transfection by PLL is typically lower than other cationic polymers that possess a buffering capacity such as poly(ethylene imine) and to cationic lipids. Extensive modifications aiming at improving the transfection efficiency of PLL have been performed, including the partial modification of the PLL side chains with histidine and imidazole groups, to enhance endosomal buffering and escape, the addition of PEG to enhance polyplex stability, the addition of targeting ligands to enhance internalization and targeting, and the addition of covalent bonds within the polyplex to enhance its stability and polyplex unpackaging. Furthermore, peptides containing multiple lysines have been synthesized such as Cys–His–$(Lys)_6$– His–Cys, which enhances endosomal escape, while providing covalent stabilization of the polyplexes via disulfide bonds.

PLL and its derivatives have not been as extensively used *in vivo* as other cationic polymers to deliver therapeutically relevant genes; however, they have found some success in systemic delivery to the liver and matrix-based delivery to enhance angiogenesis.

Cationic dendrimers

Dendrimers are polymers that branch out from a multifunctional core in a symmetric fashion. After each subsequent monomer addition (a generation), the number of attachment points increases symmetrically generating more branches. Cationic dendrimers have an attractive architecture for gene transfer because their well-defined structure and robust chemistry enables the synthesis of many generations of protonatable amines. Dendrimers such as poly(amidoamine) dendrimers and poly(propylenimine) (PPI) have been shown to be capable of mediating gene delivery *in vitro* and *in vivo*. PAMAM is commercially available and is synthesized from either an ammonia or ethylenediamine core by successive addition of methyl acrylate and ethylenediamine. PPI is also commercially available and is synthesized from a butylene-diamine core by successive addition of acrylonitrile to a primary amino group followed by hydrogenation of nitrile groups to primary amino groups. The surface charge and diameter of the dendrimers is determined by the number of synthetic steps (i.e., number of generations). The generation of PAMAM used to complex DNA determines particle size and transfection efficiency. Complexation of DNA with fifth-generation (G5) PAMAM dendrimers produces monodisperse condensates with a radius below 200 nm . At charge ratios (+/–) above or equal to one, no free DNA is observed. Although PAMAM dendrimers of generations 3 (G3) to 10 (G10) can form stable complexes with DNA, the higher generations of dendrimers (G5 to G10) can transfect cells at higher efficiencies. Transfection efficiency of PAMAM is enhanced by partial degradation of the dendrimer structure, forming a less homogeneous structure with a higher density of primary amines. The partially degraded PAMAM dendrimer has resulted in the transfection reagent Superfect. Cationic dendrimers have been used *in vivo* to deliver nucleic acids locally to the cornea, tumors, heart, and lung and systemically to the lung, liver, spleen, and tumors.

Polysaccharide containing polymers

Chitosan is composed of 2-amino-2-deoxy β-D-glucan and is prepared from naturally occurring chitin via alkaline deacetylation. Unlike other cationic polymers chitosan is nontoxic and biodegradable, making it an ideal candidate for therapeutic applications. Although the density of positive charges of chitosan is lower than for other cationic polymers, it has been shown to form particles with DNA, which protect the DNA from degradation. Chitosan/DNA complexes have been found to be in the order of 100 nm with a spherical shape. Like other cationic polymers, chitosan has been chemically modified with a variety of ligands or other functionalities to enhance its transfection efficiency. Chitosan has been recently used to deliver DNA mainly intranasally to the lungs for genetic immunization applications. After intranasal administration, DNA/chitosan complexes encoding for RSV antigen could attenuate pulmonary inflammation and reduce viral titer and viral antigen load. Recently dextran grafted with spermine (D-SPM) has been investigated to mediate DNA delivery. D-SPM are synthesized via reductive amination and can form aggregates with plasmid DNA and mediate efficient gene transfer *in vitro* and *in vivo*. Interestingly, the addition of hydrophobic domains, N-oleyl (ODS), to D-SPM (D-SPM–ODS) enhanced the stability of complexes in serum containing media. Furthermore, the addition of ODS groups achieved high transfection in the presence of serum similar to that achieved with linear PEI. These results suggest that the hydrophobic nature of the complexes may be another strategy to improve transfection in the presence of serum. However, the addition of the ODS groups also increased the toxicity of the D-SPM–ODS when compared with D-SPM, but the toxicity was similar to linear PEI and branched PEI.

Cyclodextrins (CDs) are cyclic, cup-shaped molecules with a hydrophilic exterior and a hydrophobic interior, which allows them to form inclusion complexes with hydrophobic molecules. Inclusion complexes are bimolecular complexes in which the "host" forms a cavity into which the "guest" molecule binds through noncovalent interactions. CDs are composed of six, seven, or eight glucose units, termed α, β, and γ, respectively; are water soluble; and are U.S. Food and Drug Administration (FDA) approved as solublizing agents for hydrophobic drugs. Davis et al. have investigated cationic molecules containing CDs as gene delivery vectors since 1999. Cationic CDs could form stable complexes with DNA with sizes in the 100-nm range. More recently CD–PAMAM and CD–PEI have been investigated and were found to efficiently transfect cells and be less toxic than their parent molecules. Furthermore, both CD–PAMAM and CD–PEI have been successfully used *in vivo*. Furthermore, cyclodextrin containing polymers have been recently used to deliver siRNAs to inhibit tumor growth. As mentioned for other cationic polymers, modifications to include targeting functionality are often desirable of a gene delivery formulation. A key advantage of cyclodextrin containing gene delivery formulations is that functionality can be added through inclusion complexes without covalent modifications. Therefore, targeting molecules, which contain a hydrophobic molecule bound to them, can be "tethered" to the polyplex via cyclodextrin. This approach has been used to introduced PEG, galactose, transferring, and insulin to cationic cyclodextrin formulations.

Cationic lipids

One of the most investigated approaches for condensing nonviral DNA for efficient gene transfer is the use of cationic lipids. Felgner et al. and Bennett et al. for ON used cationic lipids for the first time to deliver DNA and ONs. More recently, siRNA has been delivered to mammalian cells using commercially available lipids. Although some cationic lipids are used individually to deliver nonviral DNA (e.g., DOTAP), many formulations of cationic lipids also contain a zwitterionic or neutral colipid, such as DOPE or cholesterol, to enhance transfection. Formulations of cationic lipids have been widely applied for *in vitro* nucleic acid transfection, and more than 30 products are commercially available for this purpose, including Lipofectin (a 1:1 mixture of DOTMA and DOPE), Transfectam, Lipofectase, Lipofect-AMINE, and LipoTaxi.

The main components of a cationic lipid are a hydrophilic lipid anchor, a linker group, and a positively charged head group. The lipid anchor is typically either a fatty chain (e.g., derived from oleic or myristic acid) or a cholesterol group, which determines the physical properties of the lipid bilayer, such as flexibility and the rate of lipid exchange. The linker group is an important determinant of the chemical stability, biodegradability, and transfection efficiency of the cationic lipid. Biodegradable lipids are being developed, which can be metabolized by various enzymes (e.g., esterases and peptidases) to minimize toxicity. The linker can also provide sites for the introduction of novel side chains to enhance targeting, uptake, and trafficking. The positively charged head group on the cationic lipid self-assembles with the negatively charged DNA and is a critical determinant of the transfection and cytotoxic properties of liposome formulations. The head groups differ markedly in structure and may be single- or multiple-charged as primary, secondary, tertiary, and/or quaternary amines. The synthesis of novel cationic lipids from libraries of building blocks has provided insight into some structure-activity relationships. The hydrophobicity of the lipid moiety has a crucial effect on *in vitro* gene transfer. Multivalent head groups, such as spermine, in a "T-shape" configuration tend to be more effective than their monovalent counterparts at facilitating gene transfer. Generally, increases in the linker length correspond to increases in the gene delivery activity. Continued progress toward a comprehensive relationship among lipid structure, complexation with DNA, and subsequent interaction with the biological environment (e.g., cell membrane and extracellular membrane components) is necessary to facilitate the design of cationic lipids with optimal properties.

Mixing of DNA and cationic lipid results in the collapse of DNA to form a condensed structure (lipoplex), in which nucleic acids are buried within the lipid. The thermodynamic driving force for association of the DNA and lipid is the entropy increase from the release of counter-ions and bound water associated with DNA and the lipid surface. Liposome association with DNA has resulted in tube-like bilayers, multilameller complexes, as well as structures containing non-bilayer elements. Multilamellar organization, in which DNA is intercalated between cationic lipid bilayers, has been reported for lipolexes resulting from the interaction of DNA with unilameller vesicles of a cationic lipid, such as DOTAP and DODAB, respectively, combined with DOPE and cholesterol. Both of these studies used x-ray scattering to show that a periodicity of 6.5 nm occurs in the lamellar structure. The cationic lipid bilayer thickness was 3.9 nm, and the thickness of the water layer was 2.6 nm, which is sufficient to include a hydrated DNA double helix with a total diameter of 2.5 nm. A second periodicity was observed, which was attributed to a DNA–DNA correlation, which ranged from 2.45 nm to 5.71 nm as the concentration of helper lipid was increased. These lamellar complexes can be converted into hexagonal complexes with DNA confined in inverted lipid micelles by changing the membrane spontaneous curvature or the membrane flexibility. This hexagonal arrangement has demonstrated increased transfection, which is attributed to the relative instability of the complexes due to rapid fusion with anionic vesicles and subsequent DNA release. X-ray diffraction studies and microscopy have illustrated the high degree of variability in lipoplex structure and the need to understand and control the parameters that govern the organization of these structures.

The colloidal properties (e.g., size and stability) of the lipoplexes are principally determined by the cationic lipid/DNA charge ratio and not the composition of the lipid or the helper lipid. The charge ratio (+/–) is typically defined as the number of amines on the cationic lipid relative to the number of phosphate groups on the DNA. A neutral charge ratio (1:1 charge ratio for lipid/DNA) is typically avoided because it results in the formation of large aggregates (>1 μm). Lipoplexes prepared at a positive charge ratio and a negative charge ratio likely represent structures with different lipid and DNA packaging. At a positive charge ratio, large multilamellar vesicles (LMVs, diameter 300–700 nm) transfected cells more efficiently than the small unilameller vesicles (SUVs, diameter 50–200 nm). These observations were consistent whether the structures were formed as LMVs or as SUVs that aggregated to form LMVs. The order in which DNA and lipid are mixed is critical and significantly affects the lipid and DNA packing. For the addition of DNA to lipid, a gradual increase in size was observed. When adding lipid to DNA, the particle size remains roughly constant until the amount of lipid positive charge exceeds the nucleic acid negative charge, whereupon the particles grow rapidly in size.

The net charge on the lipoplex affects its interactions with other components present *in vivo* and *in vitro* (e.g., media, serum, extracellular matrix glycoproteins, and mucosal secretions), which can limit the transfection efficiency. A positive charge ratio, which facilitates interactions with the cell membrane, is frequently used for *in vitro* studies (3:1), whereas *in vivo* studies may require the charge ratio to be altered because of interactions with components of the physiological environment. The charge ratio of the complex determines the zeta potential, which ranges from -55 mV to +55 mV as the charge ratio is increased. Multivalent anions present in the serum or media can facilitate fusion of the lipids causing an increase in the size of the particle. Polyanions with adequate anionic charge density (e.g., heparin) release DNA from the complex by binding the cationic lipid. Serum can be a complicating factor for positively charged complexes, possibly causing premature release of the DNA from the complex and enhancing degradation by nucleases. For ON: lipid complexes, the various components of serum (e.g., BSA, lipoproteins, macroglobulin) interact with the complexes and alter the complex diameter, zeta potential, and interfere with cellular uptake and nuclear trafficking.

Aggregation of lipoplexes in polyelectrolyte solutions occurs rapidly, which can result in loss of activity in less than 24 hours; thus, strategies are being developed to stabilize the particles and prolong their shelf life. To improve lipoplex stability, PEG–PE has been incorporated into the cationic liposome. PEG containing liposomes are prevented from aggregating and interacting with serum components, which increases their stability. Alternatively, new preparation methods are being developed in which a detergent is present in solution with the cationic lipid and DNA. Removal of the detergent by dialysis allows the formation of uniform complexes. This process yielded a lipid/DNA suspension that was able to transfect tissue culture cells up to 90 days after formation with no loss in activity. Lyophilization, which is a common approach used for many pharmaceuticals, is also being applied to lipoplexes to increase their shelf life. Cryoprotectants (e.g., sucrose and trehalose) are typically added to prevent aggregation and fusion of plasmid/lipid complexes during lyophilization. Complexes lyophilized in the presence of 0.5-M sucrose or trehalose maintained transfection rates and the sizes of rehydrated complexes as compared with nonlyophhilized controls.

Cationic polymers such as poly(amino acids) have also been used in combination with liposomes. DNA is initially complexed with polylysine (PLL) at low charge ratios and cationic lipids are subsequently added to completely condense the DNA. Alternatively, the PLL condensed DNA containing a net positive charge can subsequently be complexed with an anionic lipid. Precondensation with polylysine has been shown to reduce serum inhibition and to enhance the transfection efficiency. Catinic polymer formulations have been extensively used to deliver nucleic acids *in vivo* for the treatment of cancer and cystic fibrosis as an antiinflammatory agent and to prevent or reduce viral infections.

Matrix-based Delivery

Matrix-based delivery has been proposed to enhance gene transfer *in vivo* by delaying clearance from the desired tissue, protecting the nucleic acid from degradation, and extending opportunities for internalization. Furthermore, matrix-based delivery can provide sustained delivery to maintain the vector at effective levels within the target tissue. Many of these properties have been observed for controlled release systems that deliver proteins. Gene transfer from tissue engineering matrices may increase the number of cells expressing the transgene along with the extent of transgene expression, while minimizing the quantity of vector used. Additionally, matrix-based delivery may reduce the number of dosages or the required cumulative dose. Matrix-based delivery of nucleic acids can be divided into two delivery approaches: (1) direct encapsulation and release, where naked DNA, polyplexes, or lipoplexes encapsulated into the matrix for later release; and (2) matrix-tethered delivery (also called substrate-mediated or solid phase delivery), where polyplexes or lipoplexes are immobilized to the matrix for release after matrix or tether degradation. To date most matrix-based delivery approaches involve the encapsulation of naked DNA and its subsequent release to transfect surrounding cells. Polymer encapsulation strategies can shield the vector against degradation, clearance, and an immune response. Drug release from the matrix into the tissue can be designed to occur rapidly, as in a bolus delivery, or over an extended period of time, which may affect the local concentration and cellular internalization. For rapid release, levels would be expected to quickly rise and decline as the DNA is cleared or degraded. For sustained delivery, the concentration may be maintained within an appropriate range by adjusting the release rate (e.g., through the polymer choice). Release of DNA from tissue engineering scaffolds has been observed for times ranging from hours to several weeks. Variations in the polymer composition and physical form, which includes properties such as porosity, mass, and size, affects the diffusion of DNA from the vehicle and hence the release rate.

Tethered delivery approaches aim to significantly slow down release kinetics by immobilizing polyplexes or lipoplexes directly to the matrix. Because the polyplexes are immobilized to the matrix, the matrix must also support cell adhesion and infiltration by the surrounding cells rather than function as a nucleic acid reservoir. Internalization of the immobilized polyplexes results after the tether between the polyplex and the matrix is degraded, the matrix is degraded or the affinity of the polyplex for the matrix is reduced due to environmental changes. The release kinetics of the polyplexes in this case depends on the chemistry used for polyplex immobilization and the chemistry of the matrix. Biotynilated polyplexes immobilized to a NeutrAvidin coated substrate was the first example of matrix-tethered delivery. This matrix-tethered delivery strategies resulted in a 100-fold increase of transgene expression compared with bolus delivery, likely due to an increase of the polyplex concentration at the cellular microenvironment. Furthermore, immobilization of polyplexes to the material surface has shown to enhace the stability of the polyplexes in polyelectrolyte solutions, preventing their aggregation. The strength of the tether bond or the number of tethers affects both the density of immobilized polyplexes as well as the transfection efficiency. A high density of tethers results in high surface densities of DNA with low ability to transfect, probably due to the polyplex being too tightly bound to the matrix. More recently, matrix-tethered strategies rely on electrostatic interactions between poly or lipoplexes and the matrix to immobilize the complexe.

Matrix-based delivery has been investigated mostly for regenerative medicine applications. Regenerative medicine aims to regenerate tissue by implanting biocompatible and biodegradable scaffolds at sites of injury or disease. The implanted scaffold must provide the mechanical support for the growing tissue and the bio-active signals needed for proper tissue formation while allowing for cell attachment and growth. Delivery of nucleic acids from tissue engineering scaffolds could be used as the bioactive signals needed to recreate the environments needed for tissue formation allowing for direct manipulation of cellular gene expression patterns.

Direct Encapsulation and Release

Direct encapsulation and release strategies have been proposed to enhance gene transfer *in vivo* by delaying clearance from the desired tissue, protecting the DNA from degradation and extending the opportunities for internalization. Furthermore, matrix-based delivery can provide sustained delivery to maintain the vector at effective levels within the target tissue.

Synthetic polymers

Polymers composed of lactide and glycolide (PLGA) are perhaps the most widely used and recognized biodegradable synthetic polymers because these polymers are FDA approved and are generally considered to be biocompatible. Hydrolytic degradation of the polymer produces lactic acid and glycolic acid, two substances naturally involved in metabolic pathways of the body. The degradation rate can be controlled through the composition of the polymer and molecular weight of the chains. These polymers exhibit relatively even polymer chain scission throughout their bulk after being placed *in vivo*. These properties have led to the use of these materials for drug delivery and as scaffolds for tissue engineering. Drug release from these systems typically occurs by a combination of polymer degradation and drug diffusion from the polymer. Gene delivery from polymeric matrices has been applied to tissue repair and wound healing. These matrices are typically implanted at a specific anatomic location where they serve multiple roles as described previously. Initially, the matrix functions to create and maintain a space *in vivo*. However, the matrix also acts as a scaffold to support cell migration, proliferation, and differentiation of healthy cells from the surrounding tissue. As cells invade the matrix, they encounter DNA that is either released from or entrapped within the matrix.

A gas foaming/particulate leaching process can be employed to fabricate interconnected open pore structures of PLGA for controlled release of DNA. This process employs carbon dioxide to process a mixture of polymer and porogen, in order to fuse adjacent polymer particles into an interconnected structure. The DNA can be lyophilized with the microspheres or encapsulated within the microspheres. Lyophilization of DNA with the microspheres can provide large quantities of incorporated DNA, with relatively rapid release kinetics. Incorporation of DNA into the microspheres provides for a more sustained release relative to the lyophilization method, with the release kinetics dependent on the polymer molecular weight and microsphere size. DNA can be incorporated into polymer microspheres using several approaches. Subcutaneous implantation of scaffolds results in transfected cells observed within the scaffold and the tissue immediately adjacent to the scaffold, with protein production sufficient to promote physiological responses. An alternative approach to fabrication of PLG scaffolds for DNA delivery is electrospinning. Electrospinning creates nonwoven, nanofibered membranous structures that release DNA, with maximal release occurring at approximately 2 hours.

Microspheres can also be employed to deliver DNA to tissues. Microspheres loaded with nonviral DNA can be fabricated from nondegradable and degradable polymers in sizes ranging from 0.1 to 100 μm and have been used for applications such as DNA vaccines and systemic protein delivery. One of the main advantages for delivery vehicles of this size is that they can be administered in a minimally invasive manner (e.g., direct injection and oral delivery). The use of biodegradable polymers provides the additional advantage of not having to retrieve the implant after DNA release. Unfortunately, these two qualities (size and degradability) make removal of the devices difficult, should the therapy need to be terminated prematurely. The loading of DNA into the polymer ranges from 0.1- to 10-μg DNA per milligram of polymer using various techniques based on either an emulsion or phase inversion process. A double emulsion process has been used to incorporate aqueous solutions of nonviral DNA, both supercoiled and complexed with poly-L-lysine, into polymer. Incorporation efficiencies ranging from 20% to 80% have been obtained, although the typical incorporation efficiency is approximately 30%. When supercoiled DNA is incorporated using this procedure, the incorporated DNA is structurally intact with 39% of the DNA in the supercoiled conformation. Protecting the DNA by either condensation or using a cryogenic approach can be used to increase the DNA present in the supercoiled form to more than 80%. DNA polyplexes have been encapsulated and released from polymer microspheres, which may enable these microspheres to be fabricated into matrices using an approach such as the gas-foaming procedure. PLL/DNA complexes have been incorporated into PLG microspheres using a double emulsion process. DNA is incorporated with efficiencies ranging from 30% to 45%, is released over approximately 35 days, and retains its integrity. Alternatively ONs complexed with PEI have been incorporated and released from PLG microspheres. The release profile of the ON/PEI complexes depended on the size, loading, and pore structure of the microspheres. The sustained release of ON/PEI complexes resulted in improved intracellular penetration of the delivered vector as compared with uncomplexed DNA. PLG/DNA scaffolds have successfully been used *in vivo* to enhance matrix deposition, angiogenesis, and bone formation.

Synthetic PEG hydrogels have been extensively investigated as cell transplantation vehicles and as tissue engineering scaffolds. Synthetic hydrogels allow for the complete engineering of the extracellular environment given that they lack direct cellular interactions and have limited protein absorption. Thus, every aspect of the extracellular matrix environment must be engineered, including integrin binding sites, growth factors, and other bioactive signals. DNA delivery from synthetic hydrogels based on PEG have shown that the release rate can be modulated depending on the degree of cross-linking and degradation rate of the hydrogel. Naked DNA encapsulated in photo-cross-linked PEG hydrogels could modulate the release profile of the DNA ranging from linear to a delayed release profile. Naked DNA encoding for transforming growth factor beta-1 encapsulated in thermosensitive hydrogel scaffolds resulted in reepitelization of wounds in diabetic mice if applied at early stages during wound healing.

Natural polymers

Collagens are the major component of mammalian connective tissue and thus have been widely investigated as a biomaterial for cell growth and drug delivery. At least 14 types of collagen are distributed throughout the body. The most abundant is type I collagen. Type I collagen is found in high concentrations in tendon, skin, bone, and fascia, and thus, these tissues are sources for its isolation. After isolation, typically from bovine or porcine sources, collagen is preserved using techniques such as fixation with aldehydes or other chemical preservatives, gamma-irradiation, or lyophilization. Collagen can be lyophilized to form a spongy product or can be formed into a hydrogel by using its natural ability to self-assemble at neutral pH and body temperature (37°C) or by covalently cross-linking it using aldehydes or carbodiimides.

Collagen has been used as a matrix for numerous tissue engineering applications, including bone, skin, nerve, and cartilage. The collagen serves as a scaffold for the migration of repair cells into the matrix and serves to either retain the DNA within the scaffold or provide gradual release. Collagen-based release may limit vector degradation and can induce transgene expression for up to 40 days. Naked DNA delivery from collagen matrices has been employed to promote tissue formation by transfecting invading fibroblasts. Transfected fibroblasts within DNA-loaded collagen scaffolds, also termed gene-activated matrices (GAMs), subsequently act as bioreactors for localized production of tissue inductive factors. Matrices were prepared by lyophilization of type I collagen and subsequent immersion in a DNA solution. For applications in tissue engineering, collagen/DNA constructs have been implanted into an adult rat femur and a canine bone defect model. Matrices loaded with 1 mg of DNA were capable of transfecting cells *in vivo*, which resulted in protein production for up to 3 weeks postimplant. For the canine model, however, regeneration required 100 mg of plasmid delivered from the matrix for regeneration. Atelocollagen/DNA constructs have also been used for therapeutic applications, including implanted constructs in the muscle to increase platelet number, and in the rabbit ear to aid in would healing. Furthermore, atelocollagen/siRNA constructs have been delivered intratumorally to suppress tumor growth.

DNA complexed with cationic lipids or cationic polymers can also be incorporated and released from collagen-based matrices, while maintaining their activity. Naked DNA delivery produces substantial transgene expres-sion *in vivo*, but it results in low levels of transgene expression *in vitro*. DNA complexes can transfect cells *in vitro*; thus, the ability to release DNA complexes can extend the applicability of nonviral DNA release matrices to the engineering of tissues *in vitro*. Note, however, that release of DNA complexes may differ significantly from that for naked DNA, due to the different physical properties of complexes relative to naked DNA. Collagen matrices loaded with DNA by pipetting solutions of naked DNA, PEI/DNA complexes, and lipoplexes onto collagen showed different release kinetics. *In vitro* release studies demonstrated that naked DNA was rapidly released, PEI/DNA and lipid complexes were slowly released, and that PEI/DNA complexes with a protective copolymer had intermediate release kinetics. The PEI/DNA complexes with the protective copolymer gave the highest transfection *in vitro* and *in vivo*, with the highest *in vivo* expression occurring at 4 days and measurable quantities observed at 7 days. PLL/DNA complexes encapsulated in a collagen sponge have been implanted into severed rat optic nerves as a means to promote neuron survival and promote regeneration. The PLL was modified with bFGF to facilitate the internalization and intracellular trafficking. DNA was detected in the retina for up to 3 months. Nerve terminals were observed extending into the collagen, and they seemed appeared capable of transporting the DNA by retrograde transport.

Hydrogels based on agarose, fibrin, hyaluronic acid (HA), and chitosan have been employed independently as biomaterials for fabrication of tissue engineering matrices or as materials to regulate DNA delivery. Fibrin matrixes have been extensively used as tissue engineering scaffolds, sealants, and drug delivery matrices. Fibrin sealants have been employed for the delivery of plasmids to promote angiogenesis, with fibrin-based delivery providing similar responses to delivery in PBS solution.

Agarose gels have been used to encapsulate PLL/DNA polyplexes and mediate sustained release to transfect smooth muscle cells *in vitro* with an efficiency less than that obtained by freshly formed complexes, but greater than that obtained with naked DNA. Hydrogels based on fibrin and agarose primarily function to limit the release of DNA; however, hydrogels employing chitosan offer the potential to condense the DNA. Chitosan is a positively charged, naturally occurring polysaccharide that can form complexes with DNA. Chitosan/DNA complexes exhibit minimal cytotoxicity, destabilize the lipid bilayer to facilitate internalization, and produce high levels of transfection *in vitro* and *in vivo*. Tissue engineering matrices based on these hydrogels, or combinations of these materials, provide a variety of approaches to regulate DNA delivery *in vitro* and *in vivo*. HA-based matrices have not been used extensively for gene delivery, although their potential as tissue engineering scaffold has long been recognized. DNA loaded, cross-linked HA-based delivery systems have been formed in the form of matrices and microspheres.

A solution of HA and plasmid DNA was lyophilized to form a spongy material before cross-linking with adipic acid dihydrazide to form a stable three-dimensional matrix. This HA matrix demonstrated the capacity for sustained release of naked DNA, with release likely occurring after degradation of the matrix. The release rate of naked DNA from the matrices, some of which may be associated with HA fragments, could be modulated by the extent of cross-linking in the hydrogel. DNA-loaded hyaluronic acid microspheres have been formed and found to be able to deliver genes both *in vivo* and *in vitro*. The microspheres were formed using a water-in-oil emulsion and covalent cross-linking with adipic acid dihydrazide to stabilize the microspheres. These microspheres could then be implanted to mediate *in vivo* gene delivery or delivered to plated cells. In both cases, the released DNA mediates transgene expression.

HA has also been cross-linked with collagen and used as gene delivery matrices. The procedure used can be similar to that used for collagen gene delivery systems or that used to form HA hydrogels. HA is mixed with collagen and lyophilized to form a spongy material. This material is then cross-linked using carbodiimide chemistry, dehydrothermal treatment, or exposure to ultraviolet light. After cross-linking, the matrices are soaked in a DNA solution to introduce the DNA to the porous scaffolds. These matrices have been shown to mediate transgene expression *in vivo* and *in vitro*.

Matrix-Tethered Delivery

Material-tethered delivery combines cationic polymer and cationic lipid formulations with matrix delivery to generate a more efficient delivery strategy by immobilizing the polyplexes or lipoplexes directly to a matrix that also supports cell adhesion and cellular infiltration. This approach places the nucleic acid directly at the cellular microenvironment, removing the need for diffusion of the complexes to the cell membrane Matrix tethered has not been as extensively used *in vivo* as the direct encapsulation methods described above; however, it has found success mediating DNA delivery from PLGA scaffolds and hyaluronic acid and fibrin hydrogels.

Synthetic polymers

Matrix-tethered delivery approaches in synthetic polymeric matrices have focused on nonspecific interactions (adsorption) to immobilize the complexes to the matrix. PLGA scaffolds have been coated with a variety of polyplexes such as PAMAM/DNA and PEI/DNA. PAMAM/DNA complexes were dried on a porous PLG scaffold and shown to retain their activity, being able to mediate gene transfer both *in vitro* and *in vivo*, and were found to be a function of DNA concentration and charge ratio. PEI/DNA complexes were absorbed to PLG scaffolds without allowing them to dry on the surface, in contrast to the method described above. It was found that delivery of DNA via matrix-based delivery resulted in similar levels of expression compared with bolus delivery; however, a lower dose of DNA was used. The amount of DNA immobilized was dependent on the time of incubation of the polyplexes with the scaffold, the N/P ratio used, and the initial amount of DNA used. Interestingly, higher amounts of immobilized DNA did not result in higher transgene expression, with 45 ng resulting in more efficient transfection than 600 ng.

Natural polymers

Hyaluronic acid and fibrin were employed independently as biomaterials for fabrication of tissue engineering matrices or as materials to mediate gene delivery. HA has been cross-linked with a wide variety of chemistries to form stable hydrogels. DNA/PEI complexes were immobilized to hyaluronic acid hydrogels via biotin–avidin bonds. PEI was modified with biotin groups and subsequently used to complex DNA to form biotynilated polyplexes. The polyplexes were then immobilized to a HA hydrogel, which had been chemically modified to introduce neutravidin, a biotin binding protein. Fibroblasts, which were directly in contact with the polyplex/HA hydrogel, were transfected; however, those directly adjacent to the hydrogel were not, indicating that direct contact of the cell with the tethered polyplexes is essential for transfection.

The size of the tethered polyplexes resulted in different transgene expression levels and percent of cells expressing the transgene. Small complexes (~150 nm) resulted in lower levels of transgene expression compared with large complexes (~1000 nm); however, small complexes resulted in ~50% of the cells transfected, which is double that of large complexes. Futhermore, the HA hydrogels used in these studies were topographically patterned with groves and ridges, which resulted in spatially controlled gene expression along the ridges of the hydrogel surface.

Unlike HA, fibrinogen forms a stable hydrogel matrix upon thrombin activation to form a fibrin matrix. Fibrin matrices can be further stabilized by the addition of factor XIIIa, which forms covalent bonds between glutamine and lysine residues. Schense and Hubbell have used factor XIIIa chemistry extensively to bind biologically active peptides and growth factors to fibrin matrices. More recently, Hubbell et al. used the same strategy to immobilize polyplexes to fibrin hydrogels. Two different 21 amino acid peptides were designed to have a DNA binding sequences (Cys–His–(Lys)6–His–Cys) in combination with a transglutaminase substrate site (Asn–Gln–Glu–Gln–Val–Ser–Pro–Leu) or a nuclear localization site (from SV40).

The polyplexes were formed with mixtures of the two poly(amino acids) and mixed with fibrinogen, thrombin, and factor XIIIa, resulting in the covalent immobilization of the polyplexes within the fibrin matrix. Transfection of COS-7 cells in a two-dimensional (2D) sandwich assay, in which cells are plated on top of a polyplex/fibrin hydrogel and then a second gel is cast on top, resulted in ~25% of the cells transfected. These hydrogels have been used *in vivo* to deliver a mutant HIF-1α plasmid, which has the transcription factor constantly active, and resulted in enhanced wound healing in a skin wound model. Furthermore, the delivery of a HIF-1α encoding plasmid was able to result in the formation of more mature blood vessels when compared with the delivery of a vascular endothelial growth factor (VEGF) encoding plasmid.

DELIVERY LIMITATIONS AND CURRENT SOLUTIONS

The ultimate applicability of the various biomaterials for gene delivery rests on their ability to effectively deliver the nucleic acids to their target infra cellular location. An effective gene delivery system will protect the nucleic acid from degradation, target the appropriate cell population, be efficiently internalized by the cell, avoid degradative pathways, and ultimately localize to the nucleus (DNA) or cytosol (siRNA or ON). The materials under development can specifically enhance one or more of these steps in the transfection process. The following sections describe how the materials interact with biological systems and how they can be designed to overcome the obstacles to effective gene transfer.

Extracellular Limitations

Vector stabilization and fast clearance from body

Interaction of nonviral formulations with serum components results in the deactivation of the lipoplexes or polyplexes due to aggregation. Furthermore, aggregated lipoplexes and polyplexes can lead to rapid clearance of the polyplexes by phagocytic cells and the reticulocndotheial sytem. Hydrophilic polymers such as poly(ethylene glycol) (PEG), N-(2-hydroxypropyl)methacrylamide) (HPMA), and oligosaccharides have been found to stabilize complexes against salt and protein aggregation, which results in longer circulation times. The increased stability probably results from steric effects that (1) prevent interaction with serum proteins, cells, and tissue; (2) increase solubility of the complexes in aqueous milieu; and (3) prevent particle-particle interactions. Traditional cationic polymers for gene delivery such as PEI, PAMAM, and PLL have been made more biocompatible using this approach.

Targeted internalization

The plasma membrane of the cell provides a protective shell that serves to limit the transport of undesired molecules, such as DNA. However, cells must communicate with their environment and have thus developed mechanisms to transport high- and low-molecular-weight macromolecules across the membrane. Nonclathrin-coated pit internalization can occur through smooth invaginations of 150–300 nm or via potocytosis, which involves the invagination of caveolae-rich 50–100-nm-diameter vesicles from the cell surface. DNA complexes are thought to enter cells primarily through clathrin-coated pits. These pits, with diameters of approximately 150 nm, are internalized from the plasma membrane to form coated vesicles. Interestingly, recent studies using a series of inhibitors for different endosomal pathways have elucidated different mechanisms of internalization for lipoplexes and polyplexes. Lipoplex internalization and lipoplex-mediated nucleic acid delivery was strongly inhibited by potassium depletion or using chlorpromazine, indicating that clathrin endocytosis is the primary internalization pathway of lipoplexes.

On the contrary, polyplex internalization was inhibited by 25% when the caveolae pathway was inhibited using filipin or genistein and by 20% when clathrin-mediated endocytosis was inhibited, indicating that polyplexes use two internalization pathways. Gene transfer mediated by polyplexes was completely abolished when the caveolae pathway was inhibited but not when the clathrin-mediated pathway was inhibited, suggesting that internalization via caveolae-mediated endosomes leads to efficient transfection. Particle size also affects the endosomal internalization pathway used. Particles with a diameter <200 nm were found to be internalized via clathrin-mediated endocytosis and were ultimately delivered to the lysosome. In contrast, particles that were >500 nm entered the cells via caveolae and never reached the lysosomal compartment. Furthermore, multiple studies have shown that large PEI/DNA complexes >500 nm were more efficient at mediating high transgene expression than small complexes <200 nm, suggesting that it is due to mode of internalization and intracellular trafficking.

Receptor-mediated gene delivery offers a promising approach to create a specific interaction with the cell surface and to target a particular internalization pathway. Synthetic materials termed molecular conjugates are being developed and are composed of two domains: a DNA binding domain and a receptor binding domain. The DNA binding domain is in charge of linking the DNA to the rest of the molecular conjugate molecule. The DNA binding domain is typically composed of a cationic polymer or a cationic lipid, which self-assembles with DNA.

The receptor binding domain is frequently attached to functional groups on the cationic polymer or lipid before complexation with DNA; however, complexes can be initially formed and subsequently coupled to a ligand. The function of the receptor binding domain is to direct the DNA/molecular conjugate complex to a receptor and guide the complex through the internalization pathway that leads to endosomal entrapment. The intracellular fate of DNA complexes can depend on the type of endocytic process involved in its internalization. The diversity and abundance of membrane bound receptors and ligands and the high efficiency of internalization and turnover ratio makes receptor-mediated endocytosis a powerful tool for controlling uptake. Targets for which the attached ligand binds include the receptors for asialoglycoprotein, transferrin, folate, manose, galactose, lectins, integrins antibodies and EGF. The attachment of a targeting ligand to the lipoplex has been shown to increase transfection by 1000-fold as compared with lipid with no targeting ligand. In principle, any monoclonal antibody, Fab fragment of a monoclonal antibody, peptide, peptide mimetic, proteins, or peptide fragment can be added to the molecular conjugate using either a covalent or an ionic attachment.

Maximal gene delivery through the receptor-mediated endocytosis pathway requires that the design parameters be optimized, which includes properties such as the ligand binding affinity, the length of the linker between the ligand and the complex, the complex charge ratio and structure, and the number of ligands per complex. Ligand–receptor interactions can be very specific and may be negatively affected when covalently bound to a molecular conjugate. Knowing whether the receptor binding domain is interacting to its receptor with the same efficiency as the free ligand is important to achieve high gene delivery levels. In a model using an EGF–polylysine conjugate, it was found that a longer spacer arm, between the two domains, resulted in more native-like EGF–receptor binding and higher transfection efficiency than shorter spacer arms.

The presence of the ligand can alter the structure of the nucleic acid complex. Incorporation of asialoorosomucoid into PLL/DNA complexes was more efficient at condensing DNA than PLL alone, probably due to an aggregation of many PLLs around the negatively charged protein. At low charge ratios, specific (ligand mediated) and non-specific endocytosis had insignificant levels of transfection. As the charge ratio was increased to 4, the transfection efficiency by specific binding enhanced transfection by a factor of 3 over nonspecific endocytosis. Finally, the number of ligands per complex can affect the binding of the complexes to cells. An excessive number of ligands may inhibit the binding of complexes. Optimization of the parameters that affect the surface binding of the molecular conjugates improves the specificity and gene transfer efficiency for gene delivery.

Intracellular Limitations

The steps after internalization of naked-DNA, polyplexes or lipoplexes, endosomal escape, and nuclear localization are thought to be rate limiting for the transfection of many cell types. Internalization of the plasmid does not necessarily correlate to transfection. Much of the DNA that is internalized into the endosome is either retained or degraded within the endosome. The DNA that does escape the endosome and enters the cytoplasm must sub sequently avoid degradation and be transported to the nucleus for successful gene transfer. *In vitro* studies have demonstrated that although greater than 95% of the cells were positive for plasmid (>100,000 copies per cells), less than 50% of the cells were expressing the transgene. The following sections describe how the materials interact with intracellular biological systems and how they can be designed to overcome the obstacles for effective gene transfer.

Toxicity

One common drawback of efficient nonviral gene delivery strategies is that they are generally toxic. This finding is not surprising given that efficient nucleic acid delivery formulations are also efficient at getting into the cell and moving through the intracellular space most likely in an unspecific manner. For example, PEI has been found to colocalize with the nucleous and with the delivered DNA, whereas PLL has not. As reviewed, PEI is more efficient at gene transfer than PLL and PEI is more toxic than PLL. Nuclear PEI may nonspecifically interact with genomic DNA, preventing its normal transcription, thus causing toxicity. Furthermore, the efficient endosomal buffering of PEI and PAMAM dendrimers, while improving their effectiveness to deliver DNA, may also contribute toxicity by preventing the natural acidification of endosomal vesicles and degradation of unwanted endosomal cargo. Thus, can we have an efficient nucleic acid delivery strategy without some toxicity? Is it possible to have an effective therapeutic approach with absolutely no side effects? The answer is that it needs to be attempted although the blockbuster of nonviral gene delivery formulations may not be completely nontoxic. Some general characteristics of cationic polymers and lipids make them toxic such as molecular weight, density of positive charges, and lack of degradability. This section briefly outlines the most common features associated with toxicity and their current solutions.

Nonviral formulations are generally more efficient and more toxic as the polymer-to-nucleic acid ratio is increased (higher N/P ratios), suggesting a role of free uncomplexed polymer in the solution in efficient delivery and toxicity. A recent report has shown that polyplexes of DNA and PEI contain an average of 3.5 plasmids (5800 base pairs) and 30 PEI (25 kDa) molecules when prepared at N/P ratios of 6 and 10, assuming that the DNA is completely complexed. Based on these calculations, there is 86% of free PEI in the complex mixture. Purification of the PEI/DNA complexes by dialysis has shown a reduction of toxcicity; however, it also reduced transfection efficiency. Efficient gene transfer was restored when free PEI was added to the mixture.

High-molecular-weight cationic polymers are generally more toxic than low-molecular-weight polymers, most likely due to aggregation of free polymer with the cell membrane or other cellular components. Together these findings suggest that free high-molecular-weight polymer leads to efficient but toxic gene transfer. Strategies to prevent such toxicity have focused on reducing the density of positive charges (number of primary amines) without affecting the buffering capacity of the polymer and, thus, reducing its interaction with the cell membrane and other cellular components.

Another structural aspect of cationic polymers that contributes to their efficiency as gene transfer agents and their toxicity is the degree of branching and backbone flexibility. Highly branched cationic polymers form smaller particles and mediate more efficient gene transfer than low-branched polymers but are more toxic compared with low-branched or linear polymers. The high toxicity of branched polymers has been associated with polymer backbone stiffness; more flexible, hyperbranched PEI derivatives with additional secondary and tertiary groups show lower toxicity *in vitro* than commercially available branched PEI.

One approach that could reduce the toxicity associated with a high molecular weight and a high degree of branching is making the delivery formulation degradable. Degradable PEIs are of particular interest because the basic structure of PEI is not biologically or chemically degradable. Efforts to make PEI degradable typically involve the cross-linking of low-molecular-weight PEI (600–1800 kDa) with disulfide linkages or oligo(L-lactic acid cosuccinic acid) to form the higher molecular weight PEIs required to achieve efficient transfection. Furthermore, low-molecular-weight PEI has been cross-linked with PEI through a degradable ester bond. Cytotoxicity experiments showed decreased toxicity or complexes formed with degradable PEG–PEI/DNA complexes when compared with complexes formed with 25-kDa PEI. However, transfection studies showed that the degradable PEI was less efficient at mediating gene transfer than 25-kDa PEI. Although PAMAM dendrimers have been found to be three orders of magnitude less toxic than PEI (600–1000 kDa) and PLL (36.6 kDa), they still suffer from toxic effects. The toxicity of PAMAM dendrimers seems to have a different mechanism from that of toxicity caused by linear cationic polymers in that it does not cause membrane hemolysis at a similar concentration of PEI and PLL. It has been reported that primary amines are more toxic than secondary or tertiary amines for PEI-type polymers. However, for PAMAM dendrimers, this relationship was not true. Although cytotoxicity increased with generation (higher molecular weight), it was surprisingly independent of surface charge. Strategies to reduce toxicity of PAMAM dendrimers include quaternization, reducing or reversal of surface charge, and sterically shielding the surface groups by binding C12 lauroyl groups or PEG2000 Cytoxicity of PLL, although low relative to many nondegradable delivery agents, is not negligible. Dendritic PLL has been found to have cytoxicity that is much lower than that of PLL and is nearly the same as naked DNA, although the PLL itself leads to cell viability of about 80% of naked DNA as determined by 3-(4,5-dimethylthiazol-2-yl) -2,5-diphenyltetrazolium bromide (MTT) assay.

Endosomal escape

After internalization, the coated vesicle transforms into an early endosome, which is accompanied by acidification of the vesicular lumen that continues into the late endosomal and lysosomal compartments, reaching a final pH in the perinuclear lysosome of approximately 4.5. For lipoplex-mediated delivery, the interaction of the lipids with the endosomal membrane is thought to facilitate escape of the DNA to the cytoplasm before its degradation in the lysosome. Although it is not well understood, some lipoplexes preferentially fuse with the early endosome, whereas others fuse with the late endosome. pH-sensitive liposomes can take advantage of the acidification process to facilitate the release of plasmids into the cytoplasm before lysosomal degradation. Release of the DNA from the complex may occur at the wall of the endosome. Xu and Szoka proposed a model in which destabilization of the endosomal membrane causes a flip-flop of anionic lipids from the cytoplasmic facing monolayer, which diffuse laterally into the complex and form a charge neutral ion pair with the cationic lipid. This pairing results in displacement of the DNA from the cationic lipid and release of the DNA into the cytoplasm. Displacement of the cationic lipid from the DNA before it enters the nucleus is critical for the ultimate expression of the gene.

Materials containing secondary and tertiary amines that are protonated at acidic pH, and not at neutral pH like primary amines, can act as proton sponges that buffer the decrease in pH and ultimately cause DNA release into the cytoplasm. For example, PEI shows a level of protonation of 20% at pH = 7.4 compared with about 45% at pH = 5. This proton sponge effect is thought to result from the protonation of amino moieties on the polymer as the pH decreases inside the endocytic vesicle. The influx of counter Cl^- ions, which occurs to maintain electroneutrality, induces osmotic swelling and rupture of the vesicle membrane. Evidence for the proton sponge hypothesis include decelerated acidification of endosomal vesicles, as well as elevated chloride accumulation and a 140% increase in the relative volume in PEI-containing endosomes. Modifications investigated for PLL to introduce endosomal buffering include the partial modification of the PLL side chains with imidazoles or histidine. Both approaches have been found to enhance the release of DNA complexed with PLL from the endosome.

Endosomal disrupting peptides, also termed fusogenic peptides, can be covalently incorporated into DNA/lipid and DNA/cationic polymer complexes to enhance escape from the endosome. Viruses and bacteria have evolved sophisticated endosomal release pathways. Based on the viral and bacterial pathways, peptides for gene delivery have been identified from the viral fusion proteins and have been used successfully to enhance endosomal escape. The peptides range in length from 15 to 30 amino acids and form stable amphipathic α-helices primarily due to alternating hydrophilic and hydrophobic amino acids. Most peptides are amphipathic pH sensitive being only active at low pH. There are two mechanisms by which fusion peptides disrupt endosomal membranes. First, the peptide causes the rearrangement of the lipid packaging, thereby changing the membrane integrity and causing release of the endosomal contents. Second, the peptide causes pore formation within the endosomal membrane, without affecting the membrane integrity. Most peptides induce endosomal release by membrane disruption rather than by membrane fusion. For example, GALA, which was one of the first synthetic peptides to be designed and synthesized, undergoes a conformational change to form an alpha-helix at acidic pHs. The α-helix formed induces endosomal leakage by disrupting the endosomal membrane. A similar peptide, KALA, also functions to disrupt endosomal membranes but is positively charged and is capable of condensing DNA and mediating gene delivery.

More recently, a family of acid responsive polymers based on α-alkyl acrylic acids such as methacrylic acid (MAA), ethylacrylic acid (EAA), propylacrylic acid, and butylacrylic acid (BAA) and their copolymers with alkyl acrylates or methacrylates have been explored for their ability to disrupt membranes and their potential as endosomal disruption polymers. The key feature of these poly(α-alkyl acrylic acids) is that they switch from a hydrophilic to a hydrophobic character as they become protonated (pH sensitive), and the switch to a hydrophobic character has been shown to disrupt membranes. The polymer, PPAA, has been shown to be 15 times more effective than PEAA at membrane disruption and to have maximum hemolytic activity at $pH \leq 6$, which is in the range of endosomal pH. PPAA has been successfully been used to enhance lipolyplex-mediated gene transfer *in vitro* and wound healing by altering extracellular matrix organization and greater vascularization *in vivo*.

Nuclear localization

The transport of DNA from the cytoplasm to the nucleus may be the most significant limitation to successful gene transfer. Plasmids injected far from the nuclei (60–90 μm) had less protein expression than plasmids injected near the nuclei. In addition to cytoplasmic transport limitations, the size of DNA is problematic for crossing into the nucleus. The nuclear pores allow free diffusion entry of only small particles (less than approximately 70 kDa). Entry of the DNA can be facilitated by the breakdown of the nuclear membrane, which occurs during cell division. However, for delivery to nondividing cells, nuclear localization sequences (NLSs) can be incorporated into the DNA complexes to direct the plasmid into the nucleus.

NLSs are short peptide sequences (5–25 amino acids) that are necessary and sufficient for nuclear localization of their respective proteins. These sequences can be incorporated into complexes with cationic lipids and cationic polymers, or they can be directly linked to the plasmid. Some nuclear localization signals have stretches of positive charge, which has led to speculation that cationic polymers function as nuclear localization signals. The cationic polymer PEI rapidly accumulates in the nucleus of cells and to a greater extent than PLL. Nevertheless, the attachment of NLS does significantly enhance nuclear accumulation. For the transfection of nondividing endothelial cells, lipoplex trans fection resulted in 5% of the cells testing positive for transfection, whereas the incorporation of an NLS resulted in more than 80% of the cells testing positive. Examples of nuclear localization sequences include PKKKRKV EDPY (SV40), GNQSSNFGPMKGGNFGGRSSGPYGGGGQYFAKPRNQGGY (M9), importin-β (1–643aa), and MRRAHHRRRRASHRRMRGG (mu).

Vector decomplexation

Recently, vector decomplexation has been viewed as another limiting step to efficient gene transfer. Vector decomplexation involves the events that need to take place for the dissociation of the delivery formulation from the nucleic acid. This step is critical for efficient gene transfer to take place given that without it DNA cannot be transcribed and siRNA/ON cannot efficiently mediate gene downregulation. Strategies to enhance decomplexation involve the introduction of environmentally sensitive bonds (mostly disulfide bonds) and reducing the affinity of the cationic polymer for the DNA. More recently, a thermosensitive copolymer, N-isopropylacrylamide-co-vinyl laurate, was covalently coupled to chitosan and employed to enhance unpacking. At temperatures below the polymer's critical solution temperature, the polymer extended and was soluble, causing the enhanced unpackaging of the chitosan/DNA polyplexes. Furthermore, enzymatically degradable formulations (chitosan) have been used to enhance unpackaging and gene transfer by encouraging intracellular enzymatic degradation (via chitosinase) of the polyplexes.

The design and construction of ideal formulations for nonviral gene delivery will continue to focus on generating materials that are "smarter," taking advantage of the cell's natural environments and processes. One approach to the design and synthesis of smarter nonviral gene delivery formulations is to better understand the intracellular and extracellular limitations at the molecular level and to understand the role (positive or negative) of the intracellular and extracellular molecules and environments that the lipoplexes and polyplexes come in contact with during the transfection process.

The cell is a complex structure that contains a myriad of molecules and events occurring simultaneously, which result in specific cell phenotypes. How the addition of lipoplexes and polyplexes affect this harmonious environment is essential for the design and generation of nonviral formulations that are less toxic and more effective, and this design is likely to be different for different cell types. For example, recent studies have shown that the rigidity of the matrix where the cells are attached affects polyplex uptake and transgene expression, with stiffer materials resulting in enhanced uptake, unpackaging, and gene expression. Although the molecular mechanism for this enhancement was not elucidated in this study, it is clear that the cellular environment (extracellular and intracellular) and cell "state" affects the effectiveness of nonviral formulations. During the past decade, nonviral gene delivery has identified key limiting steps to polyplex and lipoplex formulations and has addressed these limitations with clever solutions such as the attachment of specific cell binding ligands, fusogenic peptides, nuclear localization sequences, and degradability. The next decade will undoubtedly come with more advances for nonviral formulations that can more elegantly bypass the different barriers encountered during gene transfer.

12

SEQUENCING HUMAN GENOME

An almost complete sequence of the human genome is available now, and progress in the sequencing of other model organisms is impressive. This sequence information provides enormous possibility for identification of disease genes. The first step for sequencing of large genomes usually is the construction of a high-resolution, long-range physical map based on sequence tagged site (STS) markers. Using this map, the contig of overlapping clones is constructed and sequenced. This strategy (hierarchical) was used by the International Human Genome Sequencing Consortium to sequence the human genome. The second approach, the whole genome sequencing (WGS) strategy, was used by researchers from Celera Genomics. This strategy, in principle, doesn't need construction of high-resolution physical map and is based mainly on shotgun sequencing of large and small insert clones.

Unfortunately, both strategies for mapping and sequencing are not appropriate for the challenge of high-throughput comparative genomics. Alternative and complementary strategies need to be developed, and the imperative now is to find cost-effective and convenient methods that allow comparative genomics projects to be performed by a wide range of smaller laboratories. Recently developed novel techniques open new perspectives for nonexpensive and fast sequencing. These novel developments can be grouped into two classes. The first type of improvement is enormous, increasing the speed and throughput of producing sequences. These techniques are based on massively parallel sequencing approaches where billions of individual DNA molecules could be sequenced simultaneously. Another type of improvements is a recently suggested completely different and efficient strategy for simultaneous genome mapping and sequencing. The approach is based on physically oriented, overlapping restriction fragment libraries called slalom libraries. Both techniques allow increasing the speed and decreasing the cost of sequencing 10–100 times. Importantly, they can be combined to increase efficiency even more.

SHORT HISTORY OF THE HUMAN GENOME PROJECT

The Human Genome Program (HGP) was suggested and widely discussed within the scientific community and public press during the mid-1980s and over the last half of that decade. In 1985, Dr. Charles DeLisi, then Associate Director for Health and Environmental Research at the Department of Energy (DOE) began to discuss an unprecedented biology project—to sequence the complete human genome. DOE funding began in 1987. The National Institutes of Health (NIH) established the Office of Human Genome Research in September 1988. The Director of this Office was Dr. James Watson. The Human Genome Initiative was proposed to the Congress of the United States in 1988 by James Watson, initiating a worldwide coordinated research activity to sequence the DNA of humans and several other test organisms. In the United States, the (DOE) initially, and the NIH soon thereafter, were the main research agencies within the U.S. government responsible for developing and planning the project. By 1988, the two agencies were working together, a relationship that was formalized by the signing of a Memorandum of Understanding to "coordinate research and technical activities related to the human genome." The initial planning process culminated in 1990 with the publication of a joint research plan.

The HGP started in 1990 as a 15-year program. One of its main coordinators was Dr. Francis Collins, Director of the National Human Genome Research Institute (NHGRI) at the NIH. Soon, the Human Genome Organization (HUGO) spread to Europe and Japan to coordinate the research performed in other countries outside of the United States. The HGP was an international research program designed to construct detailed genetic and physical maps of the human genome, to determine the complete nucleotide sequence of human DNA, and to localize the estimated 50,000–100,000 genes within the human genome. The similar analyses on the genomes of several model organisms were also planned to be performed.

The scientific products of the HGP were suggested to comprise a resource of detailed information about the structure, organization, and function of human DNA, information that constitutes the basic set of inherited "*instructions*" for the development and functioning of a human being. Achievement of the ambitious aims of HGP would demand the development of new technologies and necessitate advanced means of disseminating information widely to scientists, physicians, and others in order that the results may be rapidly used for the public good. Important for the success of the HGP was the statement that a fraction of the project money should be devoted to the ethical, legal, and social implications of human genetic research.

It was clearly recognized that acquisition and use of such genetic knowledge would have momentous implications for both individuals and society and would pose several policy choices for public and professional deliberation. The HUGO program aims at a detailed understanding of the organization of the human genome, to enable a molecular definition of the basis for normal function as well as genetic disorders affecting human cells and the organism as a whole. An intermediate aim in this program was the construction of a high-resolution physical map for the human genome. At the beginning of this work, with sequencing still slow and expensive, the HGP adopted a "map-first, sequence later strategy." In the early 1990s, two Parisian laboratories, the Centre d'Etude du Polymorphisme Humain and Genethon, had an integral role in mapping of the human genome. The laboratories' driving forces were Drs. Daniel Cohen and Jean Weissenbach.

Later the genome project constructed a higher resolution map that was used to sequence and assemble the human genome. In July 1995, a team led by Dr. J. Craig Venter published the first sequence of a free-living organism, *Haemophilis influenzae*. In October 1996, an international consortium publicly released the complete genome sequence of the yeast *Saccharomyces cerevisiae*. In May 1998, Venter announced a new company named Celera and declared that it will sequence the human genome within 3 years for $300 million. In December 1998, Drs. John Sulston, Robert Waterston, and colleagues completed the genomic sequence of *Caenorhabditis elegans* (100 Mb). The first complete human chromosome sequence—number 22 (33.Mb)—was published in December 1999, and in June 2000, leaders of the public project and Celera announced completion of a working draft of the human genome sequence. Finally, in February 2001, the HGP consortium published its working draft of the human genome sequence in *Nature* and Celera published its draft in *Science* (2.9 billion bp).

Description of the Main Types of Vectors Used in the HGP

In this section, common vectors used for everyday cloning and subcloning like plasmid and M13 vectors will not be discussed. Only vectors suitable for cloning relatively large DNA inserts will be mentioned with the exception of lambda phage-based vectors specially designed to clone cDNA.

Lambda-Based Vectors and Main Approaches to Construct Genomic Libraries

Numerous modifications have been made to bacteriophage lambda-based vectors to facilitate their handling and to extend their use for new types of biological experiments. The application of each vector is usually limited to a specific task: the construction of general genomic libraries that contain all genomic DNA fragments or special genomic libraries that contain only a particular subset of genomic DNA fragments. Among these special libraries, NotI linking and jumping libraries have particular value for physical and genetic mapping of the human genome.

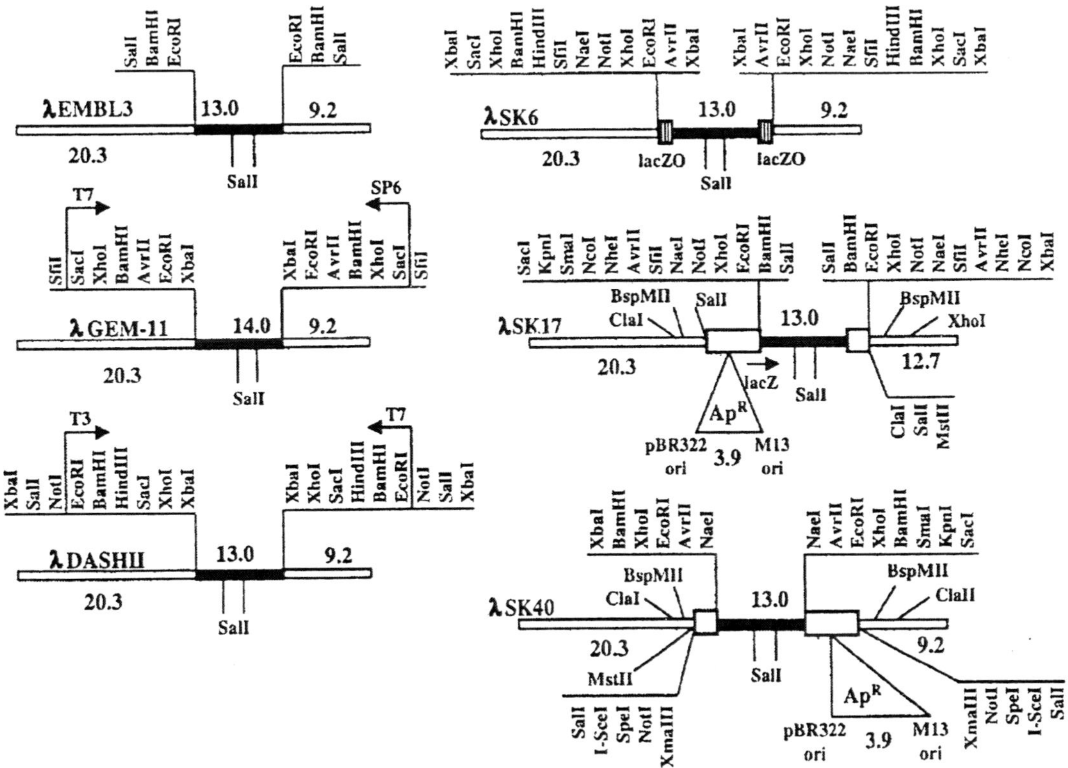

Fig. 12.1. Examples of vectors used for construction of genomic libraries.

Despite their obvious advantages for special purposes, novel vectors (YACs, BACs, PACs) cannot compete with lambda-based vectors for ease of handling, screening, amplification, and biological flexibility, due to the almost complete knowledge about phage lambda genes and biology. The easiest way to obtain a maximal proportion of recombinant molecules is to perform ligation at a high concentration of vector and insert (genomic) DNA because an elevated concentration of DNA facilitates intermolecular ligation instead of self-ligation of the vector's molecules. In this case, the main product is long DNA chains (>200 kbp) containing many copies of vector and genomic DNA fragments. Extremely efficient *in vitro* systems for packaging such DNA into lambda phage particles (10^9 plaque-forming units per microgram of DNA) to produce viable phages were developed and are commercially available. Extensive modifications of lambda phage vectors were developed that combine the features of different vector systems.

Cosmids are essentially plasmids that contain the *cos* region of phage lambda responsible for packaging of DNA into the phage particle. Any DNA molecule, containing this region and having a size between 37.7 kb and 52.9 kb, can be packaged into phage particles and introduced into the *E.*

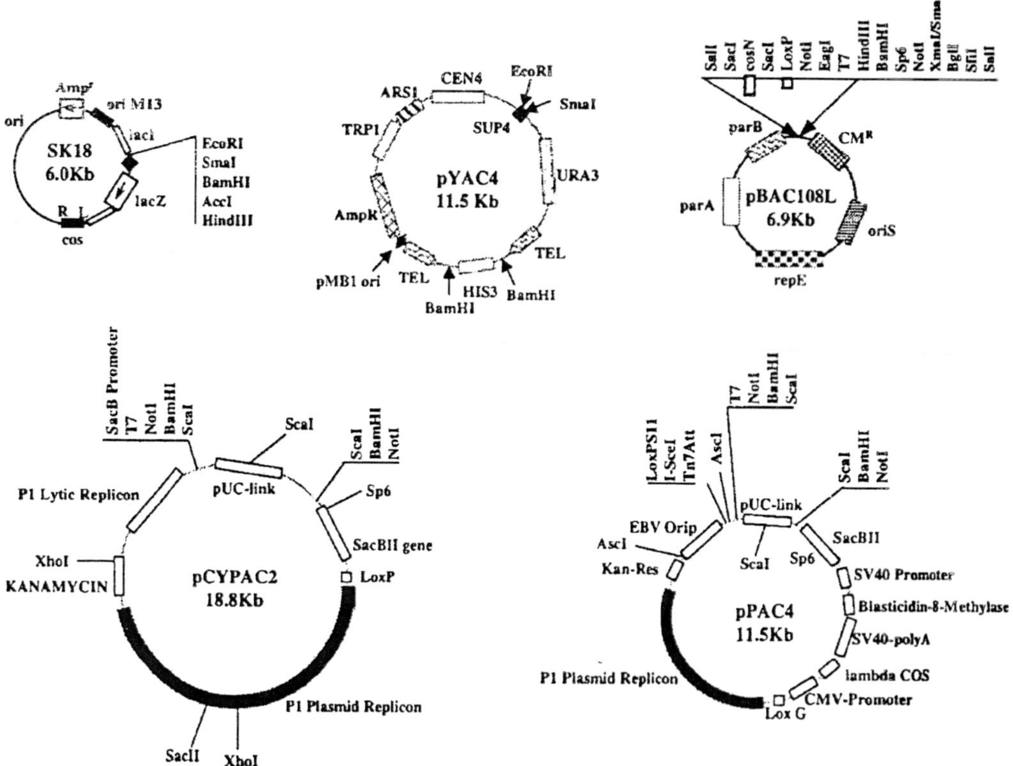

Fig. 12.2. Examples of vectors used for construction of genomic libraries (capacity more then 45 kb).

coli. The advantages of cosmids are their easy handling (as with plasmids) and big cloning capacity. As the plasmid body is usually small (3-6 kb), large DNA molecules (46-49 kb) can be cloned in these vectors.

Phasmids are lambda phages that have an inserted plasmid. They have the same basic features as lambda phage vectors, but inserted DNA fragment can be separated from the phage arms DNA and converted into a plasmid form. There are two main ways for such conversion: biological and enzymatic. In the first case, the phasmid vector contains signal sequences bordering the insert and plasmid body in the phage vehicle. These signal sequences (e.g., from P1, lambda, M13 phages) can be recognized by specific proteins (e.g., *cre*-recombinase), and the cloned DNA fragment together with plasmid body will be cut out.

The enzymatic conversion can occur if the inserted DNA fragment and plasmid sequences are placed between two recognition sequences of some rare-cutting restriction endonuclease (e.g., I-SceI enzyme that recognize 18 bp and probably does not have any recognition site in the human genomic DNA). This enzyme can be used to separate the cloned DNA fragment together with the plasmid sequences from phage arms. Self-ligation of the molecules with insert and plasmid sequences will result in the production of a recombinant plasmid that can be introduced into the *E. coli* host.

Diphasmids combine the advantages of lambda and M13 phages, and plasmids, i.e., the three main types of vectors used in everyday molecular cloning. They can be divided into two classes: (1) diphasmids that can replicate as phage lambda (a further improvement of phasmids); and (2) diphasmids that are not able to replicate as phage lambda, i.e., a cosmid that can be packaged into phage M13 particles.

In some cases, it is more convenient to work with a genomic library in plasmid than in lambda phage form. The construction of representative genomic library directly in a plasmid vector has several drawbacks and difficulties. However, these problems can be easily solved with the help of phasmid and diphasmid vectors. In this case, a genomic library is constructed in lambda phage (e.g., SK40), and then the whole library is converted to plasmid form.

Although the work with different lambda-based vectors is very similar, vectors for construction of genomic and cDNA libraries still have some special features. The major difference between cDNA and genomic cloning is the size of insert: short for cDNA and long for genomic fragments. Due to this difference, it is obvious that the enzymatic way of transferring inserts into the plasmid form is more dangerous (with the respect to the representativity of the library) for genomic libraries than for cDNA, because the probability that the insert contains a recognition site for the particular restriction enzyme increases with the length of the DNA insert. Most of cDNA vectors are "insertion" vectors, and genomic vectors are "substitution" vectors, which means that inserted foreign DNA fragments replace the stuffer vector fragment that does not have any important replicative function.

Full-length cDNAs are the most important material for the identification of all human genes. Cloning of full-length cDNA inserts has been hampered by problems related to both the preparation and the cloning of long cDNAs. Part of the difficulty associated with the preparation of long cDNAs has been overcome with the introduction of a thermostabilized and thermoactivated reverse transcriptase and the development of cap-based full-length cDNA selecting techniques. In contrast to standard cloning techniques, full-length cDNA cloning has the inherent risk of the under-representation or absence of clones corresponding to long mRNAs in the libraries, because the truncated cDNAs are usually not cloned. However, even in a perfect full-length cDNA library, cDNAs deriving from very long mRNAs will not be cloned if the capacity of the vector is insufficient. The most available cloning vectors show bias for short cDNAs: Shorter fragments are cloned more efficiently than the longer because of the intermolecular competition that occurs at the ligation and library amplification steps. To solve this problem, substitution vectors for cDNA cloning were designed.

For conversion into the plasmid form, the biochemical approach for SK-vectors was used. Some vectors, like SK16 and SK17, have a cloning capacity of 0.2– 15.4 kb and others, for example SK23, could be used for cloning of 3.7–18.9-kb inserts only. These cDNA vectors retain the most important advantages of the genomic vectors, e.g., the possibility of biochemical selection when producing vector arms and genetic selection against nonrecombinant phages. Importantly, the libraries made in some of these SK-vectors can be used as both expressed and nonexpressed libraries. For instance, libraries constructed in SK16 would be expressed only in *E. coli* strains containing *ochre*-codon mutation, and SK17 has *amber*-codon-controlled expression of cDNA.

In lambda FLC (full-length cDNA cloning), cloning capacity is either 0.2–15.4 kb or 5.7–20.9 kb. In these vectors, *cre*-recombinase mediated excision was used. The average size of the inserts from excised plasmid cDNA libraries was 2.9 kb for standard and 6.9 kb for size-selected cDNA. The average insert size of the full- length cDNA libraries was correlated to the rate of new gene discovery, suggesting that effectively cloning rarely expressed mRNAs requires vectors that can accommodate large inserts from a variety of sources without bias for cloning short cDNA inserts.

One of the most important features of a genomic library is a representativity. A representative genomic library means that every genomic DNA fragments will be present at least in one of the recombinant phages of the library. In practice, however, this is difficult to achieve. Some genomic fragments are not clonable because of the strategy used for construction of the genomic library. In other cases, genomic DNA fragments (contain poison sequences) can suppress the growth of the vector or the host cell so its cloning can be restricted to specific vector systems. The important reason for the decreased representativity is different replication potential of different recombinant vectors. Thus, amplified libraries have significantly worse representativity. Usually a library is considered to be representative if after the first plating (before amplification) it contains several recombinant clones together containing genomic DNA fragments equal to a 7–10 genome equivalent. The way in which the genomic DNA fragments are produced for cloning is also important. The more randomly the genomic DNA is broken, the more the representative library can be obtained. Clearly, the EcoRI enzyme (6-bp recognition site) will cut genomic DNA less randomly than Sau3AI (4 bp recognition). Probably, the shearing of DNA molecules using physical methods (sonication, shearing using syringe) is the most reliable way to obtain randomly broken DNA molecules. There are many different modifications to construct libraries; however, the three ways to construct genomic libraries are the most commonly used and will be exemplified below using genomic lambda-based vectors.

The classic method includes generation of sheared genomic DNA fragments using physical or enzymatic fragmentation followed by the physical separation of fragments of a particular size using, for example, ultra-centrifugation or gel-electrophoresis. The vector DNA is digested with two (or even three) restriction enzymes; those recognition sites are located in the polylinker. The arms and the stuffer fragment are purified, and on the further steps, arms/stuffer would be not able to ligate because they have different sticky ends, preventing recreation of the original vector molecules during subsequent ligation with genomic DNA fragments. In the "dephosphorylation" approach, the phage arms are prepared as described above. Genomic DNA is partially digested to obtain DNA fragments with sizes in the desired range; i.e., for the lambda vectors FIXII and SK6, it is 15–22 kb. These DNA fragments are dephosphorylated (which prevents their ligation to each other) and then ligated to the vector arms.

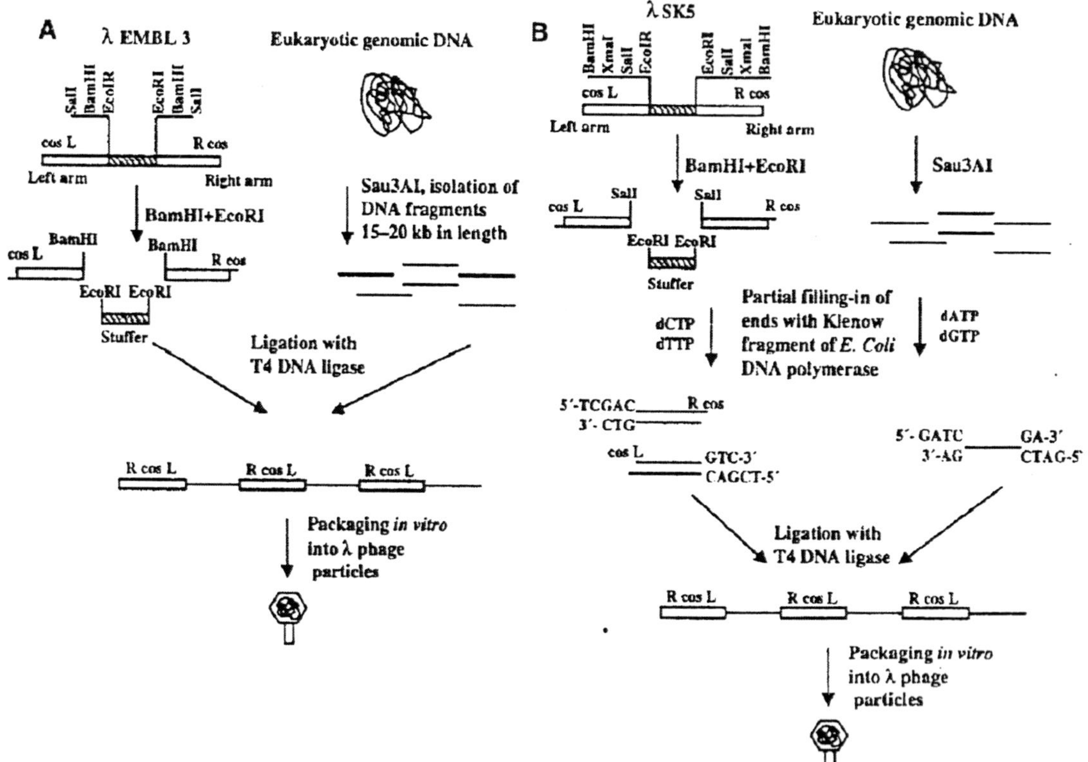

Fig. 12.3. Two main approaches for construction of genomic libraries: (a) classic method and (b) partial filling-in method.

The third, "partial filling in" method, also avoids fractionation steps. Phage arms are prepared by double digestion as described before (in this particular case, SalI and EcoRI are shown, but many other combinations can be used), and the sticky-ends produced after digestion are partially filled-in with the Klenow fragment of DNA polymerase I (or other DNA polymerase) in the presence of dTTP and dCTP. Genomic DNA partially digested with Sau3AI is also partially filled-in but in the presence dATP and dGTP. Under these conditions, self-ligation of vector arms or genomic DNA is impossible.

YACs

The mapping and analysis of complex genomes require vectors that allow cloning and work with large DNA fragments. Lambda-based vectors have many advantages as described above; however, a comparatively small size of inserts (maximum 48– 49 kb) complicates the use of these vectors for the mapping of complex genomes.

Technological improvements made the cloning of large DNA pieces possible using artificially constructed chromosome vectors that carry human DNA fragments as large as 1Mb. Such vectors are maintained in yeast cells as artificial chromosomes (YACs). YAC methodology drastically reduces the number of clones to be ordered; many YACs span entire human genes. A more detailed map of a large YAC insert can be produced by subcloning, a process in which fragments of the original insert are cloned into smaller insert vectors. YAC cloning was widespread, and many laboratories used this technique to obtain large cloned DNA fragments from different eukaryotic genomes.

One of the most widely used YAC vectors was pYAC4, and it has the main features of the YAC vectors. This vector can replicate in *E. coli* and in yeast (*S. cerevisiae*). It consists of five important genetic elements inserted into *E. coli* pBR322-like plasmid:

1. Centromeric *CEN4* sequences required for centromere function.
2. Autonomous replicating sequences *ARS1* that are necessary for replication in yeast.
3. Telomere sequences from *Tetrahymena* ribosomal DNA (rDNA) that seed the formation of functional telomeres at high efficiency.
4. Selective marker for cloning, *S UP4* (*ochre*-suppressing allele of tyrosine tRNA gene). As cloning EcoRI and SmaI sites are located inside *SUP4*, insertion of any large DNA fragment into the cloning sites will inactivate *ochre* suppression function.
5. Two yeast selectable markers: wild-type genes *TRP1* and *URA3*, which are located on opposite sides of the cloning sites.

The yeast *HIS3* gene is just a stuffer fragment to separate two arms. The general scheme of the library construction is as follows.

The pYAC4 DNA is double digested with BamHI and SmaI (or EcoRI) to generate three fragments: left chromosomal arm containing *TEL*, *TRP1*, *ARS1*, and *CEN4* and right chromosomal arm with *TEL* and *URA3*. *HIS3* gene is discarded during the cloning procedure. The two arms are treated with alkaline phosphatase to prevent self-ligation and ligated with genomic DNA (usually) partially digested. The ligation product is transformed into yeast and selected for complementation of a mutated *ura3* gene present in yeast strain by the *URA3* gene in the vector. The grown transformants are selected for complementation of a host *trp1* mutated gene by the wild-type *TRP1* gene from the vector.

This double selection is necessary to ensure the presence in a recombinant YAC of both left and right arms and inactivation of the *SUP4* gene. *SUP4* is an especially useful cloning marker because in an *ade2-ochre* host, the cells with the functional *SUP4* gene are white and those in which the suppressor was inactivated form red colonies.

Using YAC vectors, several important genes were identified and cloned, e.g., *VHL*, *CDPX1*, *GART*, *and SON*. Moreover, the first physical map covering the whole human genome was constructed with

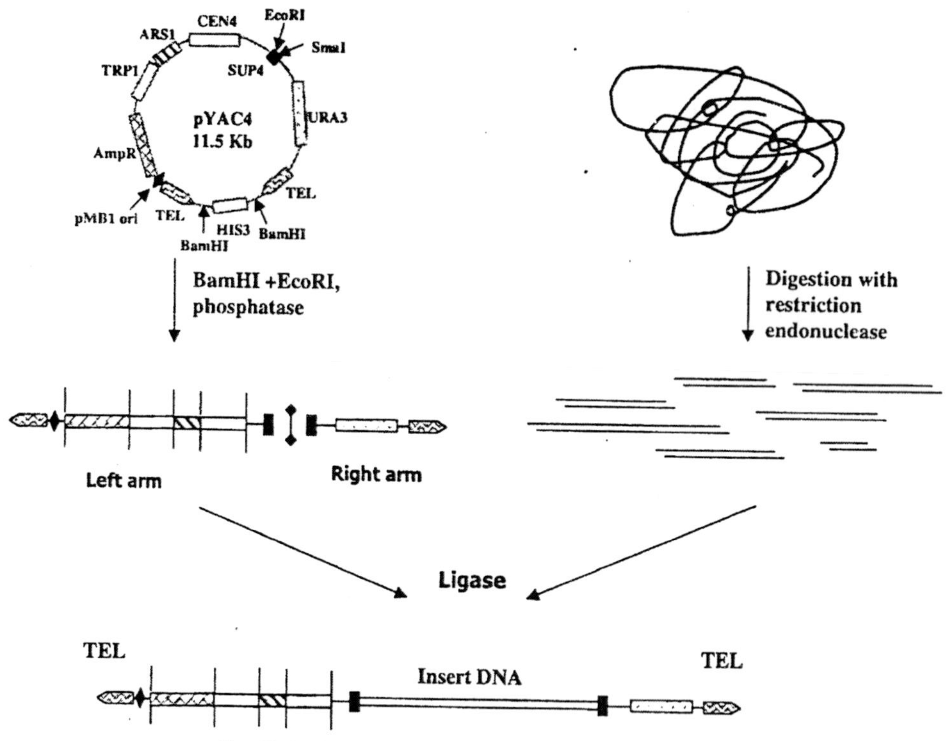

Fig. 12.4. Construction of genomic library in YAC vectors.

YAC contigs. Although YACs greatly contributed to the progress in long-range mapping of the human genome, the construction of YAC contigs is not free from problems— certain regions of the human genome are difficult to clone in YACs. Moreover, repeat rich human sequences cloned in YACs are frequently unstable in yeast. Low transformation efficiency, the presence of an abundance of chimeric clones in nearly all YAC libraries, insert instability, and difficulties in DNA manipulation relative to bacterial systems are other important limitations. Efforts to overcome the limitations of cosmids and YACs resulted in alternative large-insert cloning approaches using bacteriophage P1-based vectors and vectors based on the *E. coli* fertility plasmid (F-factor).

Bacterial (BAC) and P1-derived (PAC) Artificial Chromosome Vectors

BACs represent the state-of-the-art technology for such large-insert DNA library development. It has been demonstrated that BAC libraries are invaluable and desirable genetic resources for all kinds of modern structural, functional, and evolutionary genomics research. Genome-wide, as well as regional, physical maps of the human genome from BACs have been developed in different laboratories.

The BAC system is based on the well-studied *E. coli* F factor. Replication of the F factor in *E. coli* is strictly controlled. The F plasmid is maintained in low copy number (one or two copies per cell), thus reducing the potential for recombination between DNA fragments carried by the plasmid. Furthermore, F factors carrying inserted bacterial DNA are capable of maintaining fragments as large as 1 mega-base pair, suggesting that the F factor is suitable for cloning of large DNA fragments. Individual clones of human DNA seem to be maintained with a high degree of structural stability in the host, even after 100 generations of serial growth.

The F factor not only codes for genes that are essential to regulate its own replication but also controls its copy number. The regulatory genes include *oriS*, *repE*, *parA*, and *parB*. The *oriS* and repE genes mediate the unidirectional replication of the F factor, whereas *parA* and *parB* maintain a copy number at a level of one or two per *E. coli* genome. The BAC vector (pBAC108L) incorporates these essential genes as well as a chloramphenicol resistance marker and a cloning segment. The cloning segment includes (1) the bacteriophage lambda cosN and phage P1 loxP sites, (2) two cloning sites (HindIII and BamHI), and (3) several CG-rich restriction enzyme sites (Not I, Eag I, Xma I, Sma I, Bgl I, and SfiI) for potential excision of the inserts. The cloning site is flanked by T7 and SP6 promoters for generating RNA probes for chromosome walking and for DNA sequencing of the inserted segment at the vector–insert junction. The cosN site provides a fixed position for specific cleavage with the bacteriophage lambda terminase. The loxP site can be used similarly. In this case, P1 Cre protein catalyzes the cleavage reaction in the presence of the loxP oligonucleotide. These sites (cosN and loxP) allow convenient generation of ends that can be used for restriction-site mapping to arrange the clones in an ordered array. Restriction maps of the individual clones can be determined by indirect end-labeling and subsequent partial digestion.

PAC vectors combine the best features of the P1 and BAC systems. One of the most commonly used PAC vectors is pCYPAC2 that was constructed for the cloning of large DNA fragments using electroporation. Previously developed P1-based vectors (like pAd10SacBII) employed bacteriophages P1 or T4 *in vitro* packaging systems, enabling the cloning of recombinants with inserts in the 70–120-kb range. The pCYPAC2 vector was constructed by removing the stuffer fragment from the pAd10SacBII vector and by inserting a pUC19 plasmid into the BamHI cloning site. During the cloning process, the pUC19 sequences are removed through a double-digestion scheme using BamHI and ScaI. Religation of the pUC19 and producing of nonrecombinant clones is prevented at three levels, as follows:

1. pUC19 is cleaved into two ScaI fragments. ScaI sticky ends are not compatible with BamHI.
2. Oligonucleotides BamHI–ScaI connecting vector sequences with the stuffer fragment are physically removed from the vector and stuffer fragments.
3. pCYPAC2 fragments are treated with alkaline phosphatase to inhibit self-ligation.

NotI sites are flanking inserts that make it possible to obtain an insert that is fragment free from the vector sequences.

Different modifications of original BAC and PAC vectors were constructed, e.g., capable of replicating in human cells too. These vectors, e.g., pPAC4 and pBACe4, facilitate the use of large-insert bacterial clones for functional analysis and contain two additional genetic elements that enable stable maintenance of the clones in mammalian cells:

1. The Epstein–Barr virus replicon, *oriP*. It was included to ensure stable episomal propagation of the large insert clones upon transfection into mammalian cells.
2. The blasticidin deaminase gene is placed in a eukaryotic expression cassette to enable selection for the desired mammalian clones by using the nucleoside antibiotic blasticidin.

Sequences important to select for loxP-specific genome targeting in mammalian chromosomes were also inserted into the vectors. In addition, the attTn7 sequence present on the vectors permits specific addition of selected features to the library clones. Unique sites have also been included in the vector to enable linearization of the large-insert clones, e.g., for optical mapping studies. The pPAC4 vector has been used to generate libraries from the human, mouse, and rat genomes.

Libraries constructed in lambda-based, BAC, and PAC vectors are widely used now in different laboratories, and almost nobody is currently working with libraries constructed in YAC vectors.

Mapping of the Human Genome

As mentioned in the Introduction, mapping of the human genome was a major step in achieving the complete human genome sequence. Human genome maps were also important by themselves because they led to the isolation of many disease genes. The 3 billion bp in the human genome are organized into 24 distinct, physically separate microscopic units called chromosomes. All genes are arranged linearly along the chromosomes. The nucleus of most human cells contains two sets of chromosomes, one set given by each parent. Each set has 23 single chromosomes—22 autosomes and an X or Y sex chromosome. A normal female will have a pair of X chromosomes; a male will have an X and Y pair. Chromosomes contain roughly equal parts of protein and DNA, and chromosomal DNA contains on average 150 million bases.

In general, all maps can be divided in two main classes: genetic and physical. The genetic map is based on the frequency of recombination between two genetic markers on the chromosome. In fact, such a map just shows how these two markers are "linked" in respect to the frequency of recombination. Physical maps are based on physical distances between markers. Recombination frequencies define a genetic distance that is not the same as a physical distance. Two loci that show 1% recombination are defined as being 1 centimorgan (cM) apart on a genetic map. However, for distances above about 5 cM, human genetic map distances are not simple statements of the recombination fraction between pairs of loci. Loci that are 40 cM apart will show less than 40% recombination. This result reflects that recombination fractions never exceed 50% no matter how far apart are the loci. The female genetic map is larger than male due to a larger frequency of recombination. In general, for the whole human genome, the sex- averaged figure is 1 cM = 0.9 Mb, but the actual correspondence varies very significantly in different chromosomal regions. Usually there are more recombinations toward the telomeres of chromosomes and less toward the centromeres.

The value of the genetic map is that an the inherited disease can be located to the particular chromosomal region exploiting the inheritance of a DNA marker present in affected individuals (but absent in unaffected individuals), even though the molecular basis of the disease may not yet be understood nor the responsible gene identified. Genetic maps have been used to find the exact chromosomal location of several important disease genes, including cystic fibrosis, sickle cell disease, Tay-Sachs disease, fragile X syndrome, and myotonic dystrophy. Currently, some genetic linkage maps contain more than 100,000 polymorphic markers.

Different types of physical maps are based on different techniques. For instance, the cytogenetic map is based on detection chromosomal bands, and an average band has from one to several Megabase of DNA. Chromosomal breakpoint maps can be based on somatic cell hybrid panels containing human chromosome fragments derived from natural translocation or deletion chromosomes. The resolution for such maps is usually several Megabases. Monochromosomal radiation hybrid (RH) maps have a distance between breakpoints that is often several Mega- bases long. Whole genome RH maps have much higher resolution and can be as high as 0.5 Mb. The RH maps were very important for joining genetic and physical maps. They are based on *in vitro* radiation-induced chromosome fragmentation and cell fusion (merging human with other cells from other species to form hybrid cells) to create panels of cells with specific and varied human chromosomal components. Assessing the frequency of marker sites remaining together after radiation- induced DNA fragmentation can establish the order and distance between the markers.

Very useful were clone contig maps that could be constructed with YAC (or BAC, PAC) clones, and in this case, the average DNA insert has several hundred kilobases of DNA. If such a clone contig map was created using overlapping cosmid clones (average insert is 40–45 kb), the quality of such a map is signifi- cantly higher. A restriction map created with rare-cutting restriction enzymes like NotI can be very useful to check RH or clone contig maps.

A sequence-tagged site (STS) map requires prior sequence information and is based on mapping short known sequences using PCR amplification.

An expressed sequence tag (EST) map is based on STSs that were generated from cDNA. DNA fragments are called DNA markers after they were mapped to particular chromosomal regions. Such DNA markers are prerequisites for physical and genetic mapping of the genome. DNA markers are also important in the diagnosis of genetic diseases. DNA markers can be divided into several different classes depending on the way in which the markers were selected among the fragments of genomic DNA. Examples of such classes are anonymous, micro- and minisatellites, restriction fragment length polymorphism (RFLP) markers, *NotI* linking clones, ESTs, STSs, and so on. Another strategy of mapping is based on the completely different principle of NotI jumping and linking libraries. A big advantage to using chromosome jumping and linking clones is that they are small-insert vectors and mapping with these clones can be completely automated.

The basic principle of jumping is to clone only the ends of large DNA fragments rather than a continuous DNA segment. The DNA between two ends is deleted with the different biochemical techniques, and clones containing only the ends of a large DNA molecule are enriched by the mean of genetic or biochemical selection. In general, jumping clones contain DNA sequences adjacent to neighboring NotI restriction sites, and linking clones contain DNA sequences surrounding the same NotI restriction site. A NotI jumping library is a collection of cloned DNA fragments that contains the ends of large NotI genomic DNA fragments. A NotI linking library is a collection of cloned genomic DNA fragments flanking the same NotI site. Basically, a linking library in combination with pulsed field gel electrophoresis (PFGE) is sufficient to construct a physical chromosomal map. When linking clones are used to probe a PFGE genomic blot, each clone should reveal two DNA fragments, and they must be adjacent in the genome. In principle, with just a single library and digest, one should be able to order the rare cutting sites, but in reality, it is not possible because many fragments could have the same size. Using these two types of libraries, it is possible to move fast along the chromosome because the human genome contains a limited number of recognition sites for this enzyme (10,000–15,000). The easiest way to establish the order of NotI sites is a shotgun sequencing of NotI linking and jumping clones.

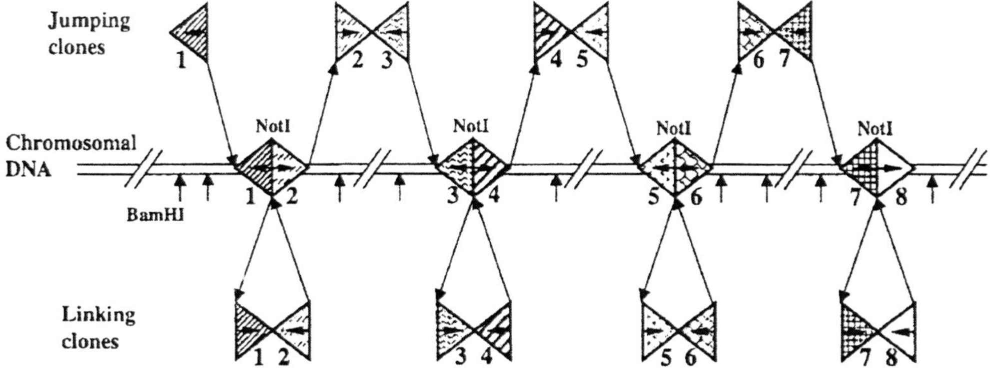

Fig. 12.5. General scheme of long-range mapping using jumping and linking libraries.

To construct linking libraries, genomic DNA is completely digested with BamHI. (Libraries can also be constructed with BglII, EcoRI, etc., but not with frequently cutting enzymes like MboI or infrequently cutting enzymes like SalI.) Subsequently, the DNA is self-ligated at a low concentration of DNA (without a *supF* marker), to yield circular molecules as the main product. To eliminate any remaining linear molecules, the sticky ends are partly filled-in with the Klenow fragment in the presence of dATP and dGTP (this is for the genomic DNA digested with BamHI; for other enzymes, partial filling-in with other nucleotides should be used). This way, all BamHI sticky ends will be neutralized and nearly all ends originated from linear molecules will be unavailable for ligation. Resulting DNA fragments are digested with NotI and cloned into λSK4, λSK17, and λSK22 vectors. These vectors permit the cloning of DNA fragments from 0.2 to 24 kb. The resulting phage particles are used to infect *E. coli* cells in which only recombinant phages could grow (spi-selection).

To construct the NotI jumping library, the same DNA and vectors can be used. However, the first steps are different. High-molecular-weight DNA is digested with NotI and circularized at very low DNA concentration (0.1 $\mu g/\mu L$). Other steps were the same.

The libraries can be converted into plasmid form, and sequences flanking NotI sites can be generated with standard sequencing primers. This sequence information can be used for generation of sequence tagged sites (STS). It was also demonstrated that the sequencing of these clones is a very efficient method for gene isolation because even short nucleotide sequences (approximately 500 bp from each side) flanking NotI sites are sufficient to detect genes. This approach was used for isolation of numerous new genes. The reason for this linkage of NotI sites and genes is the localization of practically all NotI sites in the CpG islands, which are tightly associated with genes.

A shotgun sequencing approach useful for the whole genome mapping was proposed for NotI linking and jumping libraries constructed in λSK17 and λSK22 vectors using an integrated approach. This strategy was based on the fact that NotI sites in both libraries were available for the sequencing with standard sequencing primers, and sequence information about 800–1000 bp surrounding each NotI site could be easily obtained by automated sequencing. Plasmid DNA could be isolated automatically, and thousands of clones could be sequenced. Subsequently the linear order of the NotI clones can be established using a computer program.

NotI linking and jumping libraries were very important for the mapping of two regions in the short arm of chromosome 3 and isolation of tumor suppressor genes from the AP20 and LUCA regions (*RASSF1*, *G21*, *SEMA4B*, *RBSP3*, etc.).

Main Approaches to Sequence Human Genome

Hierarchical and the Whole Genome Shotgun Sequencing Scheme (WGS)

The international public (HGP) and American private (Celera) efforts to determine the sequence of the human genome exploited different approaches. It is still not clear whether Celera's whole genome shotgun sequencing (WGC) approach was really efficient as they used publicly available data and it is not known to what extent. The major points in the hierarchical or HGP approach are as follows:

1. To construct a precise high-density STS map of the human genome. This map was integral and included not only STS but also genetic, microsatellite, FISH, and all other available mapping information.
2. To construct the clone contig of overlapping BAC and PAC clones. This contig was created and checked using a map constructed at the first step.
3. Each BAC or PAC clone was sequenced using a shotgun sequencing strategy. These sequences were assembled into the draft human genome sequence.

The shotgun sequencing approach for sequencing relatively small inserts was developed a long time ago. This method is based on the building of a complete insert sequence by randomly sequencing clones with overlapping inserts. To do this the insert DNA is subjected to partial digestion with a 4-bp cutter (like MboI) and the partially overlapping fragments are cloned at random into a suitable M13 or plasmid vector and sequenced. The sequence data obtained are fed into a computer programmed to detect overlaps between sequences and to assemble a composite sequence. Inevitably, this means a waste of efforts: The same sequence will be obtained over and over again.

Celera used a variant of this strategy that it named WGS. Central to the WGS strategy is preparation of high-quality plasmid libraries in a variety of insert sizes so that pairs of sequence reads (mates) are obtained; one is read from both ends of each plasmid insert. High-quality libraries have an equal representation of all parts of the genome and are constructed in three different sizes: 2 kb, 10 kb, and 50 kb. The method also involved end sequencing of some PAC clones that were carefully mapped. DNA fragments in these small-insert clones were generated by physical shearing of whole genomic DNA. According to the original predictions, this method requires the generation of sequences covering the whole genome not more than seven times.

The HGP and Celera announced that they have obtained a sequence of 92–97% of the human genome sequence and that a 7–10-fold genome sequence coverage is enough to generate an almost complete sequence for any human or mammalian genome. After 5 years, the scientific community understood that these estimations were overstated, and even now when more than 10-fold genome sequence coverage was achieved, the human genome sequence is far from being complete.

An important point of both approaches is that the genome should be covered by sequences at least 10 times to yield contigs covering a significant part of the genome. If the coverage is not extensive enough, then sequences and clones will represent unconnected and unordered islands. Thus, despite impressive progress, mapping and sequencing even of small genomes, like from one bacterial strain, is still expensive and laborious. As a result, genome mapping and sequencing efforts need to be concentrated to big centers, and independent work by smaller groups is seriously hampered.

Partly in view of these logistic and economic limitations, HGP and Celera approaches may not be the optimal solution, especially for several experiments addressing biocomplexity. After completion of one sequence from an organism, in many cases there will be a great demand for comparison with other individuals, related species, pathogenic and nonpathogenic strains, and so on, in the growing field of comparative genomics. Such comparisons will be highly relevant for the better understanding of health, evolution, and ecology questions but must be performed by laboratories receiving considerably less funding than those involved in the recent high-profile sequencing efforts. Another area is a sequencing of related bacterial strains and species in order to identify the genomic basis of their biological differences and their interactions within the human intestinal flora. What is a difference between pathogenic and nonpathogenic members of the gut flora?

The whole genome sequencing will be performed only for the selected organisms. However, analysis of disease genes in other species may be extremely useful for the understanding of fundamental processes, leading to development of disease.

As the body of knowledge concerning the genome structure and genes in different organisms grows, it also becomes unnecessary to collect total sequences with 10–15-fold coverage for all organisms that would be interesting to study.

One of the most perspective solutions for this problem is sequencing using microarrays. However, this approach will be not discussed here as it cannot be a strategy for the *de novo* sequencing. Two other alternative approaches that could be used for both the *de novo* and the comparative sequencing will be described below.

Massively Parallel Sequencing Approaches

The first publication using beads for massively parallel sequencing was published by Dr. Sydney Brenner et al. (2000). They described a novel sequencing approach that combined non-gel-based signature sequencing with *in vitro* cloning of millions of templates on separate 5-μM-diameter microbeads. After constructing a microbead library of DNA templates by *in vitro* cloning, a planar array of a million template-containing microbeads in a flow cell at a density greater than 3×10^6 microbeads/cm^2 was assembled. Sequences of the free ends of the cloned templates on each microbead were then simultaneously analyzed using a fluorescence-based signature sequencing method that does not require DNA fragment separation. Signature sequences of 16–20 bases were obtained by repeated cycles of enzymatic cleavage with a type IIs restriction endonuclease (BbvI), adaptor ligation, and sequence interrogation by encoded hybridization probes. The approach was validated by sequencing over 269,000 signatures from two cDNA libraries constructed from a fully sequenced strain of *S. cerevisiae*, and by measuring gene expression levels in the human cell line THP-1. This method is complicated and expensive and was used mainly for generation of SAGE tags.

Recently MPSS principles were applied for long-range sequencing. Dr. George Church and his colleagues introduced a sequencer that uses a microscope and other off-the-shelf equipment. With this technology, his team sequenced a strain of *E. coli* and could detect single-base-pair changes from an almost identical *E. coli* genome. The approach reduces sequencing costs by 90%. Dr. Jonathan Rothberg has demonstrated the power of another cost-cutting technology called "454". Using this approach, *Mycoplasma genitalium* was sequenced.

Both groups save money by eliminating the need for bacteria and miniaturizing the process wherever possible. Instead of bacteria, they attach DNA to aqueous beads encased in oil where PCR amplification was performed to produce the necessary amount of DNA. That change alone could reduce by two thirds the costs associated with space and personnel. Moreover, both perform many thousands of these sequencing reactions at once in miniature "reactors," decreasing the need for expensive chemicals. Once the DNA is ready, the two technologies diverge: The "454" technique uses pyrosequencing to identify the bases and Church's technique (MPS, multiplex polony sequencing) uses bursts of different fluorescent colors, one each to a particular base, to distinguish the bases (sequencing by ligation). Both use high-speed charge-coupled device cameras to record the labeled bases.

The "454" technique uses a novel fiber-optic slide of individual wells and can sequence 25 million bases, at 99% or better accuracy, in one 4-hour run. To achieve an approximately 100-fold increase in throughput over current Sanger sequencing technology, an emulsion method for DNA amplification and an instrument for sequencing by synthesis using a pyrosequencing protocol optimized for solid support and picolitre-scale volumes was developed. In a pilot experiment, 96% of the *M. genitalium* genome was covered by sequence contigs at 99.96% accuracy in one run of the machine. The method could potentially allow one individual to prepare and sequence an entire genome in a few days. The sequencer itself, equipped with a simple detection device and liquid delivery system, and housed in a casing roughly the size of a microwave oven, is actually relatively low-tech. The complexity of the system lies primarily in the sample preparation and in the microfabricated, massively parallel platform, which contains 1.6 million picoliter-sized reactors in a 6.4-cm^2 slide.

Sample preparation starts with fragmentation of the genomic DNA, followed by the attachment of adaptor sequences to the ends of the DNA pieces. The adaptors allow the DNA fragments to bind to tiny beads (around 28 μm in diameter). This is done under conditions that allow only one piece of DNA to bind to each bead. The beads are encased in droplets of oil that contain all reagents needed to amplify the DNA using a standard tool called the PCR. The oil droplets form part of an emulsion so that each bead is kept apart from its neighbor, ensuring the amplification is uncontaminated. Each bead ends up with roughly 10 million copies of its initial DNA fragment.

To perform the sequencing reaction, the DNA-template-carrying beads are loaded into the picoliter reactor wells—each well having space for just one bead. The technique uses a sequencing-by-synthesis method developed by Dr. Uhlen and colleagues, in which DNA complementary to each template strand is synthesized. The nucleotide bases used for sequencing release a chemical group as the base forms a bond with the growing DNA chain, and this group drives a light-emitting reaction in the presence of specific enzymes and luciferin. Sequential washes of each of the four possible nucleotides are run over the plate, and a detector senses which of the wells emit light with each wash to determine the sequence of the growing strand. This new system shows great promise in several sequencing applications, including resequencing and *de novo* sequencing of smaller bacterial and viral genomes. It could potentially allow research groups with limited resources to enter the field of large-scale DNA sequencing and genomic research, as it provides a technology that is inexpensive and easy to implement and maintain. However, this technology cannot yet replace the Sanger sequencing approach for some of the more demanding applications, such as sequencing a mammalian genome, as it has several limitations.

First, the technique can only read comparatively short lengths of DNA, averaging 80–120 bases per read, which is approximately a tenth of the read-lengths possible using Sanger sequencing. This means not only that more reads must be done to cover the same sequence, but also that assembling short reads into longer genomic sequences is a lot more complicated. This is particularly true when dealing with genomes containing long repetitive sequences.

Second, the accuracy of each read is not as good as with Sanger sequencing—particularly in genomic regions in which single bases are constantly repeated. Third, because the DNA "library" is currently prepared in a single-stranded format, unlike the double-stranded inserts of DNA libraries used for Sanger sequencing, the technique cannot generate paired-end reads for each DNA fragment. The paired-end information is crucial for assembling and orientating the individual sequence reads into a complete genomic map for *de novo* sequencing applications.

Finally, the sample preparation and amplification processes are still complex and will require automation and/or simplification.

In the MPS technique, sheared, size-selected genomic fragments (approximately 1 kb in size) were circularised with a linker bearing MmeI (type IIs restriction enzyme) recognition site (TCCRAC). Then all noncircularized material was destroyed with exonuclease and circular molecules were amplified using rolling circle amplification with random hexamers. Afterward, resulting material was digested with MmeI. MmeI digests at a distance of 18/20 or 19/21 from its recognition site. In the MPS protocol, MmeI digestion results in 17-bp or 18-bp tags of unique genomic sequence. A sharp band at approximately 70 bp was purified with 6% PAGE, and DNA ends were blunted and ligated to two adaptors of different lengths. The molecules with two different adaptors at their ends were again purified using 6% PAGE and PCR amplified. Then sharp bands at approximately 135 bp were purified on a 6% PAGE gel and emulsion PCR with 1-μm magnetic beads containing biotin labeled primer was performed. Millions of beads with amplified DNA fragments (paired tags) were immobilized in acrylamid-based gel system and a four-color sequencing by ligation was made. This method allowed to obtain 13-bp sequencing information per tag separated by a 4- to 5-bp gap (sequencing per each tag was done from both ends). Thus, 26-bp information per amplicon was obtained (2 tags $\times$ 13 bp). In a pilot experiment, this technology was applied to resequence an evolved strain of *E. coli*, and according to the estimation, this was done on less than a one-error-per-million consensus bases. In this pilot experiment, two deletion genomic fragments and several 1-bp substitutions were detected in the analyzed *E. coli* strain. Still, neither "454" nor the MPS method is up to speed yet. The accuracy of both should be improved by at least one order of magnitude. Also, to sequence mammalian genomes the length of sequence generated should be about 700 bases, but reads reported from these new approaches are between 26 and 110 bases.

Slalom Library: A Novel Approach to Genome Mapping and Sequencing

All described above sequencing approaches were based on sequencing of randomly generated DNA fragments. We recently suggested a completely different and efficient strategy for simultaneous genome mapping and sequencing. The approach was based on physically oriented, overlapping restriction fragment libraries called slalom libraries. Slalom libraries combined features of general genomic, jumping, and linking libraries. Slalom libraries could be adapted to different applications, and two main types of slalom libraries will be discussed below. This approach was used to map and sequence (with ~46% coverage) two human PAC clones, each of ~100 kb. This model experiment demonstrates the feasibility of the approach and shows that the efficiency (cost-effectiveness and speed) of existing mapping/sequencing methods could be improved at least 5-10-fold. Furthermore, as the efficiency of contig assembly in the slalom approach is virtually independent of length of sequence reads, even short sequences of 19–20 bp produced by rapid, high-throughput sequencing techniques would suffice to complete a physical map and a sequence scan of a small genome.

Two slalom libraries are used in the first type of approach. This approach allows us to construct contigs of plasmid clones covering a whole genome. However, these contigs will contain some gaps. Comparatively modest sequence information can be generated (20-25% of a genome). Using this technique, two (or more) bacterial strains (e.g., pathogenic and non pathogenic) could be quickly compared and pathogenic islands could be identified.

The main principle of the type I slalom libraries and looks similar to the computer-assisted long-range mapping with NotI linking and jumping clones. In this case, the role of NotI jumping library plays a standard EcoRI genomic (slalom "R") library that is produced by complete digestion of genomic DNA with EcoRI, and the role of a NotI linking library-EcoRI linking (slalom "BR") library. Slalom "BR" library is constructed in exactly the same way as a NotI linking library using BamHI as a second enzyme and fulfills the connecting function joining EcoRI fragments. Shortly, DNA is digested with BamHI, circularized and cut with EcoRI ("BR" library). Thus, EcoRI in this case plays the role of a NotI enzyme. Sequences from "BR" and "R" libraries are produced using standard reverse and forward sequencing primers and overlapping clones are found using a computer program. The homologies found will join the ends of EcoRI fragments in the "BR" library with the ends of EcoRI fragments in the "R" library to yield an ordered set of BamHI–EcoRI clones/STSs distributed along the genome. In reality, EcoRI sites and BamHI sites do not always alternate, and this will lead to the gaps in this set of overlapping clones, if several EcoRI or BamHI sites lie together. Thus, the genome will not be completely covered by clones because the information between some EcoRI and BamHI sites will be missing.

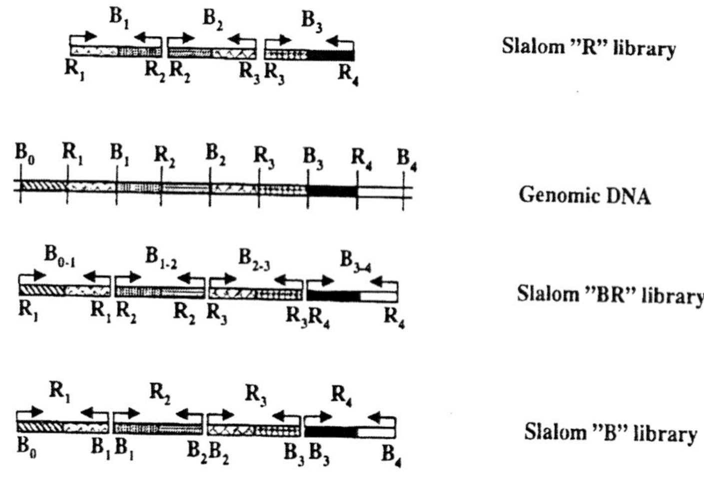

Fig. 12.6. The main idea of the slalom approach.

The problem with the gaps can be solved using the second variant of the slalom libraries (type II) where three libraries are used:

1. Standard, completely EcoRI digested (slalom "R") library
2. Standard, completely BamHI digested (slalom "B") library
3. EcoRI jumping (slalom "RBR" or connecting) library

This approach results in generation of plasmid clone contigs covering a whole genome without gaps. A large volume of sequencing information can be obtained (45–55% of a genome). The connecting library in this case is similar to a NotI jumping library. If the ultimate aim is to sequence the complete genome, then sequencing gaps could be filled-in using standard methods such as primer walking or transposon-mediated sequencing.

An "RBR" slalom library or EcoRI jumping library is prepared in the same way as a NotI jumping library using as a second enzyme BamHI. The only difference is that circularization after BamHI digestion is performed in the presence of a selective marker (e.g., Kan^R gene or oligonucleotide adaptor, etc.). The circular constructs are opened with EcoRI and cloned.

The "RBR" library can be constructed in a simpler way. Plasmid DNA isolated *en masse* from a slalom "R" library is digested with BamHI and circularized in the presence of Kan^R. Then *E. coli* cells are transformed with ligated DNA and plated on agar with kanamycin. The clones obtained in this manner will be identical in structure to the clones from an EcoRI jumping library prepared using the classic method.

By comparing the end sequences of the "B" library clones with the internal BamHI (from the marker fragment) sequences of the slalom "RBR" library clones, the BamHI clones can be positioned in relation to each other. After the comparison of end sequences in "R" and "RBR" libraries, EcoRI clones will be positioned relative to each other. Finally, EcoRI and BamHI clones will be assembled into a contig representing their organization in complete genome.

The EcoRI jumping library provides the connecting function in type II slalom libraries.

The major difference between the slalom library mapping/sequencing approach and other sequencing strategies is that the clones are generated according to a specific scheme and using complete digestion. As a result, the number of variants required to cover the whole genome decreases significantly. The preparation of libraries for the slalom approach is remarkably simple: Only complete digestion with EcoRI or BamHI is used. There is no need for size separation, agarose gel purification, or establishing conditions for partial shearing/digestion. There is no need to develop a new sequenator as any existing instrument can be used. Importantly, it is not necessary to keep all slalom clones because sequencing information can be used to design PCR primers and even large fragments (up to 40–50 kb) can be amplified by long-range PCR.

The slalom library approach differs fundamentally from the shotgun sequencing approach with respect to the efficiency of assembly (EOA). The EOA for the latter method is strictly dependent on the length of sequencing reads. The longer the reads, the higher the EOA. As the slalom approach uses nonrandom fractionation of the DNA and each start site is tightly linked with the recognition site for the restriction enzyme, even very short sequences will, in principle, be enough to create a contig of the overlapping clones. The EOA of the slalom library approach is, therefore, essentially independent of read-length. Even the short sequences generated by pyrosequencing, MPS, or MPSS should be sufficient to completely cover a genome. As one person can generate thousands of sequences a day using a pyrosequencer, the minimal set of overlapping clones covering a 4-Mb genome can be completed in a couple of days. Repeat sequences are in fact less of a problem for the slalom approach than for the shotgun sequencing approach for several reasons.

It is important to stress that the benefits of the slalom approach are most obvious in comparative sequencing experiments in combination with high-throughput techniques like pyrosequencing or MPSS (which are not com patible with the shotgun sequencing approach). Our particular experiments demonstrated that approximately 4% coverage would be enough to construct the contig of the overlapping clones and subsequently generate >20% ordered sequences with almost 100% efficiency, i.e., with 0.2-fold coverage.

Of course, closing of the gaps will be done with significantly lower efficiency. However, the finishing stages of the shotgun sequencing approach are also the most expensive and time-consuming part of the process. Lander et al. distinguished three types of gaps: gaps within unfinished sequenced clones; and gaps between sequenced clone contigs, but within fingerprint clone contigs; and gaps between fingerprint clone contigs. The first type is the simplest, and the third is the most complicated to close because constructing a contig of overlapping clones is the most difficult procedure. With the slalom approach, we already have a contig of overlapping clones, and thus, we will only suffer from the first, simplest type of gaps. It is important to mention another difference in the finishing stages of these two approaches. With the shotgun sequencing approach, sequences from different clones must be connected, and here highly related repeats, gene families, and polymorphisms will represent a major problem. These problems are nonexistent in the slalom approach, where a single insert should be sequenced.

The slalom strategy can increase several orders of magnitude the efficiency of mapping and sequencing, i.e., decrease the cost and labor, and increase the speed of sequencing project fullfillment. This strategy will allow the establishment of a physical map with a minimal set of overlapping clones that will pinpoint differences in genome organization between organisms. At the same time, a considerable sequence coverage (about 50%) of the genome at a less than onefold coverage will be achieved. This will make it possible to locate virtually every gene in a genome for more detailed study. The method makes it economically and logistically possible for a wide range of laboratories to gather the detailed information about large numbers of genomes. It offers a way to use genomics techniques for the study of biocomplexity, evolution, and taxonomy in the close future.

Identification of Genes

Many Approaches Exist for Gene Identification

The most important for the majority of research tasks is identification of genes in a particular region of the human genome. The different tissues in the body express information across a wide range, between less than 2000 (in specialized and terminally differentiated white blood cells) and more than 20,000 (in the placenta). Several methods were suggested previously for gene identification. Genomic DNA can be used as a probe to screen cDNA libraries. Different approaches were developed to capture cDNA clones using genomic DNA attached to a solid substrate (e.g., magnetic beads, nylon filters) as a target to that cDNA clones can hybridize. To identify genomic sequences that could be expressed as a special approach, exon trapping was suggested. For example, in the method of Church et al., the DNA is subcloned into a plasmid expression vector pSPL3 that contains an artificial minigene that can be expressed in a suitable host cell. The minigene consist of the following:

1. Segment of the simian virus 40 (SV40) genome that contains an origin of replication plus a powerful promoter sequence.
2. Two splicing-competent exons separated by an intron that contains a multiple cloning site (MCS).
3. SV40 polyadenylation site.

The recombinant DNA is transfected into a strain of monkey cells, known as COS cells. COS cells were derived from monkey CV-1 cells by artificial manipulation, leading to integration of a segment of the SV40 genome containing a defective origin of replication (*ori*). The integrated SV40 segment in COS cells allows any circular DNA that contains a functional *ori*SV40 to replicate independently of the cellular DNA. Transcription from the SV40 promoter results in an RNA transcript that normally splices to include the two exons of the minigene. If the DNA cloned into the MCS contains a functional exon, then the additional exons can be spliced to the minigene exons. After isolation of RNA and preparing cDNA, PCR reactions with primers specific for the minigene exons is made. Agarose gel electrophoresis can easily distinguish between normal splicing and splicing involving exons in the insert DNA. Another method to identify expressed sequences is called zoo-blotting. In this method, genomic DNA fragments are hybridized at reduced hybridization stringency against a Southern blot of genomic

DNA samples isolated from different species. This method is based on a fact that expressed sequences are usually well conserved, and for example, human DNA fragment with exons from *RB1* gene will hybridize to mouse and pig genomic DNA fragments containing *RB1* gene. However, all of these methods are laborious, time consuming, and inefficient. Currently, three approaches are the most popular for the identification of expressed sequences/genes in the genomic DNA: computer analysis of DNA sequences for possible exons, identification of CpG islands that can be done both experimentally and using bioinformatics, and large-scale sequence analysis of transcribed sequences, like sequencing of ESTs, SAGE, and CAGE.

Bioinformatic methods to identify genes will not be discussed here as special journal issues are focused on this topic, and many new programs appeared every year. In principle, these programs could be divided into two classes. One type of program predicts genes using only genomic sequences. These programs can also compare genomic DNA sequences from different organisms and search for conserved sequences. The second type of program compares different cDNA, EST, and genomic sequences to find the most possible gene sequence. This method is more reliable; however, it is important to remember that all computer programs frequently predict nonexisting genes and exons and miss really existing genes and exons. Thus, all computer-predicted genes/exons need experimental confirmation. In cases when a gene has alternative 5′ and 3′ ends and different splicing forms computer programs are not very much helpful.

CpG Islands

The dinucleotide CpG is notable because it is greatly under-represented in human DNA, occurring at only about one fifth of the roughly 4% frequency that would be expected by simply multiplying the typical fraction of Cs and Gs (0.21×0.21). The deficit occurs because most CpG dinucleotides are methylated on the cytosine base, and spontaneous deamination of methyl-C residues gives rise to T residues. Spontaneous deamination of ordinary cytosine residues gives rise to uracil residues that are readily recognized and repaired by the cell. As a result, methyl-CpG dinucleotides steadily mutate to TpG dinucleotides. However, the genome contains many CpG islands that represent stretches of unmethylated DNA with a higher frequency of CpG dinucleotides when compared with the entire genome. CpG islands are believed to preferentially occur at the transcriptional start of genes, and it has been observed that most housekeeping genes have CpG islands at the 5′ end of the transcript. In addition, experimental evidence indicates that CpG island methylation is correlated with gene inactivation and has been shown to be important during gene imprinting and tissue-specific gene expression. Thus, identification of CpG methylation is crucial for isolation of tumor suppressor genes and early diagnosis of cancer.

CpG islands are usually 1–2 kb long and are dispersed in the genome. They are called CpG (rich) islands because the %(G+C) of CpG island sequences usually exceed 60% and the human genome contains on average about 40% of C+G content. The combination of G+C richness and lack of CpG suppression means that CpG islands contain 10–20 times more CpGs than an equivalent length of non-island DNA. Altogether, there are about 30,000 to 45,000 islands in the haploid genome (the average spacing is about 1 per 100 kb). It is now clear that the majority (if not all) of CpG islands are associated with genes.

As one of the main goals of the human genome project is the isolation of all genes and the construction of a transcriptional gene map, it is clear that markers located in the CpG islands have an additional value for physical mapping. It has been shown that recognition sites for many of the rare cutting enzymes are closely associated with CpG islands. For example, at least 82% of all NotI and 76% of all XmaIII sites are located in the CpG islands. More than 20% of CpG island- containing genes have at least one NotI site in their sequence, whereas about 65% of those genes have XmaIII site(s). Summarizing the data for all genes (with or without CpG islands), we can conclude that approximately 12% of all well- characterized human genes contain NotI sites, and 43% of them have XmaIII sites. For human genome mapping this means that by sequencing DNA fragments containing a NotI site, it is possible to tag up to one fifth of all expressed genes. As discussed, the recombinant clone containing a NotI (or other rare cutting enzymes) recognition site is called a linking clone.

How many genes contain the human genome? This question is difficult, and the answer is very much dependent on the definition of a gene. According to Celera and HGP, the human genome contains approximately 30,000–35,000 genes.

However, sequencing of NotI linking clones suggested that the human genome contains 15,000–20,000 *Not*I sites, of which 6000–9000 are unmethylated in any particular cell. It means that the human genome contains 45,000–60,000 genes.

Comparison of our database containing experimentally obtained NotI linking sequences with complete chromosome 21 and 22 sequences revealed several interesting features. First, it was shown that chromosome 22 contains greater than twofold more genes than chromosome 21 (545:225 = 2.4), and we see the same ratio within the NotI flanking sequences (119:49 = 2.4). We have demonstrated that nearly all our NotI clones contained genes and suggested that 12.5–20% of all genes contain NotI sites. This correlates well with the number of genes on chromosomes 21 and 22 (168/770 = 22%). Second, according to sequencing, the two chromosomes contain 390 NotI sites. Therefore, if we assume that each NotI site is associated with a gene, then almost half of the genes contain NotI sites. This estimate seems excessive.

The human genome sequence data cannot discriminate between methylated and unmethylated cytosines. There are several algorithms for the identification of CpG islands on the basis of primary sequence. One quantitative definition holds that CpG islands are regions of DNA >200 bp with C+G content of >50% and a ratio of the "observed vs. expected" frequency of CG dinucleotides, which exceeds 0.6. The ratio for the entire genome is approximately 0.2. According to the previous data, 82% of NotI sites are located in CpG islands. It is important to note that these data were obtained either using computational methods or limited experimental datasets. Using the NotI cloning method, only unmethylated NotI sites can be isolated. Comparing the experimental NotI cloning method and computer-based identification of CpG islands, two main features are apparent: The fraction of sequences with >80% CG content is nine times higher in the NotI collection, i.e., 142 vs. 22 sequences. Another striking finding is that even NotI flanking sequences with CG content less than 50% have a very high ratio of observed versus expected frequency of CG dinucleotide: 0.71. This suggests that essentially all NotI flanking sequences generated in the study are located in CpG islands, and therefore, the computational method misses at least 8.7% of CpG islands associated with NotI sites. Thus, existing tools for computational determination of CpG islands fail to identify a significant fraction of functional CpG islands, and unmethylated DNA stretches with a high frequency of CpG dinucleotides can be found even in regions with low CG content.

SAGE and CAGE Approaches to Analyze Human Transcriptome and to Estimate the Number of Human Genes

Another approach to identify genes and analyze their expression pattern in human/ mammalian cell is large-scale sequencing of transcribed sequences. Sequencing of ESTs and isolation of full-length cDNA clones was known a long time ago and will not be discussed here. Recently two novel high-throughput methods for the analysis of human transcriptome were developed: serial analysis of gene expression (SAGE) and cap analysis gene expression (CAGE). Both methods are based on the generation of short sequence tags. Each of these tags is assumed to identify a gene transcript.

SAGE is based on two principles. First, a specific adaptor is ligated to cDNA close to the 3′ end of the mRNA (polyA tail). This adaptor contains a recognition site for a type IIs restriction aendonuclease. Originally, it was FokI, and in a recent modification (LongSAGE), MmeI was used. FokI generates 13–14-bp, and MmeI generates 20–21-bp tags. The 21-bp tag consists of a constant 4-bp sequence representing the restriction site at which the transcript was cleaved, followed by a unique 17-bp sequence derived from an adjacent sequence in each transcript. Theoretical calculations show that >99.8% of 21-bp tags are expected to occur only once in genomes the size of the human genome. Similar analyses based on actual sequence information from ~16,000 genes suggest that >75% of 21-bp tags would be expected to occur only once in the human genome, with the remaining tags matching duplicated genes or repeated sequences. Second, to optimize the quantification of transcripts, tags are ligated together to form "ditags," which are then concatenated and cloned. Sequencing tag concatemers in parallel allows the identification of up to ~30 tag sequences in each sequencing reaction. Matching tags to genome sequences identifies the gene corresponding to each tag, and the number of times a particular tag is observed provides a quantitative measure of transcript abundance in the RNA population.

CAGE is similar to SAGE in principle; however, it is based on preparation and sequencing of concatamers of DNA tags deriving from the initial 20 nucleotides from 5′ end mRNAs.

The method essentially uses cap trapper full-length cDNAs to the 5′ ends of which linkers are attached. This is followed by the cleavage of the first 20 base pairs by class IIs restriction enzymes (Mme) and then another linker is ligated. After it, PCR amplification, excision of tags, their concatamerization, and cloning of the CAGE tags was performed. CAGE tags derived by sequencing these clones are mapped to the genome and used for expression analysis, as well as for the determination of the 5′ end borders of new transcriptional units. Thus, in contrast to SAGE, CAGE allows high-throughout gene expression analysis and the profiling of transcriptional start points, including promoter usage analysis.

SAGE and CAGE concatamer sequencing is more cost-effective than a full- length cDNA library sequencing because of the much higher throughput of identified tags.

In a recent study (FANTOM 3 project), full-length cDNA isolation and 5′- and 3′-end sequencing of cloned cDNAs was combined with CAGE, gene identification signature (GIS), and gene signature cloning (GSC) ditag technologies for the identification of RNA and mRNA sequences corresponding to transcription initiation and termination sites. In this study, paired initiation and termination sites were identified and the boundaries for 181,047 independent transcripts in the mouse genome were established. In total, 1.32 5′ start sites for each 3^2 end and 1.83 3′ ends for each 5′ end are found. Based on these data, the number of transcripts is at least one order of magnitude larger than the estimated 22,000 "genes" in the mouse genome, and the large majority of transcriptional units have alternative promoters and polyadenylation sites. To extend the mouse data, two human CAGE libraries, one constructed with random primers and the other with oligo-dT primers, were combined to produce 1,000,000 CAGE tags. Mapping of these tags to the human genome identified the likely promoters and transcriptional starting site of many genes and clearly indicates that the same level of transcriptional diversity occurs in humans as in mice and is at least 10 times as great as the number of "genes."

Of the 102,281 FANTOM3 cDNAs, 34,030 lack any protein-coding sequence (CDS) and are annotated as non-protein-coding RNA (ncRNA). The function of ncRNAs is a matter of debate, but it is clear that some of them are very important for transcription regulation. Some ncRNAs are highly conserved even in distant species. According to the previous data, only 1–1.5% of the human genome is spanned by exons and 75% of the genome is non-transcribed intergenic DNA. However, FANTOM 3 data demonstrated that the majority (more than 60%) of the mammalian genome is transcribed and commonly from both strands. Analysis of the output of FANTOM 3 suggested that many more transcripts were still to be discovered and only the future can reveal the actual complexity in the mammalian transcriptome. Very similar conclusions were made in another detailed study of human transcriptome.

Was It Worth It to Sequence Human Genome?

The Human Genome Project was controversial from the beginning. Some criticism concerns scientific strategy and the ways in which it was executed. Is it important to sequence the whole human genome or only coding DNA sequences (genes)? Now it is clear that DNA sequences recognized previously as a "junk" in fact are very important for understanding how human genome functions. This "junk" DNA contains important regulatory sequences, ncRNAs, and probably the most intriguing discoveries will come from areas considered as wastelands. Many ethical questions arose during the HGP. For instance, sample collection from individuals was often done without proper consultation or explanation of the possible future use. As the HGP moved forward, commercial concerns were increasingly taking a stake in the research. Large financial investments from big companies can monopolize certain research areas, for example, sequencing of cDNA and gene identification. By subsequently seeking patents to protect their financial investments, they raised a question: Who owns the human genome?

Any major scientific advance carries with it the fear of exploitation, and HGP is not an exception. For example, knowledge of disease-associated mutations can be used for disease prevention, and at the same time, it can be used for discrimination. The comprehensive knowledge of human genome and genes can lead to biological determinism and revival of eugenics with all its negative consequences.

Another objection was that funding of the HGP would be done at the expense of other scientific directions.

The human genome map and sequence still contain many uncertainties, and only careful examination by some research group focusing on a particular genomic region can produce a reliable map and sequence. For instance, we have cloned all *Not*I sites and constructed a physical map for two chromosome 3 regions containing tumor suppressor genes. In the course of these studies, it became apparent that large-insert vectors from these regions were unstable, sensitive to deletions and rearrangements, and the original maps produced by HGP were erroneous.

It should be emphasized that the enormous efforts deployed on sequencing the human genome are extremely important; however, a critical role remains for verified, integrated maps. In sequencing, the short and long repeats spread throughout the genome are sources of numerous errors. These errors are difficult to identify with the shotgun strategy, but they become evident when mapping information is combined with the sequence. Furthermore, difficulties in sequence assembly caused by the existence of large families of recently duplicated genes and pseudogenes are easier to resolve using integrated maps.

In many cases, sequence and mapping information is duplicated, overlapping, or contradictory. One must always keep in mind that even absolutely correct and long nucleotide sequences may be localized incorrectly along the chromosomal DNA if the appropriate accompanying mapping information is ignored. For this reason, despite the vast amount of information currently available, there is an urgent need to reconcile this information in a unified framework, to generate an integrated non-controversial map for each chromosome.

The draft human genome sequence produced by HGP was estimated to cover at least 92% of the whole human genome. However, it contained only 55.7% of the *Not*I flanking sequences and Celera's database contained matches to 57.2% of the clones. The data suggest that the shotgun sequencing approach used to generate the draft human genome sequence resulted in a bias against cloning and sequencing of *Not*I flanks. Even in 2005 up to 5% of our NotI flanking sequences (that are also incomplete!) are not present in the human genome sequence available in public databases.

Several explanations can be offered to account for the low representation of *Not*I flanking sequences in the draft human genome sequences. One potential explanation is that the cloning of some *Not*I containing regions may be selected against experiments with large-insert cloning vectors. Our experience has also proven that even in small-insert plasmid vectors, some human sequences are more easy to clone than other. In our procedure, we directly selected clones containing *Not*I sites, and in a shotgun sequencing approach, such sequences could be under-represented. An alternative explanation, based on the observation that some *Not*I flanking sequences can have 100% identity over long DNA stretches, is that some *Not*I sites were incorrectly fused in the assembly process. Furthermore, our experience demonstrated that sometimes it is very difficult to read *Not*I flanking sequences because of extremely high CG content. During human genome assembling, such sequences would be eliminated as possessing low-quality data. Further experimental analysis is needed to conclusively identify the cause(s) of the bias. HGP resulted in enormous progress in automation of sequencing and other molecular biology methods.

It gives us new tools for disease-gene discovery. In fact, the information obtained during the HGP helps rather than hinders small research groups. It is still important to remember that only the euchromatin portion of the genome was sequenced, and it is not clear to what extent it was done. Many heterochromatin regions are practically not sequenced, and they most probably contain many unknown genes and other functionally important sequences. Thus, the draft human genome sequence was made, but it is a very long way to obtain a really complete human genome sequence and to understand how many genes it contains and how it functions.

13

From Gene to Product

Biotechnology and biotechnology-based methods are increasing in importance in medical therapies and diagnostics as well as in the discovery, development, and manufacture of pharmaceuticals. Biotechnologically manufactured pharmaceuticals will soon reach a market volume of more than $100 billion USD and, thus, some 20% of the total pharmaceutical market. The key step in their manufacture is the conversion of the genetic information into a product with the desired pharmacological activities by an appropriate selection, design, and cultivation of cells and microorganisms harboring the corresponding biosynthetic pathways and physiological properties.

The intention of this chapter is to give insights into the typical issues and problems encountered in the manufacture of biopharmaceuticals, to mediate general ideas and current strategies on how to proceed in the design and development of biotechnological processes, and to deliver the immediate theoretical backgrounds necessary for comprehension rather than to give detailed experimental instructions like a manual does. In focusing on gene recombinant proteins and peptidic antibiotics, the biotechnologically produced pharmaceuticals with the highest market share, representative aspects will be discussed (1) for process development and optimization approaches to increase product yield and process rentability and to ensure a consistent product quality, (2) for experimental approaches to design and to modify the molecular structure of compounds to meet specific medical needs, (3) for the replacement of chemical procedures by economically and ecologically advantageous biotechnological processes, (4) for critical issues of product purification, and (5) for specific demands in pharmaceutical production to conform to regulatory requirements. Finally, the advantage of an integrative biotechnology is emphasized, which designs the biosynthetic steps of the product in accordance with the requirements of product purification procedures already during early development stages.

Production Organisms and Expression Systems

Design and development of all microbial production processes start with the selection of appropriate organisms, strains, and expression systems enabling high yields and high quality of a desired product with defined pharmacological properties.

Industrially Established Recombinant Expression Systems

Industrially established expressions systems for production of the marketed compounds are, besides inclusion, body-forming *Escherichia coli* strains, the yeast *Saccharomyces cerevisiae* and mammalian cells like CHO- and BHK-cells. These systems were the genetically and physiologically most advanced and therefore mostly applied when recombinant production processes were starting to be developed in the mid-1980s and are now widely accepted by regulatory bodies. *E. coli* and *S. cerevisiae* can be grown cheaply and rapidly, are amenable to high cell density fermentations with biomasses of up to 130 g/L, possess short generation times, have high capacities to accumulate foreign proteins, are easy to handle, and are established fermentation organisms.

However, because gene recombinant pharmaceuticals continuously gain an increasing importance in medicine and are expected to help curing diseases that are not yet treatable today, new expression systems have to be exploited enabling the production of such pharmaceuticals with innovative properties that simultaneously meet key criteria like consistent product quality and cost effectiveness. Of particular interest in this regard are expression systems enabling the secretion of correctly glycosylated and folded proteins into the culture broth. Such secretory systems offer advantages in terms of simple and fast product purification procedures and the avoidance of costly cell rupture, denaturation, and refolding processes and thus conform to the requirements of an integrated production process.

Even though animal and plant systems (molecular pharming) and secretory plant cell culture systems have received a great deal of attention, their commercial feasibility is still under investigation, particularly with respect to their slightly different posttranslational modification modus leading to an altered pharmacological behavior and to allergenic properties. Established in the pharmaceutical industry as production organisms are, besides the above-mentioned systems, further prokaryotic and yeast species as well as filamentous fungi, which are already employed for the manufacture of natural products.

The suitability of the most prominent secretory systems among these organisms from the viewpoint of an integrative process design for the manufacture of recombinant proteins will be evaluated in the next section by discussing their potential productivity and their physiological properties.

Evaluation of Secretory Expression Systems for Pharmaceutical Purposes

Escherichia coli

As *E. coli* lacks fundamental prerequisites for efficient secretion, the marketed pharmaceuticals manufactured by *E. coli*-systems are mostly produced as inclusion bodies. Due to the membrane structure, the low chaperone and foldase level and the high periplasmatic protease concentration *E. coli*-secretion systems allow only comparably low product yields, making them suitable only for compounds marketed in small quantities like orphan drugs. Genentech, for instance, has patented a secretory *E. coli*-system for the preparation of human growth hormone. The secretory potential of *E. coli* is indicated by exceptional high product titers in the range of several grams per liter, which were reached in a system developed for secretion of hirudin using the alpha-cyclodextringlykosysl-transferase signal sequence as a leader und secretor mutants deficient in their membrane structure. Titers of human-insulin-like-growth-factor or human-epidermal-growth-factor were reported to be as high as 900 mg/L and 325 mg/L, respectively.

Most of the reached and published data, however, refers to processes leading to a periplasmatic product concentration (e.g., 2 g/L of a human antibody fragment, 700 mg/L of a monoclonal antibody) or stays below 100 mg/L, a value that generally is not considered to be in a competitive and economic range. Efforts are thus undertaken to condition *E. coli*-strains to efficient secreters. The main strategies to enhance secretion efficiency comprise (1) employment of well-characterized secretion pathways like the alpha-hemolysin system or components of such pathways like efficient signal sequences from efflux proteins or outer membrane proteins, for instance, the maltose binding protein or the TolC-protein; (2) variation of the signal peptide; (3) cocloning of and coexpression of chaperones and foldases; (4) enhancement of gene expression by employment of strong promotors and efficient transcription termination sequences; (5) generation of protease deficient mutants; (6) generation of cell wall lacking or cell wall deficient mutants; and (7) modulation of the protein primary structure that was found to exert a strong influence on productivity and secretion efficiency by influencing protease resistance, folding efficiency, and the tendency to form inclusion bodies.

Alternative prokaryotic expression systems

In addition to conditioning *E. coli*-strains to efficient secreters, alternative species, which are considered to inherently possess a superior secretion capacity, are tried to be established as expression systems. Comparably high product yields of 2 g/L and 1 g/L were reported for production of human calcitonin by *Staphylococcus carnosus* and of proinsulin by *Bacillus subtilis*, an organism that is continuously characterized and improved as a cell factory for pharmaceutical proteins. *Bacillus megaterium*, which is thought to be as efficient as *B. subtilis*, is currently developed as a secretory expression system by a Collaborative Research Center (SFB) of the German Research Community (DFG). For *Ralstonia eutropha* (formerly *Alcaligenes eutrophus*), employed at ICI and Monsanto for polyhydroxyalkanoate production at a scale of several 100 m^3 and genomically completely sequenced, 1,2 g/L of secreted organophosphohydrolase, a model enzyme proned to form inclusion bodies in *E. coli*, were reported. *R. eutropha* displays a more efficient carbohydrate metabolism than *E. coli* and is easily amenable to high cell density fermentations with biomass concentration of more than 150 g/L dry weight. This permits a lower specific productivity that in turn reduces the inclinement to form inclusion bodies and thus enables a more efficient secretion. *Rhodococcus*, *Corynebacterium*, *Mycobacterium*, actinomycetes, and streptomycetes are also considered to be potentially suitable for the development of efficient secretion systems.

A comparative study with recombinant alpha-amylase demonstrated that final yields as well as enzyme activity were considerably higher when produced by *Streptomyces lividans*, by which it was completely secreted than by *E. coli* in which it was concentrated periplasmatically. The yields reported so far, however, are still below costefficient ranges. A system developed by Hoechst/Aventis for insulin production yielded around 100 mg/L, and the yields of correctly folded human CD4-receptor sites are in the range of 200 mg/L. Attached as signal proteins were the prepeptide of the alpha-amylase inhibitor from *S. tendae* (tendamistat) and the signal sequence of a protease inhibitor (LTI) from *S. longisporus*. In the course of these studies, it was found that the choice of the linker and its length strongly influences secretion efficiency. The comparably low yields, however, demonstrate that still a lot of fundamental research is necessary to render streptomyces systems competitive. A general focus of research will be the detailed exploration of the twin arginine translocation (TAT) pathway, which has been recently discovered in addition to the conventional prokaryotic secretory (sec) pathways and enables the export of proteins with cofactors in a fully folded conformation. It evidently plays a more important role in *Streptomyces* species but might also be useable in other species.

As the potential and capacity of prokaryotes for prosttranslational modification appear to be quite limited and the knowledge about the pathways is quite scarce, the employability of most of the known prokaryotes usually is restricted to the preparation of proteins that are naturally not glycosylated, such as insulin, hirudins, or somatotropins, or to natively glycosylated proteins that are pharmacologically also active without glycosylation, like various cytokines (tumor necrosis factor, interleukines, interferones). For production of proteins that are pharmacologically active only with an appropriate modification pattern, eukayotic cell systems are more suitable.

Yeasts

Besides possessing complex posttranslational modification pathways, they offer the advantage to be neither pyrogenic nor pathogenic and to secrete more efficiently. Species established in industrial production procedures are *Saccharomyces cerevisiae*, *Kluyveromyces lactis*, *Pichia pastoris*, and *Hansenula polymorpha*, which will be dealt with more in detail in this section. Whereas *S. cerevisiae* is the best genetically characterized eukaryotic organism at all and still is the prevalent yeast species in pharmaceutical production processes, *P. pastoris*, first employed by Phillips Petroleum for single-cell-protein production, is currently the most frequently used yeast species for heterologous protein expression in general. Whereas only just a few proteins were expressed by *Pichia* species at the beginning of the last decade, the expression of more than 400 proteins have been meanwhile reported now. *P. pastoris* is considered to be superior to any other known yeast species with respect to its secretion efficiency and permits the production of recombinant proteins without intense process development.

The highest yields were reported for murine collagen (15 g/L), tetanus toxin fragment C (12 g/L compared with 1 g/L in *S. cerevisiae*), human serum albumin (10 g/L compared with 3 g/L in *K. lactis* and to 90 and 150 mg/L in *S. cerevisiae*), and human interleukin 2 (10 g/L). The highest reported yields for *H. polymorpha* relate to phytase (13,5 g/L) and to hirudin (g/L range) and for *K. lactis* to human serum albumin (3 g/L). Even though *S. cerevisiae* offers a high secretory potential as evidenced by some 9-g/L secreted *Aspergillus niger* glucose oxidase, such data document a general inferior secretory capacity, the reasons for which are numerous. For the methylotrophic species *Hansenula* and *Pichia* and the lactose using *K. lactis*, natively strong promoters are available that derive from the methanol and lactose assimilating pathways and their enzymes (e.g., alcohol- and methanol oxidase, lactose permease, galactosidase).

As the enzymes of these pathways account for up to 30% of the total protein content, the metabolic efficiency with respect to the secreted protein is significantly higher as documented by Buckholz and Gleeson: Only one or a few gene copies are sufficient in *P. pastoris* to gain the same yields as with 50 gene copies in *S. cerevisiae*. Furthermore, proteins with a molecular mass of above 30 kD are retained in the cytoplasma of *S. cerevisiae*, whereas *H. polymorpha* efficiently secretes proteins with a molecular mass of up to 150 kD, like the glucoamylase of *Aspergillus niger*. Further reasons for the differing secretion rates among the species are the specific proteolytic activities and the specific degrees and patterns of glycosylation. Besides having an impact on the protein's final pharmacological activity, glycosylation also exercises an influence on the folding and secretion efficiency. Among the discussed species, *S. cerevisiae* was shown to possess, besides a higher enzymatic activity in the secretion vesicles that leads to a reduced portion of intact secreted proteins, also the highest glycosylation capacity leading to a hyperglycosylation of the protein and a reduced secretion rate. Both the degree and the pattern of glycosylation are dependent on the genetic background of the species and strains employed as well as on the sequences of the expressed protein and adjacent regions.

By employment of the natively highly glycosylated alpha-mating type factor as a secretion signal, the extent of the glycosylation of the product can be diminished or completely avoided as shown for human interleukin 6. NovoNordisk reported leader sequence-dependent insulin yields in *S. cerevisiae* and in *S. cerevisiae* and *P. pastoris*: The sequence and therewith the degree of glycosylation of the leader influences the efficiency of the multistage cleavage and folding processes as well as the insulin glycosylation rate and secretability. Further enhancement of the secretion efficiency can be achieved by (1) mutating secretion enhancer genes, (2) suppressing secretion blocking functions, and (3) reducing proteolytic activities in secretion vesicles. So-called supersecreter strains of *S. cerevisiae* have, for instance, been generated by inactivation of the PMR1 (SSC1) function and suppression of the secretion blocking ypt1-1 gene: the yields of non-glycosylated human pro-urokinase, of human serum albumin, and of human plasminogen-activator have been augmented to a factor of up to 10. The traditional approaches pursued for enhancement of gene expression are gene amplification, employment of strong promoters, and enhancement of the transcription and translation rate.

A high amplification of the gene copy number usually is achievable with episomal vectors, which however do not reach the mitotic stability of integrative systems like the transposon (e.g., Ty-element) mediated embedment of reiterative, dispers repetitive sequences in *S. cerevisae*. Transcription rates were reported to be enhanced up to 100 times through cotransformation with transcription activators and enhancers, which evidently are limiting factors for overexpression of foreign proteins. Translation efficiency can be enhanced by preventing an accelerated degradation of transcripts and the yeast typical random transcription termination through modulation of the recognition sequences. Prevention of the random transcription termination led to an increase of tetanus toxin fragment C yields in *S. cerevisiae* by a factor 2000–3000 to 1 g/L and 3% of the total soluble protein fraction.

Table 13.1. Typical sequence of biotechnological production process steps

Step	*Method/approach*
Selection/design/engineering/development of an appropriate species/strain/expression system	*Criteria*: pharmacological activity and properties of the compound, productivity, process behavior, suitability for downstream processing steps, spectrum and and pharmacological activity of side products to be removed, experimental experience with the respective system, biological and medical safety, acceptance by regulatory bodies
Strain improvement	Mutation/selection, strain recombination (e.g., breeding/protoplast fusion), directed genomic alteration/ metabolic engineering/enhancement of gene expression rates
Biosynthetic product structure modification	Amino acid exchange/combinatorial biosynthesis/precursor directed biosynthesis
Fermentation optimization	Empirical optimization of culture conditions (media components, pH, oxygen supply), clarification of the influence of process parameters on growth, productivity and side product formation
Fermentation scale-up	Detailed process characterization for reduction of stress exposure, insurance of homogenized reaction conditions, and identification of suitable scale-up parameters (e.g., with the help of chemometric modeling, computational fluid dynamics)
Downstream processing	
Cell separation and harvest, removal of particulate matters	Centrifugation (decanter, disk-stack separator, (semi) continuous centrifuges), filtration (dead-end, tangential flow filtration)
Cell rupture	High-pressure homogenization, bead mills, sonication, enzymatic treatments
Product capture	Filtration (micro-, ultra-, nano-filtration), precipitation, solvent extraction, ion exchange, size exclusion, affinity chromatography
Product purification/polishing	Hydrophobic interaction/reversed-phase chromatography
Clearance of contaminant agents (e.g., viruses, endotoxins)	Nano-filtration, heat, pH, chemical inactivation, ultraviolet, gamma irradiation
Drying	Heat, freezing, vacuum
Galenic preparation/filling	Addition of galenic excipients, supplements, stabilizers, and adjuvants

Despite their physiologically advantageous properties and natively high expression and secretion capacity, just one industrial application is reported for each of the alternative yeast species: *H. polymorpha* is employed for hepatitis B vaccine production at Rhein-Biotech. *K. lactis* for bovine prochymosin production in a 40-m^3 scale at Gist-Brocades, and *P. pastoris* for production of recombinant carboxypeptidase B and trypsin at Roche. For pharmaceutical application, it has to be considerered that the methylotrophic yeasts in contrast to *S. cerevisiae* and *K. lactis* are not used in the production of foodstuffs and therewith have no GRAS (generally regarded as safe) status according to the U.S. Food and Drug Administration (FDA) criteria and have to be grown in expensive explosion-proofed equipments when the above- mentioned native induction systems are used. The employ-ability of yeasts in some cases however might reach a limit, particularly when the pharmacological activity of the product is impaired by the glycosylation pattern. In *K. lactis*, for instance, which usually does not hyperglycosylate, an exceptional high glycosylation of human interleukin 1â has been observed, reducing the biological activity to 5%. In such cases, a postsynthetic chemical modification has to be considered or the employment of higher developed organisms.

Filamentous fungi

Filamentous fungi are higher organized than yeasts and consequently have a more complex posttranslational modification apparatus more similar to mammals. Some proteins like t-PA in *Aspergillus nidulans* are produced with the natural human glycosylation pattern. For recombinant protein production, species are prefered, which are broadly employed in industry for production of enzymes, acids and antibiotics and thus possess GRAS-status: *A. nidulans*, *A. niger*, *A. sydowii*, *A. awamori*, various *Fusarium* and *Trichoderma* species, *Penicillium chrysogenum*, and *Acremonium chrysogenum*. Their productivity and secretion potential, which is in the range of 30–40 g/L for homologous enzymes like cellulases and amylases, is considered to be superior to any other system, but unfortunately could not be converted into corresponding yields of recombinant products, even when these were fused to such homologous enzymes. The highest yields are still obtained with heterologous fungal enzymes: 4-g/L *Fusarium* protease in *A. chrysogenum* and 4.6-g/L *A. niger* glucoamylase in *A. awamori*. The highest yield of a mammalian protein was reported for human interleukin 6 in *A. sojae* in a range of 300 mg/L. The yields of most human proteins like t-PA and various interferons, however, were reported to be below 1 mg/L.

Possible reasons for these incompetitive yields are restrictions in posttranslational metabolic steps like intracellular transport, folding, and processing. Even though filamentous fungi are industrially used now for decades, they are not adequately characterized on the physiological and genetic level. Little is known about details of the modification and secretion metabolism, and efficient gene transformation is hampered by degradation of foreign DNA, low transformation rate, and therefore, low copy numbers of the transferred genes and random genomic integration. Expression rates are restricted by a high RNA turnover, incorrect processing of the foreign messenger, and incomplete folding and secretion, which are, as in yeasts, both influenced by the glycosylation pattern. Proteins not completely or incorrectly glycosylated and excreted are rapidly degraded as shown for human interleukin 6. Currently, filamentous fungi cannot be regarded as a serious alternative for the production of pharmaceuticals. To fully exploit the potential of filamentous fungi, their physiology, particularly the glycosylation metabolism, thus has to be investigated and clarified in more detail.

Insect and mammalian cell cultures

Animal cell cultures are the systems with highest similarity to human cells with respect to the pattern and capacity of posttranslational modifications. However, their cultivation is more complicated and costly and usually yields lower product titers. Among the known systems, insect cells transformed by baculovirus vectors have reached a comparable popularity as *Pichia* among yeasts because they are considered to be more stress resistant, easier to handle, and more productive compared with mammalian systems and are thus frequently employed for high-throughput protein expression. The highest reported yields refer to human collagenase IV in *Trichoplusia* (300 mg/L). Yields reported for non-insect cultures were 80 mg/L for human apolipoprotein A1 in chinese hamster ovary (CHO)-cells and 1 mg/L for human laminin in human embryonal kidney cells.

For commercial application scale-up, related questions have to be clarified, particularly concerning oxygen supply and carbon dioxide accumulation, stability of the cell line, and the bioreactor type to be employed. Further deficiencies of insect cells are observed in (1) an inefficient processing and an impairment of the folding and secretion capacity due to the baculovirus infection; (2) the high, in part baculovirus encoded, protease activity and the resulting necessity to routinely employ protease inhibitors in the culture media or to develop protease deficient vectors; (3) an insufficient expression strength; and (4) deviations of the posttranslational modification pattern, which could act immunogenic. For optimization, the construction of new innovative vectors and the coexpression of chaperones, foldases, and folding factors such as canexin have been suggested as has been the broader development and application of alternative systems like *Drosophila*. Preferably applied in pharmaceutical production processes are mammalian systems like CHO- and baby hamster kidney (BHK)-cells. These systems are generally considered to be genetically more stable and easier to transform and to handle in scale-up processes, grow faster in adherent and submerged cultures, and are more similar to human cells and more consistent in their complete spectrum of modification, which minimizes the risk of the formation of structurally altered compounds with immunogenic properties.

In some cases, mammalian systems can be the only choice for the preparation of correctly modified proteins. Studies of Tate et al. comparing the expression of a rat serotonin transporter in various expression systems demonstrate that biologically active transporter was only synthesized in mammalian cells, whereas it was partially degraded in *E. coli*, not correctly folded in *Pichia* and not correctly glycosylated in insect cells. CHO- and BHK-cells further have the advantage to be recognized as safe regarding infectious and pathogenic agents and therefore to have a higher acceptance by regulatory bodies, which accelerates or at least does not delay approval procedures.

Criteria for the Choice of Recombinant Expression Systems

In summary, the criteria for the choice of an expression system in pharmaceutical production are the existing expertise, the available physiological and genetic know-how and tools, the patent situation, and to avoid delays of product launch and commercialization, regulatory aspects like the acceptance by the approving authorities.

The overall decision criteria, however, is the pharmacological activity profile of the yielded protein in context with the posttranslational modification pattern followed by rentability.

For production of non-glycosylated proteins and proteins that are natively glycosylated but pharmacologically active also without glycosylation, prokaryotes, which usually lack metabolic pathways for glycosylation, theoretically are the most suitable organisms, offering two alternatives: Either *E. coli*-strains are conditioned to efficient secreters, or efficient native secreters like *Bacillus*-species are accordingly developed. To fully exploit the secretion capacity of fungal species, a deeper understanding of their posttranslational modification physiology will be necessary to steer the degree and pattern of glycosylation, which influences both folding and secretion efficiency. Insect and mammalian cells display posttranslational modification patterns more similar or identical to humans, but in view of the entailed expenditures, their employment can only be justified if their modification machinery is required to ensure a desired pharmacological activity.

E. coli, *P. pastoris*, and Baculovirus-based systems are currently preferred in fundamental research for structural and functional analysis of proteins and are employed as high-throughput-expression systems but will certainly find their ways into production processes in the near future. None of the systems, however, can be considered to be generally superior to any other. For each product, the most suitable expression system has to be identified and optimized individually both on the genetic and on the fermentative level by taking into account the properties of the product, the organism, and the expression cassettes, which suggests to always have a set of accordingly developed expression systems available.

Table 13.2. Features and characteristics of expression systems

Property	*Bacteria*	*Yeast*	*Insect and mammalian cell cultures*
Growth	Fast	Fast	Slow
Nutrient demand	Minimal	Minimal	Complex
Costs of media	Low	Low	High
Possible product yield	High	High	Low
Secretory capacity	Limtited	High	Medium
Glycosylation capacity	Limited	High	High
Modification capacity	Limited	High	High
Risk of retroviral Contamination	Low	Low	High
Risk of pyrogens	High	—	—
Scalability	Good	Good	Low
Process robustness	Good	Good	Low

Once an expression system has been selected, the respective strains are continuously submitted to improvement programs to render fermentation processes more efficient by increasing strain productivity and by modifying physiological properties and process behavior to enhance process economy. This does not only apply to the fermentation process, but also to parts of downstream processing, thus requiring an integrated strain selection and process design.

Enhancement of Productivity

Secretory Recombinant Expression Systems

In terms of downstream processing efficiency, secretory expression systems indeed offer potential advantages for production of recombinant proteins compared with inclusion body-forming cytosolic systems, but most of the potentially available secretory systems are not yet fully competitive for high-volume therapeutics like insulin and therefore still require intensive improvement efforts.

Current strategies to improve productivity and secretion efficiency comprise (1) enhancement of gene expression rates, (2) optimization of secretion signal sequences, (3) coexpression of chaperones and foldases, (4) creation of protease deficient mutants to avoid premature product degradation, and (5) subsequent breeding and mutagenesis.

Natural Products

Completely different is the situation faced in the production of the so-called natural products, which are mostly secondary metabolites and therewith the endproducts of complex biosynthetic pathways of filamentous bacteria and fungi and thus require different approaches. With few exceptions like the antidiabetic drug acarbose or the chosterol-lowering drug lovastatin, such fermented pharmaceuticals of natural origin currently belong for the most part to the class of antibiotics.

Enhancement of the productivity is achieved at first by rounds of random mutation and selection and, if possible, by breeding, and/or by DNA injection or fusion techniques like protoplasting and at further stages, after a com prehensive characterization of the usually complex biosynthetic pathways, directed genomic alterations and metabolic engineering. These approaches, developments, and states in industrial strain improvement and pathway characterization will be illustrated for some of the best characterized organisms, namely the two fungal species mainly employed in industrial β-lactam antibiotic production, the penicillin producing *Penicillium chrysogenum*, and the cephalosporin C producer *Acremonium chrysogenum*.

Characterization of biosynthetic pathways

The productivity of *Penicillium chrysogenum* could have been augmented impressively during the last decades: Penicillin titers have been increased by a factor of 50,000 from a very few milligrams/ Liter in the 1940s to more than several 10 g/L by now and also some several 10 g/L cephalosporin are currently gained.

This development, however, has come to a halt during the last couple of years. As these titers have been reached through conventional mutation and selection and no further significant increase in productivity could be noted, the tools of genetic engineering were more and more included into the improvement programs. To gain a profound basis for directed genomic alterations, studies were conducted at various corporations and universities to elucidate the mechanisms and genes involved in β-lactam biosynthesis to characterize the respective biosynthetic pathways.

Cephalosporin C synthesis in acremonium chrysogenum

Biosynthesis starts with the polymerization of L-α-aminoadipic acid, L-cysteine, and L-valine to the linear tripeptide L-α-aminoadipyl-L-cysteinyl-D-valine (ACV-peptide). This reaction is catalyzed by the ACV-synthase (MW about 420 kD) through the following steps: (1) the ATP-dependent activation of these amino acids to bind them as thiolesters, (2) the epimerization of L-valine, and finally (3) the condensation by a thiotemplate mechanism.

Cyclization of the ACV-peptide to the bicyclic isopenicillin N (IPN) occurs under oxygen-, Fe^{2+}-, ascorbate-, and α-ketoglutarate-dependent action of the IPN-synthase (IPNS), which has an MW of about 38 kD. Inhibitory to IPNS activity are cobalt ions and glutathione.

Further pathway reactions are as follows:

1. IPN-epimerization to penicillin N (IPN-epimerase).
2. Penicillin N conversion to deacetoxycephalosporin C (DAOC) by expansion of the five-membered thiazolidine ring to a 6 C-dihydrothiazine-ring (DAOC-expandase).
3. Formation of deactylcephalosporin C (DAC) by dehydroxylation and oxidation of the methylgroup in C3-position (DAC-hydroxylase).
4. The acylation of DAC to cephalosporin C (DAC acetyltransferase).

DAOC-expandase and DAC-hydroxylase activities in *A. chrysogenum* are exerted by the same enzyme (MW 41 kD), which like the IPNS belongs to the group of α-ketoglutarate-dependent dioxygenases.

The first two enzymes, ACV- and IPN-synthase, are encoded by the *pcbAB*- and the *pcb C* gene, respectively. Both genes are linked to each other on chromosome VI by a 1.2-kb intergenic region carrying the putative promotor sequences from which they are divergently transcribed. The *pcb C*-promotor seems to be about five times stronger than the one of the *pcbAB*-gene. The *cefEF*-gene and the *cefG*-gene encoding for the bifunctional expandase/hydroxylase and the DAC-acetyltransferase, respectively, are located adjacent to each other on chromosome II. Again the genes are separated by an intergenic region of 938 bp, which is supposed to harbor the promotors from which they are transcribed in opposite directions. The *cefG*-gene has been proven to contain two introns. Due to an extreme *in vitro* lability, no information is yet available on the epimerase converting IPN to penicillin N as well as its putative *cefD* gene. Until recently, the structure of the *cefD* gene could have not been elucidated. Meanwhile, data could have been obtained indicating the existence of two reading frames (*cefD1* and *cefD2*) containing all characteristic motifs of mammalian acyl-CoA ligases and a-methylacyl-CoA racemases.

Regulatory studies demonstrated that the early functions are expressed simultaneously, whereas the later pathway genes *cefD* and *cefEF* seem to be induced sequentially.

In contrast, the penicillin biosynthesis genes in *P. chrysogenum* are considered to be expressed completely concomitantly.

Penicillin formation by penicillium chrysogenum

The first reactions of the penicillin biosynthetic pathway are identical to the ones in *A. chrysogenum*. IPN, however, is not epimerized to penicillin N; instead it is converted to 6- aminopenicillanic acid (6-APA) by removal of the L-α-aminoadipic acid side chain, which is substituted by a hydrophobic acyl group. Both steps are catalyzed by the same enzyme, the acyl coenzyme A: IPN acyltransferase (IAT). The enzymatic activity of IAT is believed to be the result of the processing of a 40-kD monomeric precursor into a dimeric form consisting of two subunits with MWs of 11 and 29 kD. Due to the broad substrate specifity of IAT, various penicillin derivatives are synthesized naturally by attachment of different acyl-CoA derivatives to the 6-APA-core. For industrial purposes, to facilitate extraction by organic solvents, synthesis usually is directed to the less hydrophilic penicillin V or penicillin G. This is by addition of phenoxyacetic acid or phenylacetic acid, respectively, as precursors to the culture broth.

The IAT encoding *penDE*-gene (also named *aatA*) is located on chromosome I and organized as a cluster together with the ACV-synthase and IPN-synthase encoding genes *pcbAB* (also named *acvA* in *Penicillium*) and *pcbC* (*ipnA*).

The enzymes involved in penicillin biosynthesis are distributed at different sites of the cell: ACV-activity was found to be bound to vacuole membranes, IPN-synthase occurs dissolved in the cytoplasm and IAT-activity is microbody associated.

Approaches and Goals for Further Strain Improvement

Analysis and comparison of strains

To get hints for more rational strain improvement approaches, (1) highly mutated production strains were gene tically and physiologically compared with their less-productive ancestors, (2) concentrations of pathway intermediates were determined to identify potential pathway bottlenecks, and (3) regulatory mechanisms were investigated.

In the course of such studies, high-performance strains of *P. chrysogenum* turned out to possess amplified copies of single genes like the *pcbC* gene or even copies of the whole cluster as well as increased steady-state transcript levels of pathway genes. In some strains, the amplifications were shown to be organized in tandem repeats, which presumably were generated by a hot-spot TTTACA hexanukleotide. Comparison of promotor strengths of these genes from high and low productive strains did not reveal any differences. This indicates the involvement of additional unknown trans-acting factors, as the amounts of increased mRNA did not correlate with the degree of gene amplification. Also a high specific activity of IPN synthase was reported in a more evolved *Penicillium* strain, which was independent from transcript amounts and probably due to a higher enzyme stability.

In *A. chrysogenum*, no amplification of the relevant genes could be detected. Nevertheless, transcript amounts in production strains are significantly increased.

Also chromosome rearrangements could be detected in high titer strains, but their causative influence on productivity remains unclarified for the moment.

Directed genomic alterations

Enhancement of gene expression

Considering these findings, the experiments conducted so far to improve productivity mainly concentrated on enhancing the pathway gene dosages and on enhancing promotor strengths to remove presumed pathway bottlenecks. For instance, the *cefEF*-activity was generally believed to constitute a potential rate-limiting step in view of the high accumulation of penicillin N in various strains of *A. chrysogenum* and accordingly amplified.

Such approaches resulted in partially significant increases of productivity in low and medium titer strains: Improvements of the final yields by 50% have been reported.

However, all improvements achieved so far with high-performance production strains remained with a 5% maximum in the range of normal statistical deviations.

Also more exotic approaches like the (presumed) improvement of the intracellular oxygen supply through cloning and expressing of a bacterial hemoglobin gene from *Vitreoscilla* failed to increase productivity in high titer strains.

The reasons for these failures are manifold:

1. As both direction and site of integration of the imported DNA cannot be controlled sufficiently and transformation efficiency is still quite low, the probability of finding new, higher producing mutants even in a large-scale screening is rare.
2. Most of the data available are from studies performed at academic institutions with original strains. Even when sharing the same ancestral strain, the high-performance strains employed in industries have an individual genealogy and mutation-selection history, so that their physiological behavior and properties differ drastically. Data and knowledge obtained with a particular strain thus cannot always be generalized and transfered to other strains. Even among industrial strains, significant differences have been revealed. For instance, the expression of the *cefG*-gene and the acetyl transferase activity was reported to constitute a possible rate-limiting step in Panlabs-strains. Studies conducted on other industrial strains, however, could not confirm this observation.
3. The genetic instability and drift rises with the degree of genomic alterations, particularly during long-term vegetative propagation with numerous generation cycles in industrial large-scale fermentations.
4. The complex interdependence with other metabolic areas is not yet completely investigated. Consequently, after removal of an obvious β-lactam pathway bottleneck, unknown reaction steps of the linked and preceding pathways might become flux limiting. To overcome such flux limitations, one of the most exciting recent discoveries in molecular biology, namely RNA interference (RNAi), might play a major role in the future.

Possible impact of RNAi in strain improvement

The mechanisms of post-transcriptional gene silencing, generally summed up as RNAi offer potential approaches for the specific shut down of any gene of interest: Native genes can be silenced by triggering the RNAi cascade through introduction of homologous genetic sequences. As a result of these possibilities, RNAi has already revolutionized fundamental research in molecular biology, particularly in functional genomics, and will substantially contribute to novel therapeutic approaches in medicine. For fungi, which evidently were among the first organisms in which RNAi and associated phenomena were observed, this RNAi triggered cosuppression phenomenon has been termed "quelling" and bears an enormous potential with respect to the study of biosynthetic pathways and the improvement of metabolic productivity.

On the one hand, the implication of RNAi may supply an explanation for observations made in the course of strain improvement programs of *Penicillium chrysogenum* and *Acremonium chrysogenum*, according to which antibiotic productivity can decrease drastically upon amplification of genes involved in antiobiotic biosynthesis.

The characterization and inactivation of these cosuppression mechanisms thus might help to overcome such limitations as does an application of fungal RNAi tools for silencing of pathway blocking or metabolic flux limiting genes, e.g., by the use of a novel vector system consisting of dsRNA viruses.

To fully realize the potential for further enhancement of productivity, which is generally assumed to be in the range of some 300% and to fully exploit the potential of RNAi, current and future studies thus aim at filling the actual gaps of knowledge and will be focused on

1. The exploration of regulatory mechanisms and circuits on the transcriptional, translational, and posttranslational level.
2. The determination of the specific intermediate turnover rates resulting from specific enzyme activities, enzyme titers, and enzyme stabilities.
3. The detailed investigation of linked and preceding pathways.
4. The investigation of product secretion mechanisms.

However, as no great leaps in productivity are currently reached, strains emerging from the development programs are also selected for beneficial alterations of genetic, physiological, and morphological properties that contribute to an enhanced process economy.

Improvement of process behaviour

Among the desired alterations are:

1. A decrease of side products, which (i) consume metabolic energy at the expense of the desired main product, (ii) hamper the final product purification, or (iii) even can be inhibitory to the production organism. For instance, a significant reduction of DCPC concentrations has been reached through knocking out esterases that hydrolyze cephalosporin C to DCPC during fermentation. Esterase inactivation was by conventional mutagenesis as well as through gene-disruption and by introduction of anti-sense genes.
2. Increase of the tolerance toward toxic side products and fed precursors like phenyl- or phenoxyacetic acid.
3. Further reduction of feedback inhibition by endproducts and metabolites (see below).
4. Further reduction of catabolite repression.
5. Enhancement of genetic stability.
6. Enhancement of viability, stress resistance, and life span.
7. Accelerated product formation and enhancement of time-specific productivity to shorten fermentation time.
8. Enhancement of the strain-specific productivity to reduce the amount of biomass to be processed and disposed.
9. Increase of product secretion rate.
10. Improvement of the fermentation behavior like (1) higher efficiency of substrate/precursor consumption, (2) diminished oxygen demand, and (3) diminished shear sensitivity.
11. Improvement of filterability.

The in-depth characterization of physiological properties and biosynthetic pathways not only aims at improving process behavior and process economy, but also it relates to modifications of the inherent biosynthetic pathways (pathway engineering) to create innovative, novel products with improved properties and enhanced therapeutic values, e.g., to overcome the antibiotic resistance problem, a major global health-care problem of today.

Biosynthetic Structure Modification

Although the metabolic engineering of beta-lactams by combining β-lactam encoding genes from various sources is still in an explorative state, the study of polyketide pathways and the creation of polyketide antibiotic derivatives is more advanced.

Combinatorial Biosynthesis

Compounds emerging from the polyketide pathways are the classic subject of metabolic engineering and for creation of novel structures. To create novel antibiotics, the natural biodiversity of polyketides is trying to be enhanced artificially by modifying and newly combining the biosynthetic pathway steps and enzymes involved. Polyketide synthases are multienzyme systems, which due to their modular structure and the occurrence of their encoding genes as clusters, are considered to be most amenable for directed alterations, genetic intervention, and heterologous expression in foreign hosts with different metabolic pathways. Concepts and strategies that are currently being pursued for creating novel and un-natural polyketides comprise (1) creating block mutants at various biosynthetic levels to accumulate intermediate metabolites; (2) elimination of unwanted groups; (3) modification of polyketide synthases to further broaden substrate range, eventually combined with a precursor-directed biosynthesis; (4) formation of new structures by deleting or intro ducing additional modules; (5) modification, addition, or elimination of postsynthetic modification steps like glycosylation, lactonization, and amidation; (6) the cloning and combination of various polyketide synthase genes in heterologous hosts to construct hybrid pathways and antibiotics; and (7) linking and combining routes of polyketides with pathways of nonribosomal peptide synthesis to create hybrid peptide–polyketide compounds.

As the microbial nonribosomal peptide synthases share many structural and catalytic properties with polyketide synthases like their organization into catalytic modules and domains, they are also envisaged as ideal subjects for metabolic engineering by creating large sets of modules and subsequently combining them artificially. The rapidly growing body of patents makes evident that an increasing number of companies are working on the field of combinatorial biosynthesis. However, it also becomes evident that, despite their promising prospects, these strategies of combinatorial biosynthesis are still in an initial state and need further intense research to elucidate the required genetic and physiological details.

This is just in contrast to another approach of modifying the molecular structure of peptidic compounds on the biosynthetic level, namely the directed biosynthesis of the desired compound structures by feeding of appropriate biosynthetic precursors or stimulating agents during fermentation, as it is routinely performed for production of penicillin V und G by the addition of phenoxyacetic acid or phenyl- acetic acid, respectively, as precursors to facilitate penicillin extraction from the culture broth.

Precursor Directed Biosynthesis

Microbial peptidic compounds can be modified not only in their peptide structure by direct incorporation of amino acids supplemented during fermentation but also, if present, in their fatty acid moiety. The possibilities of precursor-directed derivatization of cyclic peptides cores and fatty acid moieties by amino acids will be illustrated for three compound complexes with unique modes of action and outstanding spectra of activity against multidrug resistant germs, which were developed by Aventis, Eli Lilly, and Cubist Pharmaceuticals. The complex A1437 of Aventis is synthesized by *Actinoplanes friulensis*, which originally produced a mixture of altogether eight lipopeptides, classified according to the exocyclic amino acid position and the type of their fatty acid chains. Through addition of L-valine and asparagines, the biosynthesis could be directed toward the production of the desired D-peptide, which exhibited superior pharmacological properties in preclinical trials and is characterized by an exocyclic asparagine and an iso-C14 fatty acid moiety. The A54145 complex from Eli Lilly exhibits the noteworthy characteristic, that a built-up resistance was immediately lost in the absence of this compound. It consists of eight lipopeptides produced by *Streptomycesfradiae* containing four similar peptide nuclei in combination with three different fatty acid acyl side chains. The nuclei differ in their valine/isoleucine and glutamate/3-methylglutamate substitutions at one or both of two locations of the peptide ring.

The composition of the peptide nucleus as well as the percentage of branched-chain fatty acid acyl substituents could be directed by supplementation of either valine or isoleucine. Likewise, the complex A21978 from *Streptomyces roseosporus*, also developed at Eli Lilly, can be influenced in its composition by modification of the fatty acid chain. Precursing with valine results in an enhanced formation of the compound C2, whereas the compound C1 was preferably built upon feeding of isoleucine. Compound C1 was inlicensed as daptomycin by Cubist Pharmaceuticals for clinical development. However, due to rhabdomyolytic activities and a slight haemolytic potential, it has been approved by the U.S. Food and Drug Administration in 2003 as Cubicin salve for topical use only. Despite such disadvantageous properties, peptides in general, including those that are from nonmicrobial sources and ribosomally synthesized, are currently considered to be among the most promising compound classes for development of novel antibacterials.

However, it has to be taken into account that amino acid and precursor incorporation as well as regulation mechanisms of biosynthetic pathways also depend on growth phases, on environmental influences, and thus on the conduction of the fermentation process during which the cells are propagated.

A prerequisite for a successful fermentation are controlled and homogenous environmental conditions for the cellular reactions. However, the ensurance of controlled reaction conditions, particularly in large production scales, has been turned out to be one of the most critical issues of industrial biotechnology, as will be illustrated in the next section.

Fermentation Optimization and Scale-Up

The scale-up of fermentation processes as a central problem in biotechnology was first recognized and described during industrial penicillin production at the beginning of the 1940s and has been studied in more detail in *E. coli* and recombinant protein production.

Reduced Mixing Quality and Enhanced Stress Exposure

Fermentation scale-up is aimed at the manufacture of larger product quantities, if at all possible, with a simultaneous increase or at least consistency of specific yields and product quality. The changed geometric and physical conditions in larger scales, however, has lead to a less favorable mixing behavior and to impaired physiological reaction conditions, which in turn may lead to a decreased process constance and reproducibility, to reduced specific yields, to an increase of unwanted side products, and thus ultimately, to a diminished batch-to-batch consistency and product quality, which are all key issues in industrial production processes.

The problem of reduced mixing quality in larger scales is aggravated with increasing vessel sizes: The opposite substrate and oxygen gradients along the vessel height that are formed as a result of the conventional fermenter design, according to which substrate feed usually occurs from the top and aeration from the bottom, are more pronounced in larger reactors due to (1) longer distances to be covered leading to larger substrate and oxygen depletion zones, (2) larger volumes of culture broth to be stirred and therewith longer mixing times, and (3) stronger hydraulic pressure gradients influencing the oxygen transfer rate. Cells at the fermenter top are exposed to excess glucose concentrations and simultaneously suffer from oxygen limitations, whereas those at the bottom are exposed to glucose starvation. Excess glucose concentrations (threshold value for *E. coli* at 30 mg/L) result in acetate overproduction (overflow-metabolism), and a simultaneous oxygen limitation further induces the formation of ethanol, hydrogen, formiate, lactate, and succinate (mixed acid fermentation). The produced acids can become reassimilated in oxygen-rich zones but in any case first lead to a temporary acidification of the microenvironment and later eventually of larger regions. Combined with a decreased transportation and elimination of carbon dioxide, detrimental metabolites, and surplus heat generated by agitation and metabolic processes, resulting in zonal overheating, the lower mixing rates in large scales thus lead to the formation of zones with enhanced stress conditions. The subsequent activation of stress genes only partially protects the cell against detrimental stress effects. For instance, despite activation of heat stress genes like *E. coli* dnaK and clpB, reducing misfolding and aggregation of heat-sensitive proteins, metabolic changes and damages such as translocation of proteins and membranes have been observed upon heat exposure. The evidently unavoidable detrimental effects of the repeated and cyclic passing of different stress zones and the subsequent continuous activation and shut down of the corresponding stress genes are believed to lead to a completely altered physiology with metabolic shifts, which ultimately reduce growth and productivity and increase byproduct formation.

Altered physiology

Changes in respiratory states like the switch from aerobic to anaerobic conditions and the imposed stress conditions, increased by induction and overproduction of the recombinant protein, lead to shifts in the coupled amino acid biosynthesis, an altered composition of the amino acid pools and changes in the protein biosynthesis machinery. Even though translation processes are considered to be generally performed precisely, the resulting shifts in the amino acid pool in turn lead, due to the inherent inaccuracy of the translation machinery (unspecificity of aminoacyl-tRNA-synthases, "wobbling" of tRNA), to aminoacid misincorporations in freshly synthesized proteins, particularly in phases of high protein production rates, which are characterized by amino acid shortages. Muramatsu et al. report the incorporation of β-methylnorleucin instead of isoleucin into recombinant *E. coli* hirudin in positions 29 and 59. A misincorporation of norvalin instead of leucin and methionine into human recombinant hemoglobin in *E. coli* has been published by Apostol et al. and Kiick et al. Amino acid misincorporations are thus a cause for an increase of byproducts at the expense of the desired main product yields.

Reduced plasmid stability

An essential prerequisite for high product yields particularly in larger scales, in which cultures pass a higher number of generations due to larger culture broth volumes and longer inoculation chains from the cell bank to the production stage, is the stable propagation of plasmids to daughter cells. Plasmid stability is influenced by the plasmid properties, including size and nucleotide sequence; by the genetic background of the host; as well as by process parameters like temperature, growth rates, and substrate concentrations. Lin and Neubauer show that rapid glucose oscillations favor plasmid stability and recombinant protein production rate, whereas high glucose concentrations diminish plasmid stability. Plasmid stability and plasmid numbers are thus negatively influenced, more difficult to control, and less easy to be maintained in larger scales.

A concept to render plasmid stability and expression rates more independent from such physiological influences is the application of runaway-plasmids, the replication of which can be induced separately from growth in the desired fermentation phase, enabling copy numbers of up to 1000 in the expression phase and, due to the separation of their replication and expression from the growth phase, simultaneously a more precise replication and amino acid incorporation. Further possible measures to enhance the accuracy of metabolic processes are a reduction of the generation time and numbers throughout the process and a deceleration of the metabolic speed, e.g., through reduction of temperature, and the development of more stress-resistant microbial strains.

A prioritized goal of process optimization and scale-up thus consists of an appropriate process design that improves the physiological conditions and the metabolic accuracy by minimizing microbial stress exposure.

Process Characterization

To identify process-specific stress factors and to understand the physiological responses to the vessel-specific physical conditions, the mutual influences and interactions of the various physical and physiological parameters have to be analyzed in detail. An overview on the analytical methods currently applied and yet in development is given in the following.

Analytical methods

Among the physiologically most relevant parameters are, besides the pH as discussed, biomass, cell viability, the concentrations of substrates, metabolites and products, the partial oxygen and carbon dioxide pressures in culture broth, and the composition of the exhaust gas, giving information about respiratory states as indicated, e.g., by the respiratory quotient. Established analytical methods and tools are colorimetric procedures, chromatography, mass spectroscopy, enzymatic and electrophoretic methods, hybridizing techniques, biochips, or flow cytometry. Multiparameter flow cytometry permits, in addition to the analysis of usual metabolites, also the analysis of the cellular DNA-, RNA-, and protein content, cell viability, membrane potential, intracellular pH, cell size, and cell development stages.

In general, the data are, if possible, preferably captured as real-time values by in situ online measurements as occurring for physical parameters to avoid falsified or gappy data due to time differences between sampling and analysis. *Ex situ* methods can be designed as real-time procedures in combination with robust automated sampling and sample preparation methods like ultra-filtration and flow injection analysis (FIA). An online FIA glucose analysis method of the native culture broth without prior sampling and filtration has been presented by Arndt and Hitzmann and Kleist et al. For their robustness, *in situ* measurements of biological parameters are preferably performed by optical probes (optodes), working either on a physical base, e.g., by refractional or spectroscopic measurements, chemically as by ion exchange reactions or enzymatically by gel-embedded biocatalysts, the activity of which can be measured by means of pH-changes or by fluorophores (chemo- and biosensors). The hitherto employed enzymes have restricted their application mostly to the analysis of sugar compounds, whereby the most frequent applications are reported for glucose. However, despite intensive research, only a few concepts practically applicable for industrial purposes could have been developed.

Broader applications are physical optodes enabling the simultaneous measurement and quantification of several parameters and metabolites through continuous scans or excitations and subsequent absorption and scattering measurements within defined wavelength ranges like (1) 2-D-fluorescence spectroscopy as shown for the determination of NAD (P)H concentrations through excitation at 350 nm and the fluorescence measurements at 450 nm; (2) near-infrared-spectroscopy (NIR), which has been employed as a 700–2500-nm scan in the antibiotic fermentation at Pfizer for the measurement of nutrient and product as well as side product concentrations; or (3) measurements in infrared, ultraviolet, or visible wavelength spectra. By means of capacitance measuring electrodes, viable cell counts can be performed by seizing the electric capacitance and conductivity of cells with intact membranes in a generated electric field.

To gain a picture as comprehensive as possible by enhancing the amount of analyzable substances, multichannel arrays with parallel employment of various analytical procedures monitoring several parameters simultaneously have been established and new concepts like artificial noses and electronic tongues currently being integrated into fermentation technology, allowing the analysis of a large number of analytes by cross-talking semi-specific sensors that act in analogy to the human olphactory sensoric system. The realization of this concept will be facilitated by a further miniaturization of the sensors and chips employed as it has been achieved with biochips developed for the pharmaceutical natural product screening, onto which the needed number of reactants is fixed in smallest space or is brought together in microchannels and the analytes are separated in microcapillars (lab-on-a-chip-technology).

Process Optimization

For analysis, interpretation and correlation of the obtained signals and data through chemometric modeling, neural network—tools—seem to have gained an increasingly important role. Despite inherent limitations, adequately trained neural networks are capable of recognizing and revealing nonlinear, highly complex, and even nonobvious, hidden relations among a multitude of various physical, biochemical, and physiological process parameters and to design the according process models. Hooked up to expert systems, they allow immediate and short-term reactions to process deviations by anticipating physiological drifts and their influences on product yield and quality and to change the according set points and process profiles. In this way, neural network tools help to optimize process control and to facilitate the identification of suitable strategies for process optimization and scale-up, e.g., with respect to an optimized glucose-oxygen equilibrium.

As the maximum glucose and oxygen uptake rates are not constant but depend on growth phases and rates and get reduced by induction of product synthesis, Lin et al. established an integrative kinetic model combining these parameters with the aid of the simulation program SCILAB (Inria, F) enabling the determination of the maximum glucose and oxygen uptake rates through determination of the time that passes between glucose pulses and subsequent changes of partial oxygen pressure (pO_2) and biomass concentration. Such a model thus allows the alignment of the glucose feed meeting the maximum uptake capacity and therefore avoiding overflow metabolism. The observed pattern of glucose oscillation even can serve as a key parameter condition in later scale-up stages. The equilibration of carbohydrate and oxygen supply thus constitutes a key component of process control and optimization.

Further strategies aiming at the avoidance of oxygen limitation and glucose overflow metabolism consist of the employment of alternative carbon sources like glycerol or galactose and of a drastic glucose restriction. Wong et al. report that minimal concentrations of glucose and yeast extract yielded the highest concentrations of 0.5 and 1 g/L of a recombinant K99 antigen. Yim et al. achieved constant yields of 4.4 g/L of human granulocyte colony stimulating factor during scale-up from 2.5 to 30 L by limiting glucose feed and keeping the growth rate at the minimum ($\mu = 0.116\ h^{-1}$). Besides the above-mentioned parameters like the maximum uptake capacities, the various different physiological or directly measurable physical process parameters like pH, ammonium consumption, pO_2, OTR, or the growth parameters can be applied as a reference parameter for glucose feed in a closed-loop design. Dantigny et al. describe a biomass controlling feed depending on the ethanol formation rate and RQ for *S. cerevisiae*. To achieve a more uniform glucose distribution in large-scale tanks, Larsson et al. and Bylund et al. suggested a glucose feed at the dynamic zones of the fermenter bottom together with the injected air. A step ahead in this regard would be a further enhancement of the mixing quality by a reactor and process design permitting a multilevel injection of both air and substrates into high turbulence zones.

A supportive approach for comprehension of the large-scale hydrodynamic and reaction conditions to ensure homogenous reaction conditions and to reduce both the size of stress zones and the zonal residence times is the depiction of these zones through transfer into small reactors (scale-down) or through high-performance computing computational fluid dynamics (CFD). Whereas the sort and amount of parameters that can be simulated by the scale-down approach appear to be restricted, CFD is meanwhile broadly applied, e.g., the flow modeling software tools of Fluent Inc., Lebanon, NH. A simulation of the trajectories and distributions of gas bubbles and mass transports enables the determination of zonal pO_2 values and oxygen transfer rates. The combination with parameters like substrate concentrations and gradients, the residence times in the respective zones, population dynamics, and metabolic fluxes (structured metabolic models) leads to integrative models (integrated fluid dynamics, IFD), which permit the prediction of physiological effects and reactions. Even though it is emphasized that the integration of CFD and structured biokinetics currently requires a deeper understanding of the dynamics of metabolic and regulatory networks and cascades of signal transduction triggered by microenvironmental fluctuations and thus further research, it will most likely contribute long term to a realistic modeling of the interplay between physics and physiology and thus will facilitate the identification of key parameters influencing product yield and quality the most and therewith of suitable scale-up parameters and strategies.

Physical Scale-Up Parameters

Suitable for employment as physical scale-up parameters are all known process parameters and coefficients exerting known physiological effects, particularly those affecting oxygen supply; heat transportation and mixing, sueh as power input, aeration, and agitation rate; mixing time; pO_2; OTR; oxygen mass transfer coefficient; and biocalorimetric variables like heat fluxes and heat transfer coefficients. Biocalorimetric measurements were found to be in definite correlation with metabolic activities and with OTR and are employable as growth phase indicators; the calculations, however, require a precise measurement and knowledge of heat fluxes and sources, energy inputs, and the temperature distribution in the vessel. In most cases, however, it is, depending on the scale-up factor, not, or only restrictedly, possible from the physical viewpoint to keep physical parameters constant throughout the scale-up. Constance of even a single specific parameter mostly leads to an uncontrolled and unpredictable change of other variables into dimensions that are technically not realizable. Classic examples are (1) the mixing time, which inevitably increases in larger vessels due to the larger volumes to be stirred and that cannot be unlimitedly compensated and kept constant by increasing stirrer speeds and energy inputs, and (2) the volumetric energy input P/V. A constant volumetric power input has indeed been successfully applied as a scale-up parameter for the early industrial penicillin fermentations (1 hp per gallon, equivalent to 1.8 kW per 1 m^3) and in fermentations with low energy inputs, but it is limited in fermentations requiring high energy inputs, like recombinant *E. coli* cultures.

For this reason, mathematically driven approaches are pursued for both process and reactor scale-up by forming dimensionless coefficients, which are kept constant by an appropriate choice and adjustment of the relevant influencing process and fermenter parameters. Well-established examples are, among many others, the dimensionless power number, Reynolds number, gassing number, and the modified dimensionless power number and the modified dimensionless mixing time. The comparison of the latter two coefficients and of the corresponding curves enables the identification of appropriate types of stirrers capable of exerting the desired mixing performance at a given stirrer speed with a minimum of energy consumption and therewith to compensate the above-mentioned limitations of volumetric energy inputs at larger scales. (A quantum leap in stirrer technology in this regard seems to be the Visco-Jet of Inotec, which possesses cone-formed short tubes instead of blades and pretends to exhibit the best mixing performance with a minimum of power input and shear stress without foam generation.) The performance of further various types and designs of stirrers is presented and discussed by Junker et al. Stirrer performance coefficients and curves are thus crucial scale-up aids.

Furthermore, any of these parameters and coefficients can be combined with other variables to set up and create new, process-specific parameter correlations, coefficients, terms, groups, and characteristic curves. This relates also to the k_La—value, which currently is the most applied physical scale-up variable because it includes the relevant parameters influencing oxygen supply like agitation (via energy input) and aeration as superficial gas velocity and that, as a component of dimensionless terms, is also frequently employed for reactor scale-up.

Taking into account the limitation of a k_La-oriented scale-up in the form of a limited power input, OTR, and tolerable shear stress, Flores et al. integrated the backpressure *p* by maintaining the product of $k_La \times p$ constant through a variation of pressure, agitation, and aeration for scale-up of *Bacillus thuringiensis* fermentations. Although the specific growth was reduced and the biomass production and sporulation efficiency remained constant, fermentation time could be shortened and toxin yields were increased. Wong et al. successfully scaled-up *E. coli* fermentations from 5 L to 200 L by keeping constant the product of k_La and aeration rate (vvm) under variation of power input, working volume, and aeration according to the Wang–Cooney equation, which reflects these parameters in dependence of the fermentation scale. Diaz and Acevedo argue that the oxygen transfer capacity, indicated by the k_La value, is not the most process-relevant parameter, but the effective oxygen transfer rate as a product of k_La and mass transfer potential is, i.e., the difference between the pO_2-values in the gas and the liquid phase, and suggest an OTR-based scale-up strategy. A common, simple and robust method is the maintenance of a constant pO_2 in the culture broth by variation of stirrer speed and aeration rate. To avoid shear stress and to keep the energy input (P) at the lowest possible level, the pO_2 is steered at the minimum limit. Riesenberg et al. employ a stirrer speed and glucose-feed steered pO_2 of 20% for interferon α-*E. coli*-fermentations in 30-L and 450-L scales. These examples demonstrate that, for each process, appropriate variables and coefficients and therewith scale-up strategies have to be identified individually.

Development of Fermentation Models and Strategies

Despite the central role of the scale-up issue in biotechnology and the comparably large body of literature, no common, generally applicable strategy seems to be established. For each product, process, and facility, a suitable scale-up strategy has to be elaborated. A wholistic scale-up strategy consists of a comprehensive and detailed process characterization to identify key stress factors and key parameters influencing product yield and quality the most, and of an appropriate process control and process design ensuring optimum mixing and reaction conditions, supported by appropriate knowledge and data-driven models as well as computational tools. It should be kept in mind, however, that any approach and any model will always be approximative and that a compromise in the process-related knowledge will always be gappy and that the known mathematical methods and relations cannot completely reflect the highly complex interactions and relationships of the physical conditions governing the fermentation process. As a matter of fact, it seems, that, in view of the high complexicity of the fermentation parameters influencing each other and the only rudimentary and fragmentary reflection of the reality any model can deliver and finally the different layouts of vessels and facilities that rarely are designed according to strict scale-up criteria, successful scale-up in most cases will not be the result of a conclusive and straight-lined experimental strategy but will be the outcome of an independent optimization on each scale that highly depends on the experience, skill, and last, but not least, intuition of the experimentalist. To a lesser extent, this also holds true for the design of procedures aimed at the isolation and purification of the compounds from the culture broth. As these purification steps follow upon the biosynthetic steps and the upstream processing in the bioreactor, they are usually referred as "*downstream processing*."

Downstream Processing

Product Recovery and Purification

Biopharmaceutical products consist of a multitude of compounds and structures with most having different physical and chemical properties and derive from a large variety of sources like human and animal tissues, body fluids, plant material, and as illustrated above, microbial fermentations. Accordingly, purification strategies have to be developed individually and empirically that reflect the physicochemical properties of the product, of the product source, and of potential contaminants by finding appropriate sorts, sequences, combinations, and operation modes of the respective downstream processing steps to finally achieve high purities and high recovery rates while maintaining the pharmaceutical activity of the molecule.

Traditionally, downstream processing steps are roughly subgrouped into operations related to cell harvest, cell rupture in case of intracellularly occurring products, product capture, product purification, and product polishing to manufacture a drug ready for galenic preparation and consist of a sequence of solid–liquid separation and solvent and solid-phase extraction steps. Large-scale cell harvest usually occurs by preparative centrifugation, e.g., in a decanter or in disk stack separator or by filtration to simultaneously separate existing suspended particles from the surrounding broth. Fragile mammalian cells are usually separated by filtration methods only.

If the value product occurs intracellularly, the slurry is taken up in washing buffers of appropriate ionic strength for preparation of the cell rupture, which occurs, e.g., by high-pressure homogenization, sonification, bead milling, or enymatic procedures.

Product capture is defined as the first product extraction and purification step aimed at a product concentration by volume reduction and partial purification, whereas polishing constitutes the final purification step, which removes persistent residual minor impurities like denatured, aggregated, or nonfunctional isoforms of the product, and which follows the preceding (intermediate) purification steps aimed at the removal of contaminating solutes like host cell proteins, DNA, and media components. Product capture usually starts with precipitation, solvent extraction, and/or a cascade of ultra-filtration and nano-filtration steps before the first ion exchange or size exclusion chromatography. Antibodies and antibody derivatives, which account for about 20% of the biopharmaceutical products currently in development, are preferably bound to affinity matrices by natural immunoglobulin-binding ligands such as the *Staphylococcus aureus* membrane and cell wall protein A or the streptococci surface protein G. To broaden the availability of specific structures with suitable binding properties, synthetic ligands with enhanced stability and resistance to chemical and biochemical degradation are continuously attempting to be developed, supported, e.g., by computer-aided design. The development of synthetic ligands with enhanced selectivity and stability, tailored to specific biotechnological needs and product structures, will lead to more efficient, less expensive, and safer procedures not only for purification of antibodies but also for other proteins at manufacturing scales. Also, antibodies can be employed as a means for protein purification in the form of immunoaffinity chromatography. A novel emerging technology is the use of synthetic single- stranded nucleic acid molecules (aptamers) as affinity ligands, which fold up into unique three-dimensional structures specifically binding to the desired target structure as it has been shown for the purification of thyroid transcription factor or selectin receptor globulin.

The subsequent purification steps including polishing are mostly performed on hydrophobic interaction resins and/or on reversed-phase matrices.

Downstream Processing Optimization and Economization

Mostly due to the tremendous costs of sometimes several thousand per liter for chromatographic resins and production scales of up to several hundred liters column volume and due to the prices for the columns themselves of up to hundreds of thousands of U.S. dollars, downstream processing expenses account for the largest part (50–90%) of the total production costs and are therewith a focal area for process economization attempts. One of the many criteria for the choice of a resin is its shelf life. Bearing in mind that every downstream processing step coincides with a minimum product loss of 5–10%, the removal of a particular step not only helps to save the respective capital investment, but concomittantly to increase the final product yields, and thus to render the whole production process more economical in several respects. To reduce the number of required steps, a selection has to be made for resins exhibiting excellent separation, resolution, and yield with respect to a given product and the contaminants, i.e., for resins exhibiting excellent product binding selectivity and capacity. Likewise, the operation mode of the column has to be optimized with respect to the specific product load, adjustment of the physico-chemical operational conditions like pressure, temperature, pH(- shift), ionic strength, and sort of buffers and eluents (e.g., evaluation of continuous vs. step gradients).

A further approach is the combination of the solid–liquid separation and product recovery into a single step, e.g., by expanded bed adsorption, which permits the direct initial purification from culture broths without the need of prior removal of suspended solids. In contrast to the conventional column operation, the mobile phase is pumped upward through the column bed from beneath. The bed thus starts to expand at a liquid flow rate above a critical value, and the gaps between the sorbent beads expand. The controlled distribution of bead size and bead weight results in a stable expanded bed in which the beads oscillate around a steady position and thus avoid clogging of the column. Whereas preparative liquid chromatography methods have become a well-established separation and purification method in the pharmaceutical industry, techniques like two-phase system partitioning and its variant reverse micellar extraction, which also potentially offer advantages like the possibility of a direct extraction from the culture broth through partitioning of the compounds into two immiscible phases, need further developmental activities for economic large-scale applications in the production of biopharmaceuticals and are less common. A further criterion for the choice and design of a downstream processing procedure is thus its scalability.

Downstream Processing Scale-Up

Comparable with the scale-up of fermenters and fermentation processes, the scaleup of downstream processes, particularly of column and column operation, is not simply a matter of increasing size. Increasing column diameters, reducing the stabilizing wall effects, and increasing resin bed heights may lead to an altered settling behavior of the beads, to channel formation through shrinking and swelling of the packed matrix, to column clogging with a concomittant reduction of the flow rates and an increase of the column back pressure, to altered hydrodynamic behavior and residence times of the process fluids, and to an altered pattern for the product/ contaminants adsorption/desorption pattern. To avoid the resulting quality impairments and deviations, resins with a suitable scale-up behavior have to be selected and the resin bed height is tried to be kept constant as far as possible as is the flow rate as key scale-up parameters, which requires an appropriate experimental design in early laboratory development stages. As this, however, is only possible to a limited extent, downstream processing scale-up also is the result of an optimization of the respective operation conditions on each scale. A procedure that has been optimized for decades and scaled-up to dimensions of several cubed meters is the commercial β-lactam purification.

Downstream Processing of β-Lactam Compounds

As most of the product is secreted and is thus concentrated in the culture broth, the recovery process starts with filtration, usually with a rotary vacuum filter, followed by a cascade of solvent and solid-phase extraction steps.

Common penicillin extraction solvents are amyl- and butyl-acetate or methylisobutylketone. As penicillin is extracted as a free acid at pH 2–2.5 and the molecule is instable at this pH, extraction occurs in a counter-flow using Podbielniak- and Luwesta-centrifugal extractors to shorten the contact time with the solvent and to prevent product decomposition. Purification is through subsequent and repeated crystallization from an aqueous solution after alkalization.

In contrast to penicillin, the hydrophilic cephalosporin is more suitable for solid- phase extraction. For high yield and purity extraction, a combination of several, different chromatographic steps is used.

Hydrophobic interaction chromatography on neutral polyaromatic resins like Amberlite XAD4, 16, 1180, or Diaion HP20 is widely used in combination with weak basic anion exchangers like Diaion WA-30 or strong acidic cation exchangers like Amberlite XAD 2000 and Diaion SK-1B. The mentioned resins are recognized for their high sorption capacity and their long shelf life.

Whereas the improvements on the extraction level are less spectacular, significant progress over the last few years can be noticed with respect to side-chain cleavage to 6-aminopenicillanic acid (6-APA) and 7-aminocephalosporanic acid (7-ACA) in switching from chemical to enzymatic procedures.

Postsynthetic Structure Modification

Most antibiotics in therapeutic use are synthesized or modified exclusively by the means of chemistry and are derived from the established compound classes, which have been known for decades. Chemical derivatization thus has also been applied to substances that are of microbial origin and that therefore are termed semi-synthetic.

Among the most recent semi-synthetic antimicrobials are Aventis' streptogramin derivative Synercid and the erythromycin derivatives clarithromycin (Klacid) from Abbott and roxithromycin (Rulid) and the brand new ketolide telithromycin (Ketek), both from Aventis.

Despite these recent successes and increasing efforts, the yields of therapeutically useful entities emerging from such chemical derivation programs are continuously decreasing.

For this reason, large-scale derivation methods (combinatorial chemistry) are integrated in the search for innovative antibiotics as are biotechnological approaches for structure modification. Biocatalytic procedures, which have been shown to be useful for generating novel antibiotic structures like Loracarbef, a novel β-lactam compound from Eli Lilly highly active against various β-lactamase producing species, are also about to replace continuously chemical production processes. At several universities and corporations, screening studies have been initiated to find appropriate enzymes for compound conversions, as it has been successfully established in production processes for penicillin and cephalosporin.

β-Lactam Side-Chain Cleavage

6-APA and 7-ACA as the key intermediates for the production of semisynthetic penicillins and cephalosporins are obtained by removal of the acyl side chains.

There is a large body of patents existing for chemical and enzymatic splitting procedures, but enzymatic processes have been more successful for economical as well as for ecological reasons.

Enzymatic 7-ACA splitting procedures have been developed and commercialized by companies like Asahi Chemical, Hoechst, and Novartis. The replacement of the hitherto employed chemical deacylation processes like the imino ether or the nitrosyl chloride method resulted in a cost reduction of 80% and a decrease of the waste volume by a factor 100 from 31 t to 0.3 tons per 1-ton 7-ACA. Chlorinated hydrocarbons like dimethyl aniline and methylene cloride as well as heavy metal ions can be completely avoided. Instead of zinc salt formation, multiple silylation, formation of the imino chloride, imino ether, and finally an imino ether hydrolysis, the side chain is removed in two enzymatic steps.

Cephalosporin C is first oxidized and deaminated by a D-amino acid oxidase (DAO), which can be obtained from various fungal species, like the yeasts *Trigonopsis variabilis* and *Rhodotorula gracilis* or the ascomycete *Fusarium solani*. The resulting α-keto-adipyl-7-ACA, upon decarboxylation, is converted into glutaryl-7-ACA (G-7-ACA). DAO is a flavoenzyme containing flavin adenine dinucleotide as the prosthetic group and catalyzes oxidation of D-amino acids to their corresponding keto acids. In a second step, the glutaryl side chain of G-7-ACA is deacylated by a glutarylamidase from *Pseudomonas diminuta*. The molecular data of other potentially suitable enzymes and genes from various sources are given by Isogai. It is noteworthy that the enzymatic splitting process could have only been rendered economical and therefore commercially employable through a significant increase of glutarylamidase yield on the fermentation level by using a gene-recombinant *E. coli*-strain.

A recombinant amidase from *E. coli* is also the most commonly employed enzyme for 6-APA production by deacylation of penicillin G, a process that has been established now for decades. With an annual turnover of 30 tons, the *E. coli* penicillin amidase is one of the most widely used biocatalysts, despite the discovery of further similar acting enzymes from various microbial sources, including penicillin V acylases from the basidiomycetes *Bovista plumbea* and *Pleurotus ostreatus*; from the ascomycete *Fusarium*; or from the yeast *Cryptococcus*.

A significant milestone in economization of enzymatic β-lactam production has been reached by enzyme immobilization permitting a preservation and multiple use of the cleavage enzymes. The currently most employed resins in industries for this purpose are epoxyacrylic acids and silica gel derivatives. The general economic criterion for the preparation of a biocatalyst is production costs in relation to yield, turnover rate, storage stability, and operational/mechanical stability. Further criteria are outlined in the *Guidelines for the Characterization of Immobilized Biocatalysts* by the European Federation of Biotechnology. Application criteria are filterability, sedimentation velocity, and particle firmness. Operational and storage stability as well as the activity of this biocatalyst and the quality of 6-APA with respect to color are improved by sulfur reducing compounds. As pointed out, the ensurance of product quality and drug safety is a key issue in pharmaceutical production processes.

Quality Issues

According to regulatory requirements, pharmaceutical production facilities and processes have to be proven to function properly across the entire range of process critical parameters by a qualification of the facilities and equipment, which consists of the steps design qualification (DQ), installation qualification (IQ), operational qualification (OQ), and performance qualification (PQ) and which results in a validation of the production process to substantiate that the complete system is capable of manufacturing the respective product reproducibly in a consistent quality as expected within preset specifications and in compliance with all laws and guidelines, like the cGMP (current good manufacturing practice) regulations, among others, issued by regulating authorities like the FDA and European Medicines Agency (EMEA).

The products have to be sterile and free of any contaminations that might derive from process material, residues of preceding production campaigns (cross- contaminations) in the case of product changes, and of the agents used for facility cleaning. To restrict the introduction of such contaminations into the repective production steps, the production facilities, equipments, and solutions are usually cleaned according to validated cleaning procedures (e.g., with 1 M NaOH) and sterilized by heat or filtration before their use. Product sterility is achieved by aseptical performance of the last manufacturing steps and by micro-filtration (0.2 μm) or, if possible, by terminal heating of the product before filling. Residues of chemical cleaning agents are removed according to validated procedures by rinsing with purified water.

As biopharmaceuticals are potentially contaminanted with possibly harmful viruses and allergenic and pyrogenic acting endotoxins as residual components of their host cell, guidelines and directions have been issued by the FDA's Center for Biologics Evaluation and Research (CBER) requesting validated procedures for virus and endotoxin removal and inactivation.

Virus and Endotoxin Removal

Endotoxins, which consist of the lipopolysaccharide fraction present in the cell wall of gram negative germs and which tend to adhere to equipment surfaces and to persist in products and product solutions, as do viral contaminants deriving from cell culture processes or from starting plasma or tissue material, can also be efficiently removed by final filtration steps. Whereas ultra-filtration with a cut-off of or below 10 kDa is sufficient for endotoxin removal, viruses need to be removed by nano-filtration steps complemented by a variety of inactivation measures like pasteurization, pH inactivation, solvent/detergent treatment, or ultraviolet and gamma ray irradiation. Usually, endotoxins and viruses are already deconcentrated to a significant extent by the chromatographic steps and the solvent exposure in the course of the normal purification procedures.

Marching in step with the technical and methodological progresses, biotechnology is gaining in increasing importance in pharmaceutical production processes by replacing chemical production procedures for economical and ecological reasons and in the development and commercialization of novel therapeutic principles.

To fully exploit the potential of biotechnological production methods, an integrated process design will be necessary considering the downstream processing requirement during the design of upstream operations and vice versa. As the fate of a compound as a pharmaceutical also depends on the prospective production costs already estimated in the development phase and production processes cannot be significantly changed after approval without running the risk of having to perform ad-ditional clinical trials, it is of utmost importance to choose and design production organisms, strains, vectors, expression cassettes, and fermentation procedures as early as possible in compliance with the prospective harvest and purification methods also to be chosen and designed according to cost criteria. Integrative biotechnology thus is not only a key prerequisite for the development of competitive and economical production processes to relieve the downward price pressure applied by generic drug makers after patent expiration and for the acceleration of market approval for new drugs in the highly competitive environment of the biopharmaceutical industry, but also it is a key technology to save and liberate capital for the development of novel drugs for the benefit of mankind.

Assigning Precise Function to Genes

The genomes of *Escherichia coli*, yeast, worm, and 18 microbes have been completely sequenced. The sequencing of the human genome is scheduled to be completed by the end of the year 2003, and the sequences of other genomes will become available in the coming decade. The emergence of genomics has changed the way that we discover and isolate genes. In the past we have proceeded from a peptide sequence or phenotype to the isolation of a new gene. Now, an investigator begins with the sequence of a key gene and searches for homologous genes in an organism of interest. Certainly, genomics will have tremendous impact on enzyme industry. However, the extent to which using genomic approach for "*enzyme mining*" actually succeeds will depend on how accurately the function of a new protein can be defined without any *a-priori* functional knowledge. Here, a broadly applicable strategy is presented that allows us to assign precise function to genes.

Orthologs, Paralogs, and Functional Prediction

Over a period of more than 3 billion years, a large variety of protein molecules have evolved as biological catalysts (enzymes) to run the complex machinery of the present-day cells and organisms. The relationships between genes from different genomes are naturally represented as a system of homologous families that include both orthologs and paralogs. Orthologs are genes in different species that evolved from a common ancestral gene by speciation and retained the same function in the course of evolution. By contrast, paralogs are genes related by duplication within an organism and have evolved a related but different function. Protein families are further connected into superfamilies, which are usually homologous, and folds which share common structural features but are not necessarily homologous. Hence, a powerful approach to predicting the exact function of a new protein is to find its characterized orthologs. Currently this is done by bioinformatics (biology with computers). Nevertheless, with incompletely sequenced genomes or large phylogenetic distances, there is always the chance that the real ortholog is not yet known and that the best match in a database hit is just a well-conserved paralog. The analysis is further complicated by the fact that a significant fraction of functional annotations in databases is wrong or dubious. Using β-decarboxylating dehydrogenase family as a model, we demonstrate that, with insight into how distinct functions of orthologs and paralogs are conferred and evolved, it is feasible to identify orthologs with high confidence.

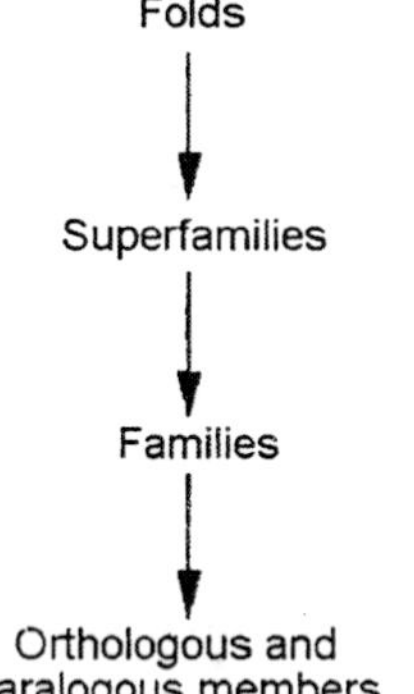

Fig. 13.1. Hierarchy in protein taxonomy.

β-Decarboxylating Dehydrogenases have Evolved Divergently from a Common Ancestral Gene

β-Decarboxylating dehydrogenases are a family of bifunctional enzymes that catalyze the Mg^{2+}- and $NAD(P)^+$-dependent dehydrogenation at C2, followed by their Mg^{2+}-dependent decarboxylation at C3 of β-substituted malate:

$$HOOC-CH(R)-CH(OH)-COOH+NAD(P)^+$$

$$\xrightleftharpoons{Mg^{2+}} HOOC-CH(R)-CO-COOH\ NAD(P)H+H^+$$

$$HOOC-CH(R)-CO-COOH+H^+ \xrightleftharpoons{Mg^{2+}}$$

$$R-CH_2-CO-COOH+CO_2$$

Three orthologs have been identified so far: NAD-dependent isocitrate dehydrogenase (NAD-IDH), NADP-dependent isocitrate dehydrogenase (NADP-IDH), and NAD-dependent isopropylmalate dehydrogenase (NAD-IMDH). NAD-IDH is limited to eukaryotic organisms and participates in the supply of NADH used for respiratory ATP production in mitochondria, while NADP-IDH is present ubiquitously in both prokaryotes and eukaryotes and involved in the generation of both NADPH and α-ketoglutarate for biosynthetic pathways. NAD-IMDH is found in bacteria, fungi, and plants. This is the enzyme that catalyzes the third step of the pathway for leucine biosynthesis. NADP-IDH and NAD-IMDH are homodimers, while all the NAD-IDHs purified so far have a hetero-oligomeric structure. The crystal structures of NADP-IDH from *E. coli* and NAD-IMDH from *Thermus thermophilus* have been solved. Both enzymes share a common protein fold that lacks the βαβαβ motif characteristic of the nucleotide-binding Rossmann fold.

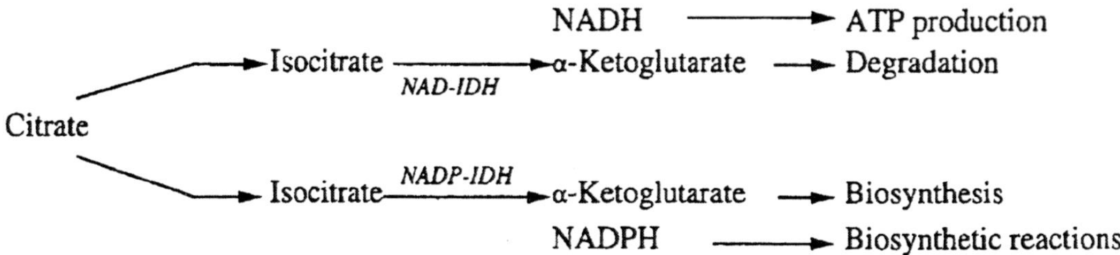

Fig. 13.2. "Division of labor" between NAD-IDH and NADP-IDH in eukaryotic organisms.

Phylogenic analyses indicate that NAD-IDH, NADP-IDH, and NAD-IMDH are homologous proteins that have evolved divergently from a common ancestral gene present in a progenitor of all extant organisms. The gene might encode the primitive enzyme that possessed a very broad specificity, permitting it to react with a wide range of related substrates that share a common 2-R malate moiety. This would maximize the catalytic versatility of an ancestral cell that functioned with limited genetic information and enzyme resources. The ancestral gene was then duplicated and acquired additional genetic information. Copies of the gene diverged via mutational modification, giving rise to contemporary enzymes with strict specificity. It has been suggested that specificity toward isocitrate may have evolved before specificity toward NADP, and that the latter evolved around the time the eukaryotes first appeared. Specialization of gene functions presumably allowed the improvement of metabolic efficiency and the evolution of new biochemical pathways.

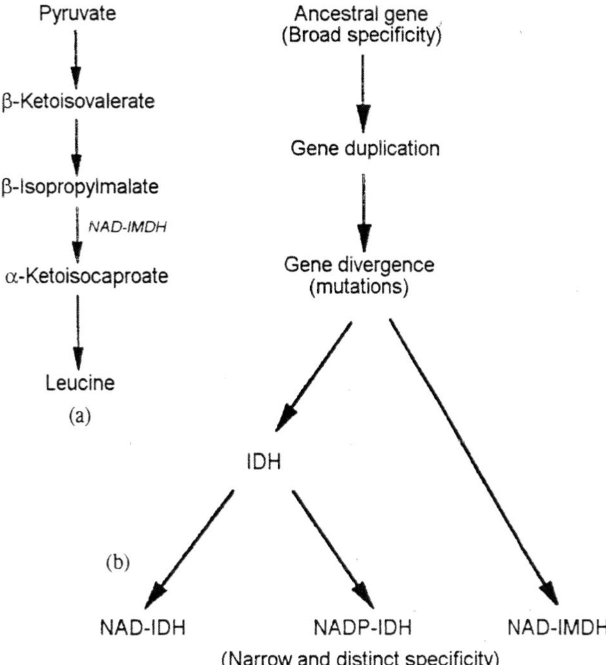

Fig. 13.3. (a) Leucine biosynthetic pathway. (b) Evolution of the β-decarboxylating dehydrogenase gene family.

Only a Few Amino Acid Replacements are Responsible for Distinct Functions of Orthologs

Over evolutionary time, a large number of sequence differences has accumulated between the members of the β-decarboxylating dehydrogenase family. The present-day phylogenies are highly divergent, and the divergence between orthologous genes approaches and even exceeds the level of divergence between paralogs within a species (our unpublished results). Thus, it is not reliable to make assignment of new protein sequences to a particular ortholog based on the best BLAST hit or similarity searches. In fact, residues critical to substrate and coenzyme binding and catalysis can rarely be aligned properly using BLAST or CLUSTAL W. This is especially the case when the sequence of *E. coli* NADP-IDH is compared to eucaryotic NADP-IDHs which share no significant identities (<17%).

The substrates isocitrate and isopropylmalate are structurally similar, i.e., $^{-}OOC(HO)CHCH(X)COO^{-}$ where X represents the γ-moiety: the $-CH_2COO^-$ of isocitrate and the $-CH(CH_3)_2$ of isopropylmalate. Coenzyme NADP differs from NAD only by a phosphate group esterified at the 2′C of the adenosine ribose. Presumably, distinct functions of NAD-IDH, NADP-IDH, and NAD-IMDH are conferred by their ability to recognize alternative substrates and coenzymes. Using protein engineering, we have demonstrated that, of hundreds of amino acid substitutions accumulated in these enzymes, only a few are involved in specificity determination.

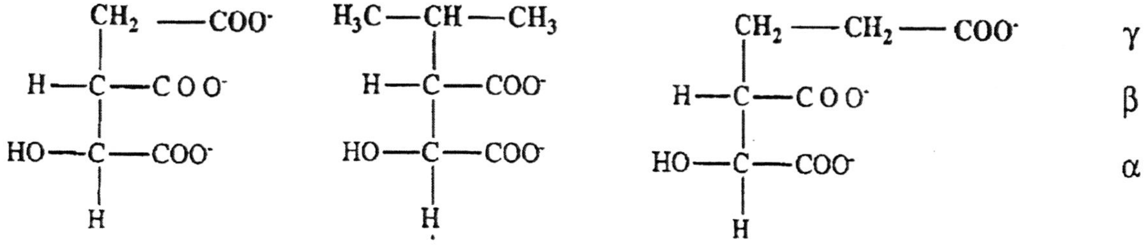

A: CH_2-COO^- / $H-C-COO^-$ / $HO-C-COO^-$ / H

B: $H_3C-CH-CH_3$ / $H-C-COO^-$ / $HO-C-COO^-$ / H

C: $CH_2-CH_2-COO^-$ / $H-C-COO^-$ / $HO-C-COO^-$ / H

γ β α

Fig. 13.4. Structures of 2R,3S-isocitrate (A), 2R,3S-isopropylmalate (B), and 2R,3S-homoisocitrate (C). α, β refers to the α- and β-carboxyl groups, respectively The unique γ-moieties are presented in bold.

Specificity Determinants in *E. coli* NADP-IDH

In *E. coli* NADP-IDH, all the residues involved in binding and catalysis have been identified by crystallographic analysis, site-directed mutagenesis, and protein engineering. The true substrate for the NADP-IDH is a Mg^{2+} -isocitrate complex which binds in a pocket, formed from residues donated from both monomers. Hydrogen bonds and some ion pairs are formed between the α-carboxylate of isocitrate and the side chains of Arg119, Arg129, and Arg153, and between the β-carboxylate of isocitrate and the side chains of Arg119, Arg153, and Tyr160. The Mg^{2+} cation is coordinated to the α-carboxylate and α-hydroxyl groups of isocitrate, the side chains of Asp307, Asp311, and Asp283′ (the second subunit). The side chain of Asp283′ acts as a base for the removal of a proton from the α-hydroxyl group during dehydrogenation, and the side chain of Lys230′ acts as an acid in the decarboxylation. The amino acid residues Ser113 and Asnl 15 on the helix δ, and the γ-carboxylate of isocitrate, are the major determinants of substrate specificity. Ser113 forms a hydrogen bond with the γ-carboxylate of bound isocitrate, which, in turn, forms a salt bridge to the nicotinamide ring of the coenzyme. Asn115 also interacts with the γ-carboxylate of bound isocitrate. The interaction has a nonideal hydrogen bond angle and is probably purely electrostatic in nature. This residue also is coordinated to the amide of NADP in the Michaelis complex. The polar environment formed with Ser113 and Asn115 is not compatible with the hydrophobic γ-isopropyl group of bound isopropylmalate. More important, this γ-isopropyl group is unable to form the binding site for the nicotinamide ring which is critical for hydride transfer. Consequently, in spite of the structural similarity of isocitrate and isopropylmalate,

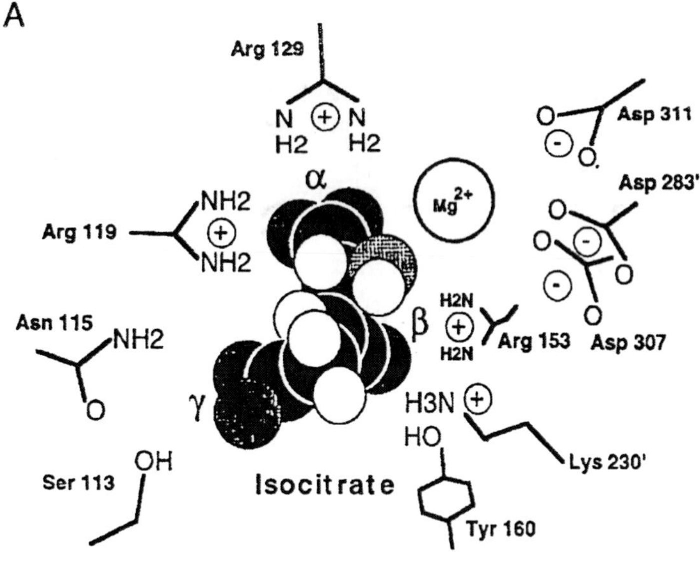

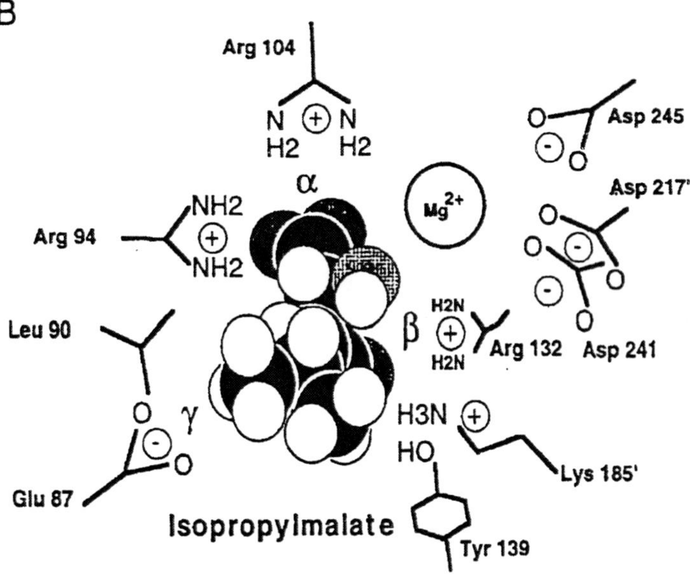

Fig. 13.5. Schematic diagram of the active site of the E. coli NADP-IDH with bound 2R,3S-isocitrate (A) and the active site of T. thermophilus NAD-IMDH with bound 2R,3S-isopropylmalate (B).

IDH does not catalyze a reaction with isopropylmalate (with reduced catalytic efficiency by a factor of at least greater than 10^8). Coenzyme specificity in the NADP-IDH is conferred by hydrogen bonds between the side chains of Arg-395, Tyr-345, Tyr-391, and Arg-2922 and the 2′-phosphate of bound NADP. The side chains of Lys344 may ion-pair with the 2′-phosphate. These interactions can not be formed with the 2′-hydroxyl of NAD. Hence, this enzyme is highly specific for NADP. Calculated as the ratio of k_{cat}/K_m, the enzyme displays a 7000-fold preference for NADP over NAD.

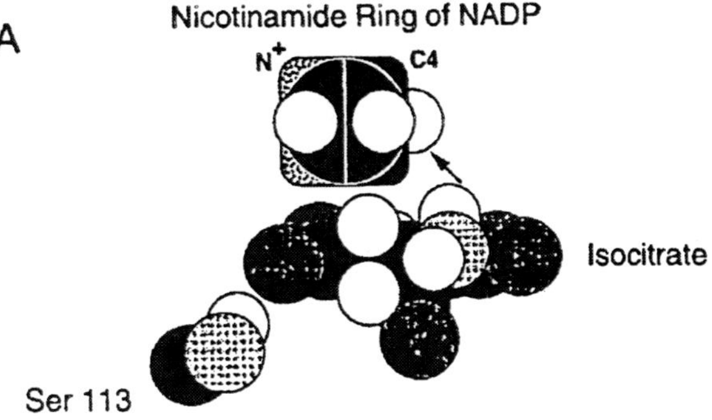

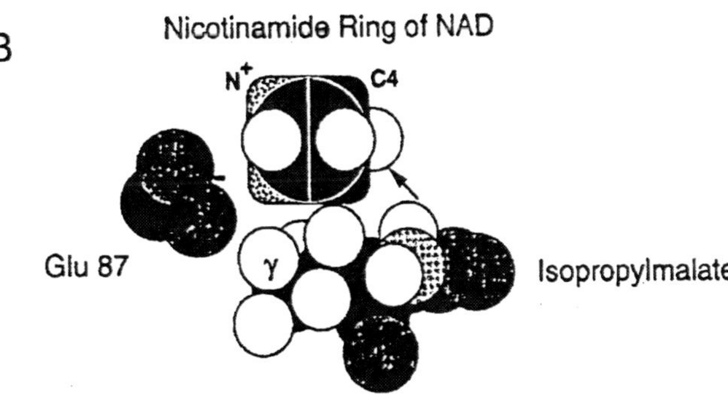

Fig. 13.6. Model for the Michaelis complex of the E. coli NADP-IDH with isocitrate and NADP bound (A) and the T. thermophilus NAD-IMDH with isopropylmalate and NAD bound (B).

Specificity Determinants in *T. thermophilus* NAD-IMDH

Despite sharing only 25% sequence identity, *T. thermophilus* NAD-IMDH and *E. coli* NADP-IDH share a common protein fold, and their tertiary structures can be superimposed. The amino acid residues involved in binding the 2*R*-malate core, common to 2*R*,3*S*-isocitrate and 2*R*,3*S*-isopropylmalate, are identical. The equivalent active residues in *T. thermophilus* NAD-IMDH are Arg94, Arg104, Arg132, Tyr139, Lys185′, Asp217′, Asp241, and Asp245. However, the two enzymes differ in the amino acid residues involved in binding the γ-moieties of substrates. In NAD-IMDH, Asn115 is replaced by Leu90, which forms hydrophobic interactions with the γ-isopropyl group of bound isopropylmalate. In addition, the helix d begins three amino acids earlier, with the consequence that the side chain of Glu87 occupies a position in close proximity to both Ser113 and the γ-carboxylate of isocitrate. The available structural data and the kinetic results suggest that the carboxyl group of Glu87 interacts with the nicotinamide ring and helps stabilize the Michaelis complex, mimicking the role played by the γ-carboxylate of the bound isocitrate in NADP-IDH. Meanwhile, this negatively charged residue lies close to an analogous position of they-moiety of bound isocitrate and thus would electrostatically repel this molecule as a substrate. Indeed, no activity is detectable with isocitrate. Consequently, Glu87 and Leu90 are major determinants of substrate specificity in NAD-IMDH. The coenzyme specificity toward NAD is mainly conferred by Asp278 (IMDH numbering), which forms a double hydrogen bond with the 2′ - and 3′-hydroxyl groups of the adenosine ribose of NAD. Meanwhile, this negatively charged residue repels the 2′-phosphate of NADP through electrostatic repulsion. As such, this enzyme is 100-fold more active with NAD than with NADP.

Specificity Determinants are Reliable Markers for Orthologs and Paralogs

NADP-IDHs and NAD-IMDHs from Other Species

The sequence of the NADP-IDHs and NAD-IMDHs from other species were compared with that of *E. coli* NADP-IDH and *T. thermophilus* NAD-IMDH. It is noteworthy that the NADP-IDH/NAD-IMDH phylogenies are so divergent that correct alignment can be made only based on detailed knowledge of the X-ray crystallographic structures of *E. coli* NADP-IDH and *T. thermophilus* NAD-IMDH. It shows that all of the binding and catalytic residues identified in *E. coli* NADP-IDH are conserved in other NADP-IDHs except Lys344, which is either conserved or replaced by a positively charged residue His. As expected. Ser113 and Asn115 are replaced by Glu and Leu, respectively, while Lys344 and Tyr345 are substituted by Asp and Ile or Leu in all known NAD-IMDHs. Hence, these major specificity determinants can be used as landmarks for predicting the exact biochemical functions of new sequences belonging to the isocitrate and isopropylmalate dehydrogenases family.

Yeast and Mammalian NAD-IDHs

No crystal structure is available for NAD-IDHs. All the NAD-IDHs purified so far have a hetero-oligomeric structure which differs from the homodimeric form of NADP-IDHs and NAD-IMDHs. Yeast NAD-IDH exists as a heterooctamer consisting of four copies of the regulatory subunit (NAD-IDH1) and four copies of the catalytic subunit (NAD-IDH2), while mammalian NAD-IDHs consist of three different subunits (α, β, and γ) having the tetrameric form of $\alpha_2\beta\gamma$. Catalytic residues are located in the α-subunit. Site-directed mutagenesis analysis suggests that the yeast NAD-IDH has an active center formed from two of the multiple subunits which is essentially identical to that of *E. coli* NADP-IDH.

Structural knowledge-based alignment shows that the catalytic subunits of NAD-IDHs retain all the active residues involved in Mg^{2+}-isocitrate binding and catalysis. Similar to NAD-IMDH, the residues Lys344 and Try345, which interact with NADP in *E. coli* NADP-IDH, are replaced by Asp and Ile in these NAD-IDH proteins. These results are consistent with their coenzyme preference toward NAD. Most of the active residues, including the residues equivalent to Ser113 and Asn115 of *E. coli* NADP-IDH, are found in the regulatory subunits of both yeast and mammalian NAD-IDHs. However, both Asp307 and Asp311, which coordinate the Mg^{2+} of Mg^{2+}-isocitrate in the *E. coli* NADP-IDH, are substituted by Asn, Ser, or Thr in these sequences. This replacement should abolish the binding with Mg^{2+}-isocitrate, the true substrate for IDHs. Indeed, only two Mg^{2+}-isocitrate sites per $\alpha_2\beta\gamma$ tetramer of yeast NAD-IDH have been observed. Meanwhile, the Arg129 residue, which binds via ionic hydrogen bonds to the α-carboxylate of bound isocitrate in the *E. coli* NADP-IDH, is replaced by a hydrophobic branched-chain residue such as Val, Ile, or Ala. This should significantly weaken the binding affinity with isocitrate. The substitutions of these important residues agree with the regulatory roles of the subunits. The residue Asp278 identified in the *T. thermophilus* NAD-IMDH is conserved in yeast IDH1 but is replaced by polar residues Gln or Ser in the mammalian β and γ subunits. Thus, identifying the critical specificity determinants is sufficient to define the function of NAD-IDH proteins as well.

Functional Misassignment can be Confidently Corrected

Insight into the structural and functional determinants for enzyme specificity allowed us to access functional assignment of β-decarboxylating dehydrogenase sequences. Of the cDNA or genomic sequences that have been published or deposited in databases, at least 20 are incorrectly annotated. Case studies are presented here to demonstrate that correct annotation can be made with certainty.

Bacterial NAD-IDH Sequence

All the eubacterial IDHs purified so far are NADP-specific, while NAD-IDHs are only found in the mitochondria of eukaryotic organisms. However, early enzymatic studies suggested that NAD-IDHs may exist in some bacteria. This prompted our rigorous search for possible eubacterial NAD-IDH sequences. Of 17 nonredundant prokaryotic IDH sequences available in the databases, the sequence from *Streptococcus salivarius* was predicted to encode a NADP-IDH protein of 391 amino acid residues. All of the substrate-binding and catalytic residues identified in *E. coli* NADP-IDH are conserved in this protein, including Ser113 and Asn115, which are the major determinants of specificity toward isocitrate. In contrast, the residues Lys344 and Tyr345 interacting with NADP in the *E. coli* NADP-

IDH are replaced by Asp and Ile, as seen in NAD-IMDH. This observation allows us to assign the function of the *S. salivarius* protein as NAD-IDH. These results demonstrate that, similar to NADP-IDH, NAD-IDH is present in both prokaryotic and eukaryotic organisms.

Plant NAD-IDH Sequences

The tomato "NADP-IDH" cDNA sequence was isolated from tomato roots and was upregulated during arbuscular mycorrhiza colonization. This sequence has been placed in the database and annotated as an NADP-IDH-like protein. Both equivalent Ser113 and Asn115 residues are found in this sequence, indicating that it is indeed an IDH protein. Nevertheless, the presence of the negatively charged Glu at residue 344 suggests that this IDH is NAD-dependent. Similar to the regulatory subunits of yeast and mammalian NAD-IDHs, the Arg129, Asp307, and Asp311 residues of the *E. coli* NADP-IDH involved in the binding of the Mg^{2+}-isocitrate complex are substituted by Val, Ile, and Asn. This leads to the prediction that the current protein belongs to a regulatory subunit. It has been shown that plant NAD-IDHs are exclusively localized in mitochondria. As such, this protein sequence can be annotated as a regulatory subunit of tomato mitochondrial NAD-IDH.

The two *Arabidopsis* cDNA clones, "NAD-IDH1" and "NAD-IDH2", were identified by homology searches from the *Arabidopsis* EST database. These sequences share 36–50% identity with yeast and mammalian NAD-IDHs and contain a typical mitochondrial import targeting peptide. However, the report concluded that it was impossible to make subunit assignments, comparable to those for mammalian and yeast NAD-IDHs, and suggested that a single-subunit form of *Arabidopsis* NAD-IDH may exist and these two clones may represent isozymes. With a careful examination of the active site residues in these two sequences, it is obvious that, like the tomato NAD-IDH protein, these gene products lack the Mg^{2+}-binding site and should correspond to different regulatory subunits of NAD-IDH. Since the binding residues equivalent to Arg129, Asp307, and Asp311 found in *E. coli* NADP-IDH are missing from these sequences, neither subunit can form an active enzyme. This is consistent with the observation the cDNA clones failed to complement yeast NAD-IDH mutants. The residues involved in the binding of Mg^{2+}-isocitrate complex must be present at the third subunit.

It is noteworthy that the N-terminal sequences of the four plant NAD-IDH proteins described here share common features of a mitochondrial transit peptide: rich in basic and hydroxylated amino acids but lacking acidic residues. Furthermore, these sequences contain basic residues at the N-terminal extremity which are characteristic of mitochondrial transit peptides and are normally absent from chloroplastic transit peptides. In contrast, the motif of Val/Ile-Arg-Ala/Cys⊥Ala (⊥ cleavage site) is frequently found at the cleavage site in the end of chloroplastic transit peptides, including the one for the chloroplastic NAD-IMDH from rape, but is absent from all the NAD-IDH sequences. Taken together, these results allow us to predict that, like their mammalian counterparts, plant NAD-IDHs must consist of three different subunits. Recently, three cDNA clones encoding different NAD-IDH subunits have been isolated from tobacco plants. Both biochemical and genetic studies of the enzyme indicated that indeed, the physiologically active form is composed of the three different subunits.

New Orthologs can be Readily Discovered: NAD-Homoisocitrate Dehydrogenase

It has been suggested that new enzyme functions are established most easily and most commonly by recruitment of proteins already catalyzing analogous reactions. NAD-IDHs, NADP-IDHs, and NAD-IMDHs are enzymes of very ancient origin. Protein engineering demonstrates that a few amino acid residue substitutions are sufficient to alter their substrate and coenzyme specificities. Such a strategy may have been used to modify these enzymes into new orthologs that catalyze identical chemical reactions but have distinct substrate specificities. An example of this strategy is discussed below.

In fungi, lysine is synthesized via an α-aminoadipate pathway. The conversion of homoisocitric acid to α-ketoadipic acid occurs due to enzyme homoisocitrate dehydrogenase (NAD-HDH):

$$\text{Homoisocitric acid} + NAD^+ \xrightleftharpoons{\cdot\ Mg^+} \alpha\text{ - ketoadipic acid}$$
$$+CO_2 + NADH + H^+$$

This reaction is clearly analogous to that of NAD-IDHs, NADP-IDHs, and NAD-IMDHs. Early studies showed that the enzyme of *S. cerevisiae* was separated from the NAD-IDH and has a different pH optimum. The molecular mass of the enzyme is 48 kDa. These results suggest that NAD-HDH is a novel member of the β-decarboxylating dehydrogenase family. In spite of a number of biochemical and genetic studies, the gene encoding the enzyme has not been identified.

The substrate homoisocitrate is structurally similar to isocitrate and isopropylmalate, where the γ-moiety is $—CH_2CH_2COO^-$. With the principles governing the relationship between structure and function in NADP-IDHs and NAD-IMDHs, we predict that all of the substrate-binding and catalytic residues shared by *E. coli* NADP-IDH and *T. thermophilus* NAD-IMDH should be conserved in NAD-HDH. What makes this enzyme distinct would be the amino acid residues involved in binding the γ-moieties of substrate. Compared to isocitrate, the γ-carboxylate of homoisocitrate is one carbon farther away from C2. This difference prevents the formation of a salt bridge between the bound homoisocitrate and the nicotinamide ring of the coenzyme in the Michaelis complex that would otherwise pull the nicotinamide C4 out of the catalytic trajectory during hydride transfer. In this enzyme, the nicotinamide ring is probably aligned with the bound homoisocitrate by the protein itself, as seen in NAD-IMDH, where the carboxyl group of Glu87 interacts with the nicotinamide ring. However, the presence of a negatively charged residue such as Glu at this position would electrostatically repel the γ-moiety of bound substrate. Hence, the residue equivalent to Ser113 of the NADP-IDH and Glu87 of the NAD-IMDH should be Tyr or Gln, which is able to interact with nicotinamide ring via hydrogen bonding. Meanwhile, the residue equivalent to Asn115 of NADP-IDH and Leu90 of NAD-IMDH is likely a nonpolar residue which interacts hydrophobically with the extra-carbon portion of the γ-moiety of the bound homoisocitrate. The genome of *S. cerevisiae* has been completely sequenced. A search of the entire genomic sequence with *E. coli* NADP-IDH leads to the identification of a candidate sequence with functional annotation as NAD-IMDH. This protein of 385 amino acid residues shares 32%, 34%, and 35% identity with the yeast NAD-IMDH and the regulatory and catalytic subunits of NAD-IDH, respectively. The molecular mass is estimated as 41 kDa. As expected, most of the substrate-binding and catalytic residues identified in *E. coli* NADP-IDH are found in this protein. Remarkably, the major specificity determinants in the NADP-IDH, Ser113 and Asn115, are replaced by Tyr and Ile, which makes this protein different from IDH and IMDH. Meanwhile, the residues Lys344 and Tyr345, which interact with NADP in *E. coli*, are replaced by Asp and Ile. This observation allows us to confidently assign the function of the protein as NAD-HDH.

Using the β-decarboxylating dehydrogenase family as a model, we demonstrate that rules for predicting the precise function of members of gene families can be established. The strategy is based on our recent findings that only a few amino acid residue substitutions in these enzymes are sufficient to change substrate and coenzyme specificities and thus alter enzyme functions. The few critical specificity determinants then serve as reliable markers for determining orthologous or paralogous relationships. The power of this approach has been demonstrated by correcting functional misassignments and discovering new genes. With the progress of genome-wide efforts to determine representative three-dimensional structures for all protein families, it is likely that the current approach will become broadly applicable. Extension of similar studies to other protein families would be much needed in order to take full advantage of the enormous wealth of biological information coming out of the EST and genome projects. In conclusion, such a powerful approach should allow us to significantly accelerate the discovery of new enzymes and related pathways in the coming years and thus herald an exciting new era for enzymologists.

14

GENOME VARIATION

In the past few years there has been significant progress towards completing the sequences and beginning to characterize the content of the genomes of several mammalian species. The most notable advances have been made in the study of the human genome. The availability of a near-finished reference DNA sequence has been most crucial in clinical genetic- and genomic-investigations because for the first time it provides a common template for comprehensive comparative studies aimed at cataloguing genotypes and their influence on phenotypic outcomes. Although much progress has been made in this endeavor (~2000 disease genes or associated variants identified) there are still some 4000 genetic diseases for which the molecular etiology is unknown. There are also numerous phenotypic traits in the apparently "healthy" population that can have a strong genetic component; one important example being genetic factors affecting drug metabolism. Genetic variation in the human genome has, until recently, mainly been studied either at the single nucleotide- or the karyotypic-level. The most common class of variation is single nucleotide (nt) substitutions. These mostly benign changes are now well studied with an estimated 11 million single-nucleotide polymorphisms (SNPs) currently described in the human population. Most of the Human Genome Project-coordinated endeavors to catalogue common variants in the genome sequence have been focused on SNPs. Small insertions and deletions are also usually grouped into this category.

Genomic variation detected by karyotyping would include larger tracts of usually contiguous DNA that can vary in copy number (*deletion* and *duplication*), distribution (*translocations* and *insertions*), or orientation (*inversions*) along the chromosomes. In most cases these large genomic rearrangements are associated with clinical outcomes. To date, there has not been an exhaustive assessment of the frequency, extent, or distribution of variants in the kilobase (kb) to megabase (Mb) size range, mainly due to lack of robust genome scanning technologies available for this resolution of analysis. However, to partially address this problem there have been recent technical advances that capitalize on the genome sequence as a reference substrate allowing rapid assessment of gains or losses of sequences along chromosomes. As the data begin to accumulate it is becoming increasingly apparent that these "so-called" large-scale copy number variants (or LCVs), often averaging hundreds of kb in size, are present in the genomes of apparently healthy individuals at a much higher frequency than originally thought.

In many cases these genomic variants partially or entirely encompass genes, which can affect their copy number. Moreover, in some cases they overlap with nearly identical segmentally duplicated DNA (called low-copy repeats or duplicons). Given that segmental duplications (and possibly LCVs) are implicated in a growing list of over 30 human diseases, which arise due to a gain, loss, or disruption of dosage sensitive genes or regulatory regions these new observations may also be relevant to other unresolved genetic diseases. In this chapter we will describe three different categories of genomic variation and discuss how each type of variation may influence human disease. We will describe what are known about genomic disorders and the mechanisms that cause them. We will then discuss how similar molecular events may underlie certain phenotypic variation and susceptibility to common complex diseases as well as influence the dynamic structuring of the human genome.

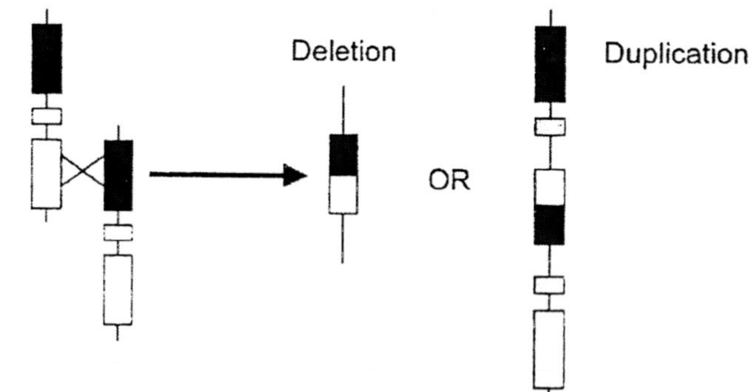

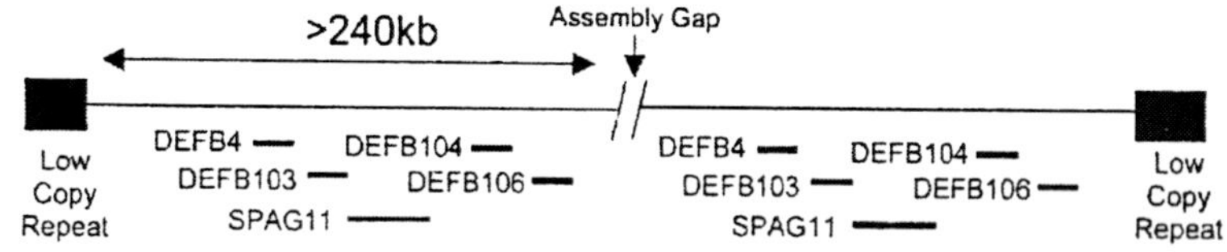

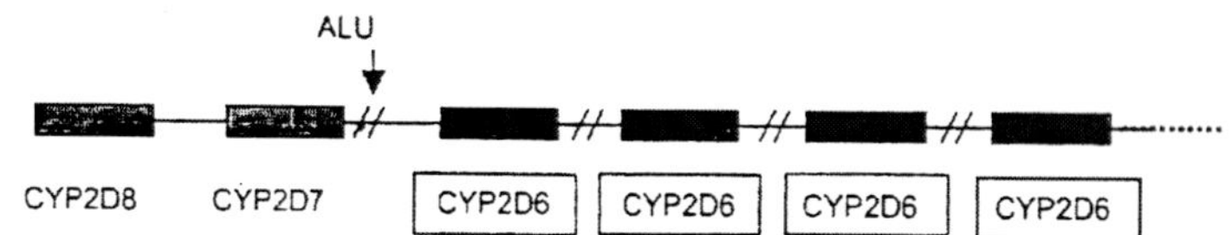

Fig. 14.1. This figure outlines the three types of genomic variation.

Mechanisms of Genome Rearrangement

There are a large number of diseases that are caused by genomic rearrange ments involving several genes and they are usually referred to as "*genomic disorders.*" In most cases genomic disorders arise due to errors occurring in the chromosomal recombination process. Molecular genetic studies have now led to the precise positioning of chromosomal breakpoints for many of these genomic disorders. While the regions affected by the rearrangements are mostly made up of unique sequence, the intervals immediately surrounding the breakpoints often show a high degree of DNA sequence similarity. These findings indicate that the majority of recurrent rearrangements are caused by misalignment of nearly identical sequences in the genome. This type of mechanism of aberrant recombination is referred to as non-allelic homologous recombination (NAHR). The rearrangements caused by NAHR include deletions, duplications, inversions, or more complex combinations of these rearrangements.

Homologous sequences have also been found :ar the breakpoints for the few known examples of recurrent translocations, suggesting that similar mechanisms exist for interchromosomal recombination. Large deletions and duplications will give rise to genomic disorders when the gene(s) located within the affected region are dosage sensitive. Inversions and translocations do not create differences in copy number of the genes in the genomic segment affected, but may cause disease by directly disrupting genes or acting on them indirectly by dysregulating their control elements in the breakpoint regions.

Recurrent Genomic Rearrangements

Large stretches of highly homologous DNA sequences usually referred to as segmental duplications or low copy repeats or duplicons have been shown to be the primary cause for NAHR. The type of rearrangement caused by segmental duplications depends on the architecture of the specific sequences involved. If the direction of the duplicated sequence is the same, it will result in either deletion or duplication, while inverted segmental duplications give rise to inversion. One of the best-studied examples of how low-copy repeat regions having a simple organization gives rise to genomic disorders is based on extensive studies of the p12 band of chromosome 17.

Rearrangements in this region can cause one of two diseases, namely, Charcot-Marie-Tooth disease type 1A (CMT1A) and hereditary neuropathy with liability to pressure palsies (HNPP). CMT1A is caused by a 1.4 Mb genomic duplication, while HNPP is caused by a deletion of the equivalent region. Molecular studies indicate that these diseases are the reciprocal products of NAHR events between two flanking 24kb segmental duplications sharing 98.7% sequence identity. Similar mechanisms cause two genomic disorders on 17p11.2, Smith–Magenis Syndrome (SMS) and dup(17)(p11.2p11.2) syndrome. In these cases a large DNA segment about 3.7 Mb in size, which is deleted in SMS and duplicated in dup(17)(p11.2p11.2) patients, is flanked by long duplicated sequences of ~200 kb arranged in the same orientation along the chromosome. However, the organization of segmental duplications is often complex with several sub-regions organized in different directions compared to the ancestral segments. Series of duplicated regions may therefore give rise to a number of different size deletions, duplications, or more complex rearrangements causing different disorders. The most studied such region is located at 22q11 and it contains a number of segmental duplications of complex organization, which are now known to be involved in deletions, duplications, inversions, translocations, and marker chromosomes.

Deletions and Duplications

The most common rearrangement caused by illegitimate recombination triggered by the presence of segmental duplications is chromosomal deletion of the unique sequence. If reciprocal exchanges occurred equally as would be predicted from modeling an equal proportion of deletions and duplications should be observed. The data indicate, however, that deletions are vastly over-represented. Disorders arising due to recurrent deletions are referred to as microdeletion syndromes. True microdeletion syndromes are caused by haploinsufficiency of several genes. One of the most common microdeletion syndromes is DiGeorge Syndrome/Velocardiofacial Syndrome (DGS/VCFS), with a prevalence of 1.3–1.5/10.000 births (7,8). The deletion is induced by low copy repeats located at 22q11.2. The frequency of de novo deletions in this region is at least one magnitude higher than de novo point mutation rates for human autosomal dominant disorders.

When large deleted regions including several genes give rise to a complex clinical phenotype, it can often be difficult to distinguish which of the genes in the segment contribute to the phenotype. Williams–Beuren syndrome (WBS) offers one such example. WBS is caused by a 1.6 Mb deletion at 7q11.2 region, which contains more than 20 genes. The phenotype ofWBS displays unique facial features, growth retardation, infant hypercalcemia, and supravalvular aortic stenosis. Patients with WBS have a distinctive personality and are highly sociable, musical, and talk remarkably well, but have severely impaired visuospatial constructive abilities. It has been shown that disruption of only the elastin gene, harbored within the region commonly deleted in WBS patients, gives rise to dominant supravalvular aortic stenosis, thus explaining part of the phenotype. Using a similar "*genotype–phenotype*" correlation additional disease contributing genes in the region are being discerned for other sub-phenotypes.

One of the most recent additions to the family of genomic disorders is Kabuki Syndrome, a form of congenital mental retardation with a phenotype that appears to be genetic in etiology. However, little evidence of a genetic abnormality, either chromosomal or Mendelian, had previously been established. Recently a duplication of a 3.5 Mb region was found at 8p23.1-p22 in six unrelated patients, suggesting that this may be the common cause for this disorder. Parkinson disease is a late-onset disease and the second most common neurodegenerative disorder after Alzheimer disease, affecting approximately 1% of the population over age 50. In 1997 kindreds with a familial form of Parkinson disease were shown to carry mutations in the alpha-synuclein gene (SNCA). A study last year reported on a family showing linkage to the SNCA locus but where no disease causing mutations could be found. Further investigations revealed that the affected family members all carried a duplication of a ~2 Mb stretch of DNA spanning the SNCA gene. This finding not only suggests a mechanism of the role of SNCA in Parkinson disease, but also that large duplications and deletions may more often than originally thought be involved in disease etiology in families where mutation screening of causative genes appears negative.

Inversions and Translocations

Genomic disorders caused by inversions and translocations are far fewer in occurrence than those arising due to deletions and duplications. In most cases, inversions and translocations normally do not cause disease by leading to a direct gain or loss of dosage sensitive genes, but the genomic lesions may disrupt genes residing at the respective breakpoints. Approximately 40% of all hemophilia A patients carry an inversion at chromosomal region Xq28. This recurrent inversion spans ~400 kb and is mediated by two inverted segmental duplications, one of which is located in intron 22 of the factor VIII gene, with two other copies being located approximately 400kb telomeric of the same gene. When the inversion occurs, it disrupts the factor VIII gene, giving rise to hemophilia A.

Recurrent de novo translocations are rarely observed in the human genome with only three so far being described in any detail. Two of these events include the region on chromosome 22q, which is also involved in causing the deletions and duplication leading to DiGeorge and velocardiofacial syndromes. The most frequent translocation is called t(11q;22q). The breakpoints on both chromosome 11q23 and chromosome 22q11 are clustered in multiple unrelated families. Both breakpoints have been shown to contain palindromic AT-rich sequences that can mediate hairpin structure formation suggesting they mediate t(11q;22q). Moreover, the same region on chromosome 22 and a similar mechanism of rearrangement has been suggested to underlie the t(17q;22q) translocation that involves the neurofibromatosis (NF1) gene on chromosome 17. This translocation has been found in a number of patients with neurofibromatosis type I. The third translocation that has been reported numerous times in the literature is the t(4;8)(p16;p23) translocation. Two pairs of olfactory receptor gene clusters are located in close vicinity to each other on two separate chromosomes (4p16 and 8p23). The olfactory clusters have evolved by gene duplication events and thus share high sequence similarity. As would be predicted the breakpoints of the translocations were found to be located within these olfactory genes in all translocation carriers identified.

Gene Conversion

Many human genes have highly related family members existing as functional genes or pseudogenes that can be clustered or dispersed elsewhere in the genome. Unequal crossing over between a functional gene and a related pseudogene can result in the deletion of the functional gene, or the formation of fusion genes with one part derived from the pseudogene. However, similar DNA sequences may also give rise to "*gene conversion*" events. Gene conversion is the nonreciprocal transfer of sequence information between a pair of sequences. For example, one (donor) sequence remains unchanged while the other (acceptor) sequence is replaced by the nucleotide content of the donor. It has been suggested that this mechanism involves mismatch repair of a heteroduplex involving highly similar sequences. The mismatch repair system identifies the nucleotide bases that are not perfectly matched in the heteroduplex and changes them such that both copies are identical. This unusual recombinational outcome has been shown to be a recurrent mutational mechanism in some diseases. A gene conversion event may include a functional gene and its pseudogene copy, which carries a premature stop codon. In this case gene conversion would transfer the stop codon mutation to the functional gene, thereby disrupting the functional copy. The classical example of pathogenesis caused by gene conversion between a gene and its pseudogene is steroid 21-hydroxylase deficiency. More than 95% of mutations causing this disease are caused by sequence exchange between *CYP21B*, and the closely related, tandemly duplicated pseudogene *CYP21A*. The same mechanism has been shown to be involved in causing Schwachman-Diamond syndrome, where stop codons are created in the SBDS gene due to gene conversion with its 97% similar pseudogene copy. In the SBDS example the gene and pseudogene are part of non-contiguous larger segmental duplications located on the long arm of chromosome 7.

Balanced Genomic Variants Can Induce Rearrangements

One interesting explanation for a few of the genomic disorders caused by deletions is that one of the parents of the proband carries a balanced genomic variant. These balanced genomic variants then appear to predispose to unbalanced chromosomal rearrangements associated with disease in the offspring. As such, in several disorders caused by large deletions, inversion of the exact same fragment that is deleted in the patient has been found in one of the parents. For example, an inversion of the 15q11-q13 region, which is deleted in patients with Angelman syndrome, has been identified in 2/3 of mothers of patients with deletions. Interestingly, this inversion is found in 9% of the general population. Similarly, an approximately 1.9 Mb inversion has been found in 1/3 of all transmitted chromosomes of the deletion that causes Williams–Beuren syndrome. This inversion is not so common (estimated at less than 5%) in the general population, but seems to predispose to deletions in the offspring. Inversions may also lead to duplications in the offspring. The recently identified duplication at 8p23.1-p22 in patients with Kabuki syndrome may also be mediated by a submicroscopic inversion. In two out of six cases, heterozygous 8p23.1 inversions were found in transmitting mothers of patients with duplications. One of the few recurrent translocations, the t(4;8)(p16;p23), may also be mediated by inversions in the transmitting parent. Heterozygous inversions at both chromosomal loci were found in all mothers of five de novo trans- location patients.

Non-Recurrent Genomic Rearrangements

Long stretches of nearly identical sequences (>90% DNA sequence identity) seem to be the primary sequence motifs inducing recurrent rearrangements in the genome. However, in many cases of genome rearrangement, the region involved is unique. The mechanisms causing these rare non-recurrent events have also been studied. In a study by Stankiewicz et al., the authors investigated whether the highly homologous regions (i.e., sequences that are 90–100% related at the nucleotide level) could be the explanation also for non-recurrent deletions and translocations. The results did indeed suggest that highly homologous sequences are often involved in large non-recurrent deletions, but are not a common cause for translocations. There are many regions in the genome that show high sequence similarities that do not fulfill the criteria normally used to describe segmental duplications. These include members of gene families, pseudogenes, and common small repetitive elements. There are a number of examples where pseudogenes or homologous functional genes are involved in recombination events creating subsequent rearrangements. One example of this is Hunter syndrome, where more than 10% of patients carry an inversion created by non-homologous recombination between the IDS gene and its pseudogene copy.

Several genetic diseases are caused by non-recurrent rearrangements. It has been speculated that these rearrangements can be caused by clusters of common repetitive elements. The most common repeat sequences in the human genome are ALU repeats, with approximately 500,000 copies in the human genome. ALU repeats are ~280 bp in length and are usually flanked by short direct repeats of 6 to 18 bp. The 45-kb low-density lipoprotein receptor gene has an ALU repeat present, on average, every 1.6kb. The very high frequency of pathogenic deletions in the LDL receptor gene has been shown to coincide with ALU repeat sequences at both breakpoints. Another disease caused by non-recurrent deletions and duplications is Duchenne muscular dystrophy (DMD). Approximately two thirds of DMD cases are caused by deletions of one or more exons of the large (>2Mb) DMD gene. Sequencing of the regions flanking the deletions in patients with DMD showed that 30% of deletion occurred at common repeat sequences (ALU and LTRs), while the remaining deletions were flanked by unique sequence. Some repeat sequences in the human genome are known to be transposable elements. This means that these elements can be copied and inserted in new genomic regions, usually via an RNA intermediate. One mechanism by which these transposable elements can cause disease is if they are inserted into a functional gene, causing a disruption of the transcript. This phenomenon is referred to as insertional inactivation. Obviously, this is more likely to occur if the gene is large, as is the case for the neurofibromatosis I and hemophilia A loci.

Segmental Duplications

It has been known for some time that a large proportion of genomic disorders arise from rearrangements in the genome that is due to aberrant recombination. As discussed above, the major cause for these recombinational errors is the misalignment of long stretches of nearly identical DNA sequences. Analysis of the human genome sequence shows that a large proportion of the genome consists of segmental duplications, also known as low copy repeats. One of the most important mechanisms for genome evolution and creation of new genes is by duplication of large segments of genetic material. Duplicated copies of genes can then mutate and obtain new or specialized functions. It is therefore not surprising that duplicated segments exist in the human genome. However, the abundance of such sequences in the human genome has only recently been appreciated. Since the completion of the human genome sequence, several analyses show that approximately 5%, or 150 Mb of the genome exists as segmental duplications having at least 90% DNA sequence identity. This statistic does not include common repetitive elements or short (<1 kb) repeated sequences, which would make the proportion of repeated sequences up to >50% of the genome. The high sequence identity indicates that these sequences have been created by recent duplications of large stretches of genomic DNA. The size of duplication segments ranges from a few kilobases to a few megabases. Importantly, it is not rare for duplication regions to contain several genes. For example, the human specific 500 kb inverted duplication on 5q13 contains six different genes, including the SMN1 gene involved in spinal muscular atrophy.

Segmental duplications are normally divided into two classes depending on their chromosomal relationship to each other (referred to as being intrachromosomal or interchromosomal). The intrachromosomal duplications are chromosome-specific and are often clustered in the same region of the chromosome and in some cases even as tandem copies. Interchromosomal duplications are found on non-homologous chromosomes and are less common than the intrachromosomal class. Interchromosomal duplications appear to cluster in pericentromeric and subtelomeric heterochromatic regions of chromosomes. Due to their high identity segmental duplications have caused problems for the successive assemblies of the human DNA sequence. Tandemly duplicated segments of very high sequence identity are especially difficult to identify. There is a strong correlation between the location of segmental duplications and the remaining gaps in the human sequence assembly, and it is expected that the proportion of segmental duplications in the genome will increase as the assembly of the "complete" genome is finalized.

Common Genomic Polymorphisms

In previous sections we have described the gain or loss of gene copies, which are rare and lead to major phenotypic effects. There are, however, a class of genomic alterations leading to gene copy number differences that lead to less significant phenotypes and which occur more frequently and in some cases in >1% of the population (indicating they are polymorphisms). Many of these variants have already been shown to be directly related to gene expression. With new techniques available to scan the genome for copy number changes, reports of large genomic variants are increasing in frequency. It seems as if the findings of such variants are no longer chance findings of very rare occurrences in the genome, but may be quite common in the normal population. Detailed studies of genes where a variable number of gene copies have been found in the normal population has shown a concomitant increase in mRNA from that gene.

The first indication that a previously unappreciated number of large- scale polymorphism exist in the human genome, as well as the genomes of other species, was a study comparing the copy number of ~29.000 genes in several primate species. The data showed a large number of gains or losses of genes that were lineage specific. A substantial number of gene copy number changes were shown to have occurred during the last 5 million years after human divergence from our closest ancestor, the chimpanzee. The data indicate that gene duplication and deletion are strong forces in shaping the genome, and that it is a process that is even more pronounced in the human genome than some of our closest living relatives. Although only five humans were included in the study, close examination of the data revealed several genes that displayed copy number differences within the human population. Using a different approach, Fredman et al. investigated SNPs in segmental duplications. By measuring the ratio between the two alleles for the SNP, they found differences between individuals that could only be explained by either copy number differences or gene conversion. The regions were then investigated using quantitative methods and it was shown that a number of the regions exhibited variable number of copies in the normal populations. Their data indicated that segmental duplications are highly dynamic regions in the genome, often involving copy number differences and recurrent gene conversion events. Although only a small number of copy number variants were verified in the study, it pointed to the fact that this type of variation is substantial.

The extent of large-scale variation in the human genome was investigated in two independent studies published in the summer of 2004. Using a method called ROMA (representational oligonucleotide microarray analysis) Sebat et al. found 80 regions that show copy number variation in healthy, unrelated individuals. The average size of these regions was reported to be 400 kb and many contain entire coding transcripts. They also showed that these variants were unlikely to be somatic variation by testing DNA from a number of different tissues from the same individuals. The only somatic changes were shown to occur in the T-cell receptor clusters and immunoglobulin related genes. Although the coverage of the human genome is very high using the ROMA method, all regions that are not unique in the genome are excluded from analysis. Since the study by Fredman et al. indicate that segmental duplication regions are likely to be the most dynamic regions in the genome, the findings by Sebat et al. is likely an under-representation of the true variation content of the human genome.

In a separate study, Iafrate et al. used CGH (comparative genomic hybridization) to investigate the extent of large-scale variation in the human genome and found 250 regions that displayed copy number variation between 55 unrelated individuals. The method is based on hybridization to genomic clones, indicating that the size of these variants are >50 kb. Many of the regions found to be polymorphic in the population were shown to occur in regions with segmental duplication or gaps in the human genome assembly, reinforcing the role these regions play in genome rearrangement and evolution. A database of large-scale genomic variants has now been created by the authors. This is a valuable resource for scientists screening for human genome rearrangements in correlation to disease or normal variation. Overall, the results of these studies suggest that the human genome is much more dynamic in nature than was previously thought. In the near future, more detailed information about the extent and frequency of large-scale genomic variants should become available. It will then be important to link these variants to variation in transcription both in the normal population and in disease.

These findings may therefore represent an important step towards the understanding of complex genetic disease.

Gene Copy Number Variation

There are several types of genes that have been shown to display copy number differences in the genome, many being highly relevant to the pharmacologic responses. One class that is conspicuously over-represented are genes involved in the defense against pathogenic or toxic agents, where a number of genes display a high degree of polymorphic variation which includes variation in gene copy number: glutathione-S-transferase (GST) genes, cytochrome P450 (CYP) genes, the complement component C4, and the defensin genes. In each case, changes to gene copy number have been shown to give rise to concomitant changes in the level of enzyme activity, with phenotypic consequences.

Glutathione-S-Transferase Genes (GST)

The GSTs are phase II enzymes involved in the metabolism of a large range of endogenous and exogenous toxic compounds. Individuals can have large variations in GST activity, which can have a major impact in the sensitivity of cells to these toxins. This is known, or postulated to result in differences in individual susceptibility to illnesses related to such substances including various carcinomas. In addition, the efficacy of therapeutic drugs is affected by individual variation in the ability of these enzymes to metabolize them with individuals being described as low or high responders. There are two families of GST genes: cytosolic and microsomal. There are at least 16 cytosolic GSTs, which are encoded by several classes of genes based on their biochemical, immunological, and structural properties, giving rise to at least 16 different proteins. A further six genes are known to encode microsomal GST. Of these, two genes display polymorphic variations in copy number (GSTM1 and GSTT1) whilst one (GSTT2) has two copies in all individuals.

Microsomal Glutathione-S-Transferase 1 (GSTM1)

The predominant GSTM1 allele is a null allele where an 18-kb fragment encompassing the entire gene is deleted following unequal crossing over between break points 5 kb downstream from the GSTM2 gene and 5 kb downstream from the GSTM1 gene. In fact, GSTM1 is found in only half of the genomes of Caucasians and Saudi Arabians, the other half of the populations exist with no copy of the gene in their genome. The lack of this gene may predispose to some cancers. Most other individuals have either one or two copies, however, some people who have ultra rapid GSTM1 activity have been found to have three copies of the gene. It is unclear if these people are more resistant to cancer, but it is likely that are more resistant to the effects of some toxic compounds in the environment. It is also likely that some individuals who have two copies of the gene may have both of those copies on one parental chromosome, having one null allele and one duplicated allele.

Glutathione-S-Transferase Theta 1 (GSTT1)

The gene for GSTT1 has a null allele, which results from deletion of a 54-kb fragment from 22q1 1.23, which includes the entire gene. The deletion occurs as a result of homologous crossover between two 18 kb flanking sequences, HA3 and HA5, which have greater than 90% sequence homology. This deletion allele is common in the population with 20% of individuals having no copies of GSTT1, while 46% are heterozygous and have a single copy of the gene, which fits the Hardy-Weinberg equilibrium. The null allele has been associated with a number of carcinomas however, other research suggests that the effects are mainly seen in sub-populations.

Cytochrome p450

Cytochrome p450 (CYP) is a superfamily of heme-containing phase 1 enzymes, which metabolize both endogenous compounds such as steroids, fatty acids, and prostaglandins, and exogenous compounds such as environmental carcinogens, pollutants, drugs, and other xenobiotics. At least three genes (CYP2D6, CYP2A6, and CYP21A2) are present in variable copy number.

The CYP2D6 (22q13.1) gene product (cytochrome P450 CYP2D6) is a highly polymorphic enzyme involved in the oxidative metabolism of many different classes of commonly used drugs, including antidepressants, antipsychotics, beta-blockers, opiates etc. About 7-10% of Northern Europeans have low CYP2D6 activity and are classed as poor metabolizers. These patients may develop adverse drug reactions when treated with standard doses of drug. In contrast, some individuals are ultrarapid metabolizers, and require higher drug dosages in order to achieve the required response. The enzyme is highly polymorphic and the alleles give widely varying enzyme activity, however, another source of variation in activity is changes to gene copy number.

A number of studies have shown that many of the alleles are duplicated in a polymorphic manner although the frequency of duplication varies considerably between populations: 1% and 7% in Caucasian and Japanese populations but 21% and 29% in Saudi Arabian and Ethiopian populations, respectively. The number of gene copies varies up to 13 and increased gene copy number results in increased gene expression and subsequent increased catabolism of drugs by the gene product roughly in proportion to the gene dosage. The mechanism for the duplication to give up to five copies of the gene has been proposed to be unequal crossover between Alu repeat sequences. Larger numbers of gene copies may have been formed following unequal segregation and/or rolling circle replication followed by homologous recombination, however, there is little evidence for this theory.

The CYP2A6 is a major hepatic member of the CYP family in humans, which metabolizes pharmaceutical agents including nicotine to the inactive cotinine. A number of reports suggest an association between smoking and null alleles including a deletion allele. The activity of this enzyme is related to the number of cigarettes people smoke; individuals with less active enzyme have more nicotine in their blood for the same number of cigarettes smoked and thus smoke less. Compared with individuals with the same CYP2A6 alleles, individuals with duplication of CYP2A6 on a single chromosome showed increased activity of the enzyme of approximately 1.5-fold and had increased blood carbon monoxide levels, the latter being a measure of the amount of tobacco smoked.

A deletion allele is very common in Japanese (20% of alleles) Korean (11%), and Chinese (15%) populations. This deletion is the result of a homologous unequal crossover between the 3′ flanking regions of the CYP2A7 and CYP2A6 genes, which result in the deletion of the entire A6 gene. This should lead to the concomitant formation of a tandem duplication of the A6 gene. Although this has been found, the frequency is not equivalent. Duplication of CYP2A6 (19q13.2) has been found in 1.7% of a smoking population and 1.3% of a normal population both of Caucasian origin. A single individual with the duplication was also found in a Chinese population (1 out 114; 0.9%). This may suggest that duplication does not occur frequently, and the deletion occurs through a different mechanism, such as the formation of a loop, or alternatively the duplication may not be detected as southern blots may not show the presence of the extra copy. A novel deletion allele, present in less than 1% of a Japanese population has been described, in which a larger section of DNA has been deleted.

The CYP21A2 gene and the C4 complement component genes (C4A or C4B) are located close together on 6p21.3 near a highly variable region. The C4 gene is highly polymorphic with at least 34 allotypes known to exist. These are grouped into two isotypes, C4A and C4B, which vary in activity; the C4A has a slow reaction rate but a long half-life while the C4B has a fast reaction rate and short half-life. Deficiency of C4 increases the susceptibility or severity of viral and bacterial infections and is also an important risk factor for autoimmune diseases, such as systemic lupus erythematosus. Conversely, excessive C4 or over-activation of C4 could aggravate an inflammatory response and render an individual more vulnerable to tissue injuries. The variable region is bounded on the telomeric side by the genes RP1 and C4 (A or B) and on the centromeric side by the genes CYP21A2 and TNXB. Within these boundaries a unit (termed RCCX) consisting of four genes, may be found in variable copy number typically 0, 1, or 2. The four genes are CYP21A1P (a pseudogene of CYP21A2), TNXA, RP2, and C4 (A or B). Thus an individual may have between 2 and 6 copies of the C4 and the CYP21A1P genes. The mechanism leading to the variations is probably unequal crossing over between C4 genes.

The CYP21A2 is essential for the biosynthesis of glucocorticoid and mineralocorticoid hormones. Gene conversion whereby either the entire active gene or part of it is replaced with corresponding sequences from the pseudogene gives rise to a defective CYP21A2 gene. Low activity CYP21 activity is the primary cause of congenital adrenal hyperplasia, the severity of symptoms being associated with the enzyme activity level ranging from androgen excess through simple iridizing down to salt wasting in the absence of the gene.

The RCCX unit almost invariably carries the CYP21A1P pseudogene and extra copies of the active gene are rare; the frequency has been assessed in a Northern European population and found to be present at a frequency of 1.6% and duplications have also been found in other populations. Although these additional copies of CYP21A2 are invariably defective, mutational analysis of this gene is often carried out as part of the diagnostic process for congenital adrenal hyperplasia and duplication complicates this analysis, as one CYP21A2 gene copy may be defective due to partial replacement with pseudogene sequence, whilst the other copy remains intact. This may lead to the misassignment of carrier status.

β-Defensin Genes

Defensin genes encode small antimicrobial peptides and are an important part of the immune system. The α-defensins are highly expressed in neutrophils, while β-defensins are expressed in a variety of epithelia, especially the airways, and have been shown to have broad antimicrobial properties. All the defensin genes are located in a cluster at 8p23.1, a region known to be frequently involved in chromosomal rearrangements. In the α-defensin family, the highly identical DEFA1 and DEFA3 genes have been shown to have variable number of copies in the normal population. The DEFA3 gene currently maps to four places near a gap in the human genome assembly. It was recently shown that three genes in the β-defensin gene cluster, DEFB4, DEFB103, and DEFB104, are located in a 240kb repeat unit that is polymorphic in the population. Individuals carry 2 to 12 copies of this repeat unit in their genomes. The highest number identified on a single chromosome was eight repeats, indicating that individuals with more than 12 copies in total are likely to be found. Quantitative analysis of mRNA from the DEFB4 gene shows that there is a direct correlation between the copy number and the level of expression of this gene. These defensin polymorphisms have been shown to be the basis for a previously described euchromatic variant in the same region.

Methods for Studying Genomic Variation

Despite its fundamental importance for molecular genetics, it is only very recently that effective methods have been developed for studies of submicroscopic gains or losses of specific genomic loci. There is still no method available for genome-wide investigation of inversion variants. Many studies require a higher resolution than what can be attained by using classical fluorescence in situ hybridization (FISH) or comparative genomic hybridization (CGH). Several human diseases have been shown to be caused by small deletions or duplications, involving single exons or parts of genes. The detection of such small copy number variants has previously been limited to quantitative Southern blot, and more recently, real-time PCR. However, neither of these methods is ideal for screening multiple loci in large cohorts of patients or control groups. Several methods have now been developed to meet the demand for techniques to perform analyses of duplications and deletions in a high throughput setting.

Array Based Methods to Identify Copy Number Differences

The Comparative Genomic Hybridization (CGH) method was originally used for identification of copy number imbalances in metaphase spreads. Two differentially labeled DNA samples are hybridized to normal chromosomes and the ratio of fluorescence intensity is measured. Differences in fluorescence are indicative of relative copy numbers in the two DNA samples. However, the resolution of the method was initially limited to several megabases only. Development of microarray technology and the subsequent adaptation of CGH to array format dramatically increased the resolution of the method. The basic principle of array-CGH is the same as the original CGH, but the DNA is now hybridized to glass slides containing DNA clones instead of metaphase chromosomes. Array-CGH has been used successfully with both cDNA and genomic clone arrays. Although the resolution of the method has improved significantly it is still limited to a lower limit in the kilobase(s) range due to sensitivity of hybridization and detection.

Commercially available genome-wide arrays have ~1 Mb resolution. Chromosome-specific arrays with contiguous coverage and 75 kb resolution have been successfully implemented. A novel approach was recently described, where oligonucleotide probes were used. This method, named ROMA (representational oligonucleotide microarray analysis), achieved an average resolution of 30kb throughout the genome using 70-mer probes on the array. It is likely that the resolution can be improved even further using oligonucleotide arrays. Until recently, CGH has predominantly been used for identification of chromosomal aberrations in tumors. With higher resolution arrays available the use of CGH technology is becoming more widespread. The major advantage of the method is that the whole genome of an individual can be analyzed for chromosomal imbalances at a comparatively high resolution in a single experiment.

Another type of array-based approach that can be used to identify deletions and duplications is to use whole genome sampling analysis of SNP arrays (e.g., the Affymetrix 10 or 100 k SNP chip). Not only can deletions be identified as contiguous stretches of homozygous markers, but also the SNP discrimination ratios and the perfect match intensities can be normalized across the chip and compared to a reference set of individuals. This way, loss and gain of genetic material can be distinguished in addition to the collection of SNP genotype data.

Quantitative Multiplex PCR

Real-time quantitative PCR is most commonly used for analysis of differences in gene expression. However, the same principles for quantification can be applied to genomic DNA. Both the 5′-nuclease assay with dual-labeled Taqman probe, and the SYBR-Green I assay formats, have been successfully used to screen for genomic DNA changes in copy number. However, neither of these approaches is well suited for multiplexing and cost becomes an issue for high-throughput screening. Several other multiplex PCR based methods have therefore been developed for the purpose of screening for copy number differences. These can be summarized by the name quantitative multiplex PCR of short fluorescent fragments (QMPSF). PCRs are designed to span the regions of interest, e.g., exons of a specific gene. In its simplest form, the forward primers are labeled with a fluorescent 6-FAM moiety, and a PCR is run for ~20 cycles until it is in the quantitative range.

The product is then purified and run on an automated sequencer and the electropherograms from the individuals to be compared are superimposed. A control sequence that is not expected to be duplicated or deleted is included as a DNA quality and quantity control. More recent versions of this methods includes the addition of chimeric primers, i.e., primers carrying an extension of nucleotides in their 5′-end, rendering the effective annealing temperatures more homogeneous in a multiplex PCR after the first few cycles. The use of chimeric primers thereby reduces the amount of optimization needed to find adequate primer concentrations to yield homogeneous fluorescent peak levels. Chimeric primers can also be used to simplify the assay and reduce cost. Normally, each forward primer has to be labeled with a 6-FAM fluorescein. However, if identical 16-mer extensions are added as part of the chimeric primer, this sequence can be used as a template for a universal 6-FAM labeled primer that is added before the last two cycles of the PCR reaction, thereby labeling all PCR products using a single FAM-labeled primer. Adding this step substantially reduces the cost of the assay.

Multiplex Probe Amplification Assays

One approach that has proved successful for identifying copy number differences in the genome is based on using amplifiable probes. The initial version of this methodology was called multiplex amplifiable probe hybridization (MAPH). The test DNA is denatured and bound to a nylon filter and hybridized with amplifiable probes, each recognizing a unique DNA sequence. All probes are of unique length and carry identical end sequences and can thus be amplified in a subsequent step using universal primers that are fluorescently or radioactively labeled. Products are then separated and quantified based on their radioactive or fluorescent intensities compared to control samples. Multiplexing has been performed with up to 40 probes in a single reaction using MAPH. A technique based on similar principles is multiplex ligation-dependent probe amplification (MLPA). This assay is performed in solution. Two probes are annealed adjacently to target regions and then ligated.

Each probe pair gives rise to a product of unique length, but has identical end sequences, permitting simultaneous PCR amplification with universal primers. One primer is fluorescently labeled allowing gel based separation and quantification. The fact that the method is dependent on ligation also makes it possible to target one specific allele when SNPs are present. The drawback of this method is the requirement for substantial optimization. However, when a set of probes has been optimized they can be used to quickly and effectively score large numbers of samples. It has been known for a long time that genetic diseases are often caused by rearrangements of large segments of genomic sequence. Many of these rearrangements occur due to NAHR between segmental duplications. The mechanisms causing recurrent rearrangements are now better understood, and this could give clues to identifying hotspots for genomic rearrangements. A wide array of new methodologies to study gain and loss of genomic sequences has led the way to genome-wide studies of large-scale variants in disease as well as in the genomes of healthy individuals.

The results of these studies indicate that the genome is much more variable between individuals than was previously suspected, with each individual carrying a number of large genomic polymorphisms. Many of the large variants encompass entire genes, indicating that this could be a primary source for variation in gene expression between individuals. This previously unappreciated source of variation has opened the door to new ways of thinking about disease mechanisms and genome evolution. In the near future we are confident that we will not only get a high resolution map a large-scale variation in the human genome, but we will also see a number of these variants being linked to specific phenotypic traits.

15

Use of Genomics for Enzyme-based Drug

Genomics has changed our view of the biological world in the past decade, providing both new information and new tools to characterize biological systems. Over the past few years, dozens of microbial genomes—including several of substantial clinical importance—have been completely sequenced, pushing the search for novel antimicrobial compounds into the postgenomic era.

Genomic information and associated new technologies have the potential to revolutionize the drug discovery process. Tremendous new opportunities exist to identify targets for therapeutic intervention, and to initiate new screens for therapeutic agents. The concurrent increase in high-throughput capacity allows the realization of the genomic potential for significant increases in drug discovery efforts. The new strategies used in antimicrobial drug discovery may have application in numerous therapeutic areas.

State of Bacterial Genomics

The development of technologies and strategies for efficient genomic sequencing and contig assembly has resulted in the completion of dozens of microbial genome sequences within the past five years. With both academic and commercial organizations engaged in sequencing microbial genomes, prokaryotic genome information is increasing rapidly. In publicly available databases, there are currently 22 completed eubacterial genomes and at least 87 in progress. Additional microbial sequences are available in commercial sequence databases, such as those offered by Incyte Genomics, Inc. and Genome Therapeutics Corp.

Coupled with a widely recognized need for new antimicrobial agents due to the rapid emergence of drug resistance, microbial genomics has been embraced by the pharmaceutical industry. Underlying the pharmaceutical interest in microbial genome sequences is the belief that target-specific screening and new targets will allow identification of new structural classes of antimicrobial agents that will inhibit the growth of microbes that are resistant to currently available chemotherapeutic agents.

Several general features of microbes and microbial genomes have emerged through the analysis of individual genomes and comparisons between them, as discussed in the following paragraphs.

1. The sizes of bacterial genomes vary over 10-fold. The smallest known bacterial genomes are those of the symbiotic mycoplasmas. These microorganisms live in close association with eukaryotic cells and characteristically lack a cell wall and possess unique sterol-containing plasma membranes. The sequenced genome of *Mycoplasma genitalium* is 580 kbp, and was predicted to encode 470 proteins, while *Mycoplasma pneumoniae* is 810 kbp and was predicted to encode 678 proteins. The largest bacterial genome fully sequenced to date is *Escherichia coli* K-12 at 4.6 Mbp, while the largest eubacterial genome sequence projects currently in progress are in *Pseudomonas aeruginosa* (5.9 Mbp) and *Pseudomonas putida* (6.0 Mbp).

2. Bacterial genomes are information-rich. Over 85% of most sequenced bacterial genomes encode protein or RNAs, with only a small fraction of the genome dedicated to control regions and noncoding features. The *E. coli* K-12 genome is relatively typical: 87.8% of the 4.6-Mbp genome is predicted to encode 4288 proteins, 0.8% encodes stable RNAs, 0.7% is noncoding repeat sequences, with the remaining 11% as regulatory sequences, undetermined, or nonfunctional DNA sequence.
3. Bacterial genes are relatively small. Due to the lack of introns, an average bacterial gene is roughly 1 kbp. Thus, the majority of information about encoded proteins and pathways can be understood without the assembly of the genome sequence into a single contig. Thus, for most pharmaceutical applications, including target identification and validation, "*nearly complete*" bacterial genome sequences provide adequate information for target identification and pathway assessment.
4. The conservation of protein sequence information among eubacteria is sufficient to recognize proteins with similar structure and anticipated function ("orthologs") among all groups of eubacteria. Typically, orthologous proteins between Gram-positive and Gram-negative species will have 30–40% amino acid identity, whereas in closely related bacterial species, such as the Gram-negative species *E. coli* and *Salmonella typhimurium*, orthologous proteins will have 75–95% amino acid identity. Currently, approximately 70% of the predicted proteins in a typical eubacterial genome have at least one ortholog in another sequenced microbial genome.
5. Related bacterial genomes differ by the addition and subtraction of genes and pathways. Numerous plasmids, bacteriophage, natural transformation, and transposable elements mediate horizontal transfer of genes between both closely related and distant microbial species, and potentially between prokaryotic species and eukaryotes. In addition, these same transposable elements can mediate chromosome rearrangements—duplications, deletions, and inversions—through legitimate and illegitimate recombination events. Comparisons of closely related species, such as *S. typhimurium* and *E. coli*, or even different strains of the same species show that gains and losses of DNA segments are frequent events in bacterial evolution.
6. Many microbial genes are of unknown function. Even in the well- studied bacterium *E. coli*, over 38% of the predicted proteins have no experimental data to support an understanding of their functional role in the cell.

Characteristics of Good Antimicrobial Target

The discovery of new chemotherapeutic agents is difficult because of the numerous safety and efficacy criteria that must be satisfied by a single compound. For antimicrobials, the hurdles are extremely high—patients are frequently in crisis, but the desired therapeutic outcome is complete cure. Thus, a good antimicrobial agent must possess a wide range of different properties: strong and rapid inhibition of microbial growth; little interaction with mammalian targets at therapeutic doses; and desirable physical, chemical, and pharmacological properties that allow appropriate formulation, sufficient residence time within the body to achieve the antimicrobial goals, and the lack of significant damage to mammalian cells, tissues, or organs. In addition, a good antimicrobial agent should have relatively low resistance development, so that the clinician can be assured of the agent's efficacy for each patient, and so that the developing pharmaceutical company can achieve a reasonable return on its research and development investment. Frequently, broad antimicrobial activity spectrum is also desirable because it allows empiric treatment and first-line therapy.

Microbial genomics has vastly increased the number of potential antimicrobial targets over the past few years, making it necessary to identify criteria to assess and prioritize the targets for subsequent screen development. A rationale can be made that certain characteristics of a chemical inhibitor will be influenced by the characteristics of the target, while other characteristics appear independent or only partially dependent on the target.

Table 15.1. Characteristics of a good antimicrobial agent

Property	*Relationship to target*
Bactericidal/fungicidal	Killing versus inhibition of growth is thought to be primarily a property of the target as is the ability to cause bacterial or fungal cell lysis.
Low resistance frequency	Certain essential genes can be bypassed by inhibition of another gene product. Such situations may result in high frequency of resistance emergenc.
Microbial breadth of spectrum	Existence or nonexistence of the target can be assessed through bioinformatics; however, such studies do not guarantee essentiality in the new species. In addition, efflux-based properties can influence a compound's breadth of spectrum.
Selectivity of inhibitors	Presence or absence of the target in eukaryotes can be assessed through bioinformatics; however, certain prokaryotic enzymes with clear orthologs in eukaryotes are the targets of successful antibiotics: trimethoprim; fluoroquinolones.
Potency of inhibitors	Intracellular amount of enzyme may influence amount of the inhibitor necessary for potency; protein concentrations in bacteria vary over at least 3 orders of magnitude.
Pharmacological properties (serum binding, distribution, clearance, half-life, etc.)	Many of these properties may be influenced by the non-specific affinity of the compound for host proteins; however, these properties are not generally predictable from target choice at this time.
Synthetic accessibility, simplicity, patentability	Size, shape, and amino acid composition of the inhibitor-binding site may influence the chemical classes of inhibitors, as well as the achievable selectivity.

Using Genomic Information in Target Assessment

Genome sequences provide a significant source of new informaion for expanding and prioritizing the set of antimicrobial targets for drug discovery. With the current state of knowledge, experimental validation of the predictions is still necessary in most cases. Fortunately, new methods have been developed to allow large-scale experimental assessment.

Predicting Efficacy

The typically desired goal of antimicrobial chemotherapy is to kill microorganisms, or at least to rapidly inhibit their growth through the chemical inhibition of one or more essential cellular processes. Proteins that will provide good antimicrobial targets must cause loss of viability or cessation of growth when the target protein is inhibited. Experimental methods have shown that most genes in microbial genomes are not individually essential for growth. Thus, many microbial enzymes will not make good therapeutic targets, and a selection process is necessary to identify those whose inhibition can provide therapeutic benefit.

In silico methods aim to identify the pharmaceutically relevant genes from genome sequence information. One computational strategy assumed that bacteria accomplished their essential functions through common mechanisms that would be evolutionarily conserved. Comparison of the completed genomes of *Haemophilus influenza* and *M. genitalium* showed that approximately 250 genes existed in both of the bacterial genomes and these were hypothesized to comprise a "*minimal genome set*" necessary to support bacterial viability. However, as additional genomes were sequenced, the set of completely conserved genes became very small, putting into question the initial assumption of the complete conservation of essential genes in bacteria.

An experimental test of the hypothesis that conserved genes were essential was made by comparing the genomes of *E. coli* and *M. genitalium*. Of 26 genes that were conserved between *E. coli* and the small *M. genitalium* genome, only six genes caused loss of viability when disrupted; 20 genes were nonessential for growth under standard laboratory conditions. Thus, selecting genes that are evolutionarily conserved among microbial species is not sufficient to reliably predict whether the genes are necessary for microbial viability.

Experimental approaches for antimicrobial target validation rely on genetic inactivation of the gene product and assessment of the resulting growth properties. These approaches use genetic methods to predict the idealized antimicrobial properties of a chemical inhibitor of the target. Experimentally, mutational inactivation of a potential target has been accomplished by gene disruption, conditional expression, or conditional-function mutations. Initial assessment is generally undertaken *in vitro*, using standard laboratory conditions; additional validation in relevant *in vivo* animal infection models can be determined in certain systems to assure that inhibition of a gene product will cause significant attenuation of an infection.

Conditional expression and conditional lethal mutants have a long history of use in identifying and characterizing essential genes in haploid organisms. This approach allows assessment of the physiological consequences of the loss of a gene's function, and often provides insight into the gene's normal physiological role, as well as its essential or nonessential character. In addition, conditional lethal mutant strains have been used for target-directed whole-cell screening strategies.

Gene disruption has been applied to individual genes to test essentiality, or in high-throughput mode to provide a genome-wide assessment of the essential genes in an organism. Most high-throughput methods use an efficient transposon system to generate a population of random insertions, then use molecular methods to display the insertion sites that remain in the population after a period of growth. Strains that carry disruptions of genes that cause inviability or slow growth are lost from the population, so that the display identifies all nonessential genes that can be disrupted without loss of viability.

High-throughput gene disruption methods led to the estimate that 265–350 genes of *M. genitalium* were essential for growth of this microorganism under standard laboratory conditions. Of these genes, approximately one-third were of unknown function. Genetic methods, based on the genetic redundancy in a collection of conditional lethal mutants, led to the estimate of 100–200 essential genes that could be identified by a conditional lethal approach in *S. typhimurium*. Both of these estimates count genes that are individually essential; functions necessary for viability that can be provided by either of two gene products will not be counted as essential in these studies.

Disruption strategies have disadvantages and pitfalls that should be recognized when interpreting data and making predictions of the essentiality of bacterial genes. The methods frequently use negative evidence—the inability to isolate a viable strain—to demonstrate essentiality. In addition, many bacterial genes exist in operons, in which disruption of an upstream gene can decrease transcription of downstream genes in the operon. Thus, disruption of an upstream gene can cause the erroneous conclusion of its essentiality, if the downstream genes are not independently assessed, or if the operon structure is not recognized. Disruption strategies designed to circumvent the problems of bacterial operons and polarity have been devised. When using disruption methods for assessing gene essentiality, it is also useful to remain cognizant of the relatively frequent occurrence of tandem duplication. In *S. typhimurium*, the spontaneous tandem duplication frequency at some loci was as high as 1% of the cells in a population; duplication of a locus can allow inheritance of the gene disruption, while still providing gene function, which could confound some assessments of gene essentiality.

Predicting Resistance Frequencies

High resistance frequencies arise in targets and pathways that have high evolutionary flexibility. An unusually high frequency of reversion in conditional lethal mutants of a potential target gene may foreshadow high-frequency resistance to chemical inhibitors of the target. The peptidyl deformylase of eubacteria removes the N-terminal formyl group from the initiator methionine of most bacterial proteins after translation. The gene, *def*, is essential in *E. coli*—a strain carrying a disruption of the *def* gene is not viable. However, disruption of the *def* gene can be inherited if cells have also lost the function of the initiator methionyl-tRNA formyltransferase enzyme (*fmt*), which transfers a formyl group onto the methionine. Inhibitors of the deformylase have been identified; as predicted by the genetic evidence, resistance to these inhibitors arises as a result of inactivation of the formyltransferase activity.

Low resistance emergence has been associated with antibiotics that inhibit more than one essential target, since it is expected that each gene will require mutation for the cell to become resistant. An excellent example supporting this contention is the highly successful beta-lactam antibiotic class, whose members inhibit bacterial penicillin-binding proteins (PBPs). In most eubacterial genomes, multiple PBPs exist, and in *E. coli*, several of the PBPs are known to be genetically essential. Resistance due to target-based mutation does not arise frequently, and the only clinically important resistance mechanisms are not target based, but rather due to beta-lactamases and efflux mechanisms.

However, choosing multigene targets does not guarantee low resistance frequencies. The fluoroquinolones are highly successful antibiotics that inhibit the two bacterial Type II topoisomerases, DNA gyrase and topoisomerase IV. These two topoisomerases are structurally related, each enzyme is genetically essential, and both of these paralogous topoisomerases are found in most eubacterial genomes. However, while commercially successful, the fluoroquinolones are subject to both target-based and efflux-mediated resistance development. Analysis of resistant isolates shows that resistance mutations arise frequently, each of which provides modest increases in resistance, but whose additive effects cause substantial increases in resistance to the organism.

Nonetheless, there are several unexploited gene families that may provide additional multigene targets for inhibitors, such as the two-component signal transduction systems, tRNA synthetases, RNA polymerase sigma subunits, and the aminoacyl ligases of peptidoglycan biosynthesis.

Predicting Breadth of Spectrum and Selectivity

Genomic information can provide a rapid assessment of the potential for broad- spectrum activity or high microbial selectivity of a target. It is relatively easy to identify orthologs in the eubacteria, because even distantly related eubacteria have orthologous proteins with over 30–40% amino acid identity. Certain publicly available tools, such as the WIT and KEGG sites, provide extensive databases of orthologous genes in sequenced genomes. These metabolic catalogs provide an invaluable tool for assessing and organizing lists of orthologous proteins in microbes.

The eubacterial DNA polymerase III enzyme is a multiprotein complex, best studied in *E. coli*. As can be observed from the table, a number of the proteins that are necessary for efficient replication in *E. coli* are not found in the genomes of other prokaryotic species. This raises questions about whether structurally dissimilar proteins provide these missing functions, or whether certain microbial systems do not require these functions. In contrast, there are examples of species that have two or more paralogs of a protein that is found in single copy in *E. coli*, such as the multiple genes encoding orthologs of the DNA polymerase III alpha subunit that are found in Gram-positive bacteria, such as *Bacillus subtilis* and *Mycobacterium tuberculosis*.

Additional factors that will affect the breadth of spectrum of an antimicrobial inhibitor cannot be predicted at present from genome information alone. Among these factors, efflux transporters may modulate the species specificity of numerous antimicrobial agents. While many classes of efflux pumps can be recognized from sequence homology, no prediction of the compounds that will be subject to efflux currently can be derived from sequence information.

Genomic information is being used to predict the potential of a target for broad antimicrobial activity spectrum and high selectivity. Within the bacterial kingdom, orthologs can be determined with relative certainty. However, the amount of sequence dissimilarity that is necessary to assure selectivity is unknown; similar three-dimensional protein structures can be determined by significantly different primary sequences, and the success of the fluoroquinolones shows that selectivity can be achieved even when the microbial target has a mammalian homolog. These factors introduce uncertainty about the wisdom of hoping for selectivity based on simple sequence analysis, and of using sequence-based selectivity arguments to eliminate otherwise good antimicrobial targets.

Are Some Proteins Better Targets Than Others?

Genomics has motivated a significantly increased effort in protein structure determination and structure prediction. The accumulation of three-dimensional protein structures has increased dramatically in the past few years. In 1999, approximately 2500 structures were added to the Protein Data Bank (PDB), a 20-fold increase over the 116 structures added to the PDB in 1989. Over 10,000 three-dimensional structures of proteins, peptides, and viruses now reside in the PDB. Of these, the number of prokaryotic proteins with structural information is significant: in *E. coli*, 771 of the 4288 predicted proteins have significant similarity to a protein with known three-dimensional structure.

In addition to increased structure determination, significant improvements have occurred in the ability to predict protein structures. The CASP3 competition to test current structure prediction methods concluded that alignment techniques—predicting structures for proteins with amino acid sequence similarity to a protein with known structure—worked very well for pairs of proteins with greater than 30% amino acid identity. Since the homology among eubacterial orthologs is generally greater than 30%, the eubacterial proteins with a known three-dimensional structure can provide strong guidance for predicting the structures of orthologous and paralogous eubacterial proteins. Such guidance could be very important for structure-based design approaches to drug discovery.

It has been estimated that only 1,000–10,000 distinct protein folds exist in all proteins, based on the decreasing accumulation of novel structures as new proteins are added to the Protein Data Bank. Potentially, one strategy for prioritizing proteins as antibiotic targets would be to select proteins with unique folds (or to avoid those with "popular" folds) in an attempt to lessen the opportunities for toxicity based on mammalian proteins with similar binding sites.

Using newly available microbial genome sequences, the protein folds in each of eight microbial genomes were predicted from genome sequence information. This analysis allowed the assembly and comparison of each organism's "*protein fold census*." From this analysis, the distribution of occurrence of protein folds was determined for each species. The top-10 folds in each eubacterial genome accounted for 34–40% of the total ORFs in that genome. Certain folds are found frequently in prokaryotes, and less frequently in eukaryotes, such as the TIM-barrel, the NTP hydrolases with P-loop, and the Rossman fold. In addition, there are numerous folds that are less common in prokaryotes, which are not predicted from the current analysis of eukaryotic genomes.

The quantity of a protein produced by a microbe may also be important in selecting a target. The amounts of proteins vary from less than one monomer per cell to over 10,000 monomers per cell. Thus, the necessary concentrations of an inhibitor could vary over several orders of magnitude, even for an inhibitor with nanomolar binding affinity.

The increasing number of co-crystals of protein with a bound ligand has improved and generalized our understanding of small-molecule binding to proteins. Such information may aid the development of additional tools for rational drug design, and increase the success of performing *in silico* screening and of biasing compound libraries for experimental screening. In addition, the development of these tools may allow the appropriate assessment of which proteins are more likely to be selectively inhibited by small molecules.

In general, small molecules bind to crevices and depressions in proteins, which can be active site locations, non-active site locations, or both. Analysis of the binding sites of over 50 proteins revealed an overrepresentation of large bulky groups, such as tryptophan and tyrosine, as well as histidine and arginine in active sites. Small molecules frequently displace well-ordered water molecules upon binding to a protein. The bulky amino acids found in active sites are thought to create "rough" surfaces that may increase binding affinity either directly, by increasing the available surface of interaction between the protein and ligand, or indirectly, through trapping and constraining the movement of water molecules that will be released upon ligand binding. Strategies for identifying rough surfaces by fractal geometry have shown success in predicting active site locations.

Genomic Methods for Enzyme-based Lead Identification

For genomics to increase its value in the pharmaceutical setting, methods must be developed to improve and accelerate steps downstream of target selection. Several new biochemical and whole-cell screening strategies have emerged that allow homogenous assay formats on an expanded range of protein targets. Coupled with improvements in liquid-handling systems, robotics, and databases, these methods have significantly expanded the ability to perform high-throughput screening on a wide range of targets.

Traditional Biochemical Approaches for Lead Identification

Traditional target-directed screening methods have employed a biochemical screen against a particular target to assure high sensitivity and specificity for the target. DNA sequence information, coupled with tagging methods and affinity purification, enable simpler methods for obtaining large quantities of a target protein from clinically relevant species.

Enzyme assay methods for screening have been augmented by new screening technologies that allow homogeneous assay formats. Scintillation proximity assays (SPA) rely on microbeads or plates that contain scintillant to provide a signal when a radioactive substance is physically nearby. Numerous binding assays have been developed, in which the receptor protein is bound to microbeads or plates, resulting in activation of the scintillant when a radioactively labeled ligand binds to the target protein. Most methods have utilized biotin-streptavidin or antibody affinity to bind the target protein to the scintillant-containing solid support. Such methods require knowledge of a specific ligand that binds the target protein, as well as the ability to obtain radioactive ligand in sufficient quantity to perform the screening.

Ligand-Binding Approaches for Lead Identification

A traditional biochemical approach to screening limits the targets to those that have well-developed biochemical assays or known ligands. Currently, this approach is limited to a relatively small subset of the pharmaceutically relevant targets, even in well-studied microbial systems. Over 25% of the essential genes identified in *Staphylococcus aureus* have no functional characterization; many of the remaining essential genes do not have biochemical assays that could be readily implemented in high-throughput screens.

Recently, methods have been developed and implemented in high- throughput screens that can differentiate ligand-bound and unbound protein, based on the increased conformational stability of a protein when it is bound to a ligand. Such methods have been applied to lead identification, using the assumption that ligands bound to the target provide a good starting point for the development of inhibitors. These methods enable screening to identify inhibitors of proteins for which there is little functional information. The ligand-binding approaches for lead identification enjoy the advantage of all biochemical assays, in their ability to provide quantitative and sensitive measures of the inhibitor's ability to bind the target protein. In addition, such assays do not require the inhibitor to overcome permeability barriers in order to be detected by the screen. Several experimental methods have been proposed to detect ligand-induced stabilization of a target protein.

Selection and enrichment methods have been used to identify peptide and oligonucleotide ligands that bind to target proteins. Combinatorial peptide libraries are often produced using phage display methods, which incorporate random nucleotides into a site on the phage genome that allows transcription, translation, and incorporation of the encoded peptides onto the surface of the phage particle. Methods have also been described for identifying folded oligonucleotide molecules that bind tightly to a target protein.

The Systematic Evolution of Ligands by Exponential enrichment technology ("SELEX") is an enrichment strategy that can identify high-affinity oligonucleotides that bind to a protein target. The peptide and oligonucleotide ligands identified by these methods can have binding affinities ranging from micromolar to subnanomolar after repeated rounds of enrichment.

Phage display and SELEX methods have been adapted to identify small-molecule inhibitors of target proteins. Peptide or nucleic acid inhibitors are not generally desirable as therapeutic agents, primarily due to their susceptibility to serum proteases or nucleases and lack of bioavailability. However, the peptides or oligomers can be used as reagents to identify small molecules that competitively inhibit binding of the peptide or oligomer ligand to the target.

Whole-Cell Approaches for Lead Identification

New genome-based whole-cell screening approaches have used genetically altered strains to create novel, target-specific phenotypes. Several of the whole-cell screening approaches use hypomorphic phenotypes created by partial loss of function or underexpression of an essential gene. Cells carrying such mutations are hypersensitive to inhibitors of the target and can detect even weak inhibitors. These screens are the chemical equivalent of a genetic search for synthetic lethal mutations.

Genetic synthetic lethality screens have shown that two mutations may be individually heritable but jointly noninheritable, either when the genes are functionally redundant or when the gene products interact physically or functionally with one another. When one cellular component is weakened by mutation, it becomes more susceptible to inhibition by chemical inhibitors of that target, creating a synthetically lethal situation. This strategy has provided the basis for whole-cell target-directed screens.

Genomics Impact on Lead Compound Characterization

New approaches evolving from genomics may aid the process of determining mechanism of action for new classes of inhibitors. Rapid and high-throughput approaches for determining a compound's mechanism of action will allow the entry of this information earlier in the drug discovery process, at the stage of lead selection as well as in the functional characterization of diverse compound libraries.

Preliminary studies have shown the value that a combination of genetic and genomic techniques can have for providing high-throughput methods for determining mechanism of action. Manipulation of the gene dosage of an inhibitor's target by twofold was found to cause hypersensitivity or resistance to an inhibitor in *Saccharomyces cerevisiae*. Similarly, mutants with weakened target function, obtained through semipermissive growth of conditional lethal mutants, were hypersensitive to target inhibitors. Several groups have now recognized that a set of strains carrying alterations in possible target genes provides a tool for characterizing the mechanism of action of inhibitors.

In addition, the ability of a transcriptional or proteomic profile to provide a biological "*fingerprint*" of the function of a compound has been shown recently. Such studies should prove useful for identifying structure–activity relationships, identifying pharmacophores, and for toxicological assessments of new lead compounds. Over the past five years, genomics has significantly changed antimicrobial drug discovery. A much larger collection of targets is available for screening, and new methods for screening have taken advantage of the large number of targets and high-throughput robotics. Further advances are clearly necessary to reap the benefits of the postgenomic era. The ability to tailor chemical diversity libraries to be more likely to identify specific target inhibitors with high selectivity is still an important future goal. Advances in mammalian genomics will help in achieving this goal, as will the numerous emerging techniques and technologies for analysis of large-scale data sets that allow biological characterization of small- molecule lead compounds.

16

GENE THERAPY

Human gene therapy (HGT) is defined as the transfer of nucleic acids (DNA or RNA) to somatic cells of a patient, which results in a therapeutic effect, by either (1) correcting genetic defects, (2) overexpressing proteins that are therapeutically useful, or (3) inhibiting the production of "harmful" proteins (e.g., by shRNA). Although it has several theoretical advantages, so far HGT has not delivered the promised results: Convincing clinical efficacy in pivotal phase III clinical trials has not yet been demonstrated in the United States or Europe (although two gene therapy products for cancer treatment have recently been approved and marketed in China). HGT is a complex process, involving multiple steps in the human body (delivery to organs, tissue targeting, cellular trafficking, regulation of gene expression level and duration, biological activity of therapeutic protein, safety of the vector and gene product, to name just a few), most of which are not completely understood.

In most applications, gene therapy represents a new, innovative drug delivery system making use of the technical and scientific advances of the last two decades in microbiology, virology, organic chemistry, molecular biology, biochemistry, cell biology, genetics, genomics, and genetic engineering. It is more than "*gene transfer*," which is only a part of the complex, multiphase process of identification, manufacturing, preclinical testing, and clinical development of gene therapy products.

The prerequisites of successful HGT include therapeutically suitable genes (with a proven role in pathophysiology of the disease either by its lack, mutation, or overexpression), appropriate gene delivery systems (e.g., viral and nonviral vectors), proof of principle of efficacy and safety in appropriate preclinical models, and suitable manufacturing and analytical processes to provide well-defined HGT products for clinical investigations.

The principle of gene therapy has specific therapeutic advantages over existing therapeutic modalities (such as small molecules or biologics) in certain disease indications. These include (1) correction of the genetic cause of a disease, (2) selective treatment of affected (diseased) cells and tissues (the cells and tissues produce their own "remedy"), and (3) long-term treatment after a single application. It may be best suited for so-called "nondrugable" targets (i.e., the modulation of target molecule is not feasible with small-molecule or protein drugs). Based on these theoretical principles, at the time of its first introduction more than 17 years ago, gene therapy promised to be an effective and safe treatment modality, which will soon cure diseases and replace classic therapies.

Over the past few years, significant progress has been made in various enabling technologies and in the molecular understanding of diseases and the manufacturing of vectors. These advances, combined with the growing experience with gene transfer in humans, promises to contribute to the ultimate success of this new class of therapeutics.

BASIC PRINCIPLES

From Nucleic Acid Delivery to Therapeutic Effects

Gene therapy consists of multiple biological processes in the body, the exact nature of which is in most cases still unknown. Gene therapy is initiated with the introduction of an appropriate vector (viral or nonviral) either into the body locally (direct tissue injection), into body cavities (e.g., peritoneum or cerebrospinal fluid), or into the bloodstream (systemic delivery). The vector needs to "find" its target tissue, after which it enters the target cell membrane and traffics through the cytoplasm to reach and enter the nucleus. Once there, the therapeutic (trans)gene needs to be transcribed and the formed mRNA needs to be appropriately translated into the therapeutic protein. The protein then acts on its receptor(s) either on the cell that produced it (intracrine or autocrine mechanism), on neighboring cells (paracrine mechanism), or at distant sites after entering the blood circulation (endocrine mechanism, e.g., erythropoietin, coagulation factors, and growth hormone). Finally, after interacting with its receptor, the protein needs to induce an appropriate biological effect that results in therapeutic benefits. For gene correction or gene knock-down approaches, the steps are similar to those outlined above, except that the last step is modification of the genome ("*gene correction*") or blockade of mRNA transcription (siRNA/shRNA) of endogenous genes, respectively.

Although the factors needed for successful gene therapy are not different from any new therapeutic modality (which include technical [gene delivery and expression], clinical [therapeutic efficacy and safety], and socioeconomic factors), the specific technical success factors are unique for gene therapy approaches. They include the choice of appropriate therapeutic gene(s) (with a proven role in the pathomechanism of the disease, specifically targeted and of sufficient potency), gene delivery systems (of sufficient targeting ability, transfection efficiency, and safety), and gene expression regulation systems to control the level and timing of transgene expression.

The therapeutic and socioeconomic success of gene therapy products includes the requirement that the benefits of gene therapy should outweigh the risks and should offer advantages over conventional (usually less expensive) treatments, before this new approach will become accepted in the general medical practice.

Essential Components and Selected Technical Features of a Gene Therapy Product

Gene delivery vectors

The goal in the discovery and development of most gene therapy vectors is to deliver and express genes at the appropriate site and at therapeutically meaningful levels in a controlled manner. The first-generation gene therapy vectors have used the ability of viral systems to deliver genetic information to human cells. Attempts are also made to develop nonviral synthetic vectors and hybrid synthetic-viral systems that are potentially safer alternatives for gene delivery. A third approach uses isolated human cells (stem cells, progenitor cells, or somatic cells) as a means to introduce the therapeutic genes into specific human cell populations where the therapeutic product is required.

Viral vectors

Viruses "acquired" numerous biological properties over millions of years of evolution that allow them to effectively recognize and enter cells, traffic within the cytosol to the nucleus, translocate into the nucleus, and express their genes in the host cell.

The most frequently used viral vectors in clinical trials so far are retroviruses and adenoviruses. Several other viral vectors are in preclinical development or are under clinical evaluation, including adeno-associated virus (AAV), lentivirus, herpes simplex virus (HSV), and others.

Retroviruses can lead to a stable integration of the transfected gene into the host genome and therefore produce long-lasting gene transfer. Replication-deficient retroviruses are produced *in vitro* in

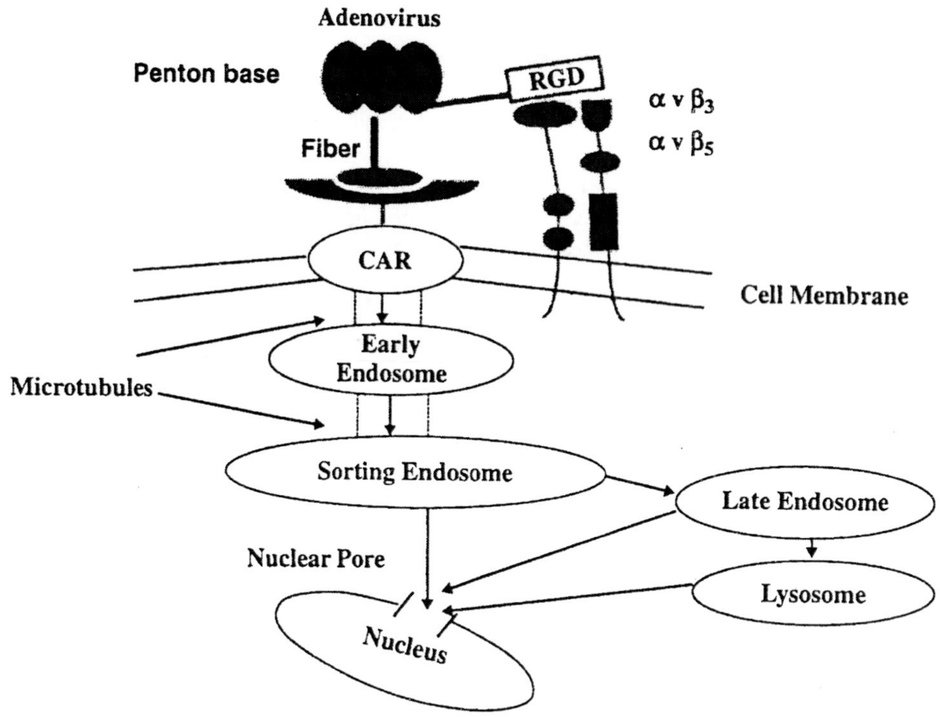

Fig. 16.1. Cellular recognition, uptake, and trafficking of adenoviral gene delivery vectors.

specific packaging cells transfected previously with retroviral genes (G, P, E) that have been deleted from the genome of the therapeutic retroviruses. Major limitations of the retroviruses are their low titers, their inability to infect nondividing cells, and the potential risk of insertional mutagenesis. The development of new pseudotyped retroviruses has increased virus titers that will permit more efficient gene transfer.

Table 16.1. Gene delivery systems (vectors) used in gene therapy clinical trials

Delivery System	*Number of Trials*
Retrovirus	254
Adenovirus	240
Naked DNA	132
Lipofection	85
Poxvirus	52
Vaccinia virus	30
Herpes simplex virus	26
Adeno-associated virus	19
RNA transfer	10

There are more than 50 known serotypes of *adenoviruses*, but until recently, serotype 5 (Ad5) and to a lesser extent serotype 2 (Ad2) (both class C adenoviruses) have been used as recombinant, nonreplicating gene delivery vectors. *Recombinant Ad5* can be produced in high titer. Ad5 vectors do not lead to stable integration of the transgene into the host genome (only at very low frequency in cell culture), and they usually remain extrachromosomal and cause only a transient transgene expression.

Replication-deficient adenoviruses are produced *in vitro* in specific packaging cells that complement gene products (e.g., *E1* and *E3*) deleted from the genome of the therapeutic adenoviruses. They give effective transient gene expression in proliferating and nonproliferating cells, but first-generation adenoviruses have the disadvantage of producing immunological and inflammatory reactions. These complications should be lessened with second-generation adenoviral vectors.

Some adenoviruses are human pathogens (wild-type Ad5, for example, causes the "common cold" syndrome), and most patients have already been exposed to them during their lifetime, resulting in the presence of various levels of circulating neutralizing antiviral antibodies (NABs). This exposure may hinder the effectiveness of their systemic application. Use of viral vectors that are not human pathogens (e.g., various serotypes of adenoviruses, AAV, or nonhuman adenoviruses) can avoid this problem. Immune response evoked by the first application of the viral vector (human or nonhuman) may interfere with their repeated application (although the immune response may depend on the route of delivery and dose used). First- and second-generation adenoviral vectors have limited cloning size (<10 kb), which prevents the use of large therapeutic genes, multiple genes, or complex gene regulatory elements. The use of "gutless" adenovirus avoids this problem, allowing a cloning capacity of up to ~30 kb, but filling the vector with "useless" DNA is a challenge, and so is the proper manufacturing of these modified vectors, which require the presence of helper viruses. *AAVs* have been used for effective gene transfer to muscle. Numerous AAV serotypes have been identified recently, with a different tissue tropism, which gives us hope for using them in a tissue-specific manner.

In addition to pseudotyping (retroviruses) or deletion of nonessential viral genes (adenoviruses), several other strategies are pursued to improve viral vectors for human therapeutic use. This is a very active field, the overview of which is beyond the scope of this chapter. Some notable activities include changing viral coat proteins (fibers, pentons, etc.) to redirect the tropism of the virus and incorporation of specific gene regulatory systems (gene-switches, tissue-specific promoters, etc.) to allow proper timing, duration, extent, and localization of therapeutic gene expression.

Nonviral vectors

The existing synthetic vectors (naked DNA, cationic liposomes, etc.) are far from being perfect delivery systems. Although they are less pathogenic and may have reduced toxicity compared with some existing viral vectors, depending on the dose injected, liposomes may aggregate in the blood and can cause severe toxic reactions. Plasmid and liposome complexes are easy to produce and are safer, but they have low gene-transfer efficiency. However, novel lipid formulations and synthe tic cationic polymer carriers have clearly improved the effectiveness of plasmid-mediated gene transfer.

In the future, the "perfect" gene delivery vector may be synthetic, incorporating many advantages of viruses (which over their evolution acquired the perfection of gene delivery to host organisms, such as dense DNA "*packaging*," cell recognition, cellular uptake, cytosolic trafficking, efficient nuclear uptake, and gene expression in the host cell nucleus), but avoiding the unwanted properties of viruses (e.g., off-target tropism, pathogenicity, cell toxicity, and immune and inflammatory reactions).

Dense DNA packaging (a prerequisite for efficient gene transfer) can be achieved by using, for example, protamine sulfate (a "trick" borrowed from sperm cells, which similar to viruses package DNA efficiently). The particle should be "shielded" from binding to plasma proteins, blood cells, or to each other to allow longer circulating plasma half-life and more efficient uptake in target tissues (e.g., at the site of leaky vessels in tumors) ("passive" targeting). They will be engineered to contain cell recognition ligands (e.g., transferring for proper "active" targeting of cancer cells), cell membrane fusion proteins, and nuclear localization signals (all "borrowed" from viruses) for efficient cellular trafficking. Chromosomal localization and insertion for long-term expression of the therapeutic gene will be achieved by adding, for example, the *rep* gene, which allows targeting and insertion of the

DNA to chromosome 19. These examples are just a few that are being tested today. However, even more sophisticated systems can be expected in the future, along with appropriate manufacturing and analytical processes, which will allow their introduction to human subjects.

Cell-based delivery of therapeutic genes

Although cell therapies have been used in medicine for several decades (e.g., blood transfusion), the use of cells manipulated *ex vivo* with therapeutic genes and then reintroduced into patients offers a new strategy by which to deliver therapeutic genes.

Human hematopoietic stem cells, mesenchymal stem cells, neuronal stem cells, embryonic stem cells, and peripheral T cells are the focus of ongoing research efforts. The panel of stem cells available for gene therapy purposes will increase as isolation and culturing procedures improve and appropriate factors are identified that can be used to drive their differentiation along distinct cell lineage pathways. Issues currently being addressed include the development of vectors (e.g., lentiviruses) for efficient stem cell gene transduction, expression and regulation of therapeutic genes during lineage progression from stem cells to differentiated cells, control of stem cell growth, expansion *ex vivo*, and engraftment and differentiation *in vivo*. Genetically engineered stem cells or less pluripotent progenitor cells are currently being tested for therapeutic angiogenesis (endothelial cell progenitors), Parkinson's disease (neuronal stem cells), bone marrow transplantation (hematopoiectic stem cells), and AIDS (e.g., hematopoietic stem cells transfected with the *RevM10* gene).

"Customized" gene delivery vectors

It is important to emphasize that there will not be a "universal" vector that is optimally useful for all indications. On the contrary, each disease target will have a specific set of technical requirements, and the "perfect" vector for a specific disease should be optimized according to these specific criteria. For example, some diseases will require local delivery (e.g., ischemia, retinitis pigmentosa, and Parkinson's disease), whereas others necessitate systemic delivery (e.g., cancer). For certain diseases, the gene of a secreted protein (e.g., coagulation factors VIII and IX for hemophilia A and B, respectively; growth hormone; and erythropoietin) can be expressed in almost any tissue of the body. Sometimes only transient, short-lived gene expression will be needed (e.g., therapeutic angiogenesis and cancer), whereas in other cases long-term (sometime lifelong) gene expression duration will be necessary (e.g., most monogenic diseases, such as familial hypercholesterolemia, hemophilia, and SCID). For certain disease targets, most, if not all, target cells need to be transfected (cancer), whereas in other cases, this will not be necessary (e.g., with most secreted therapeutic proteins).

In certain diseases, tight control of gene expression will not be important (e.g., coagulation factors), whereas in others very tight regulation of the gene expression will be essential (e.g., insulin). Some diseases will require specific targeting of the vector for efficient and safe delivery after systemic application (e.g., cancer). Other disease targets will require tissue-or disease-specific promoter elements (e.g., arteriosclerosis and cancer). In some instances, conditionally inducible gene expression regulation (gene-switch) will allow precise dosing and timing of gene expression, which will also be an essential element for safety reasons (i.e., ability to "turn off" the gene if serious side effects occur).

Most vectors optimized for a certain disease target will consist of multiple "components," each fulfilling some necessary technical, biological, or therapeutic need. As the different elements will probably be perfected (and patented) by different companies, the introduction of the optimal multicomponent vector may be difficult because of intellectual property rights and commercial obstacles.

Gene delivery targeting

The effectiveness of gene therapy is determined by a combination of the effects of gene delivery into the target tissue, the entry of the new genetic material into cells, and the expression of the transfected gene in the target tissue. When specific physical or biological targeting methods are available, they generally improve the expression of the transfected gene in the target organ and reduce gene expression in off-target tissues, which may lead to unwanted side effects.

Physical targeting

A variety of physical gene delivery methods has been introduced to achieve better local tissue targeting of vectors. An example of the effective physical targeting is catheter-mediated gene transfer to various regions of the body (e.g., feed arteries of organs, such as leg muscles, heart, and liver, or retrograde injection via veins). Intramuscular injection of plasmid DNA or viral vectors encoding angiogenic growth factors has been used in ischaemic myocardium and peripheral vascular disease. Another approach to local delivery to small arterioles and capillaries is injection of biodegradable microspheres coated with recombinant growth factors or plasmid DNA. Ultrasonography, alone or in combination with microbubbles, can also potentially be used to improve the efficiency of gene transfer. For facilitation of intramuscular, intratumoral, or intradermal delivery of naked, plasmid, or cationic liposome-carried DNA, gene gun technology and electroporation can be used. Although these delivery methods offer certain advantages in specific disease targets, they are being progressively replaced by more specific biological targeting methods.

Biological targeting

Biological vector targeting uses modification of viral coat proteins (for viral vectors) or surface properties of synthetic vectors (e.g., liposomes).

Passive targeting makes use of alteration of the pharmacokinetics of vectors by "shielding" them from binding to blood cells, plasma proteins, immunoglobulins, unwanted tissues, or to each other, allowing them to circulate for longer periods of time in the blood and accumulate in specific tissues with "leaky" blood vessels (such as tumors).

Active (vector) targeting aims at directing vector binding and uptake to specific cells in the body by selective "targeting" molecules attached to the surface of the vectors by a variety of technologies (e.g., chemical and genetic). Recent advances in the biological understanding of adenovirus structure and adenovirus receptor interactions have lead to the development of targeted adenovirus vectors. Receptor-mediated entry of adenovirus serotype 5 (Ad5) into cells has been found to depend on two of its coat proteins. The fiber knob protein mediates primary attachment to the cell via the coxsackie-adenovirus receptor (CAR) protein. After cell attachment via fiber–CAR interaction, an RGD tripeptide motif in the penton base protein binds to integrins ($\alpha_v\beta_3$ and $\alpha_v\beta_5$) that mediate cellular internalization. Other adenovirus serotypes use different cell-surface receptors (e.g., the group B adenoviruses bind to CD46), most of which have not been identified yet.

Two basic requirements are necessary to create a (re)targeted Ad5 vector: Interaction of adenovirus with its native receptors (e.g., CAR) must be first removed, and novel, tissue-specific ligands must be added to the virus. Three general approaches have been used to achieve these basic requirements. In the "two-component" approach, a bispecific molecule is complexed with the adenovirus. The bispecific component simultaneously blocks native receptor (CAR) binding and redirects virus binding to a tissue-specific receptor (e.g., to integrins using the RGD motif). In the "one-step" approach, the adenovirus is genetically modified in the fiber protein domains to remove native receptor interactions and a novel ligand is genetically incorporated into one adenovirus coat protein. The third approach is to use specific polymers to cover the entire virus and "shield" it from unwanted interactions. This method creates a truely "stealth" virus, preventing its interaction, not only with its primary (CAR, via fiber) and secondary cell-surface receptors (integrins, via penton RGD), but also with plasma proteins (including neutralizing antibodies), blood cells, and most tissue sites, providing an ideal situation for extended persistence in the circulation and *passive targeting*. The polymer coat allows covalent attachment of specific "ligands" of choice to its surface, effectively retargeting the vector to a desired tissue (*active targeting*).

Transcriptional targeting

Receptor targeting technology can be combined with "*transcriptional targeting*" approaches (by the use of cell-, tissue- or disease-specific promoters). A tissue- or disease-specific promoter will allow therapeutic gene expression only in cells that express transcription factor proteins binding to these specific promoter sites. Some tissue- or disease-specific promoters, identified and tested in animal models to date, include the promoter of the prostate-specific antigen (PSA) gene, osteocalcin gene, glucose "sensing" molecules for insulin gene delivery, and hypoxia response element (HRE) activated by hypoxia inducible factors (HIFs) in hypoxic/ischemic tissues (e.g., tumors).

Gene expression control systems

Regulating therapeutic gene expression will be necessary for both the clinical efficacy and the safety of most HGT applications. Gene therapy offers the promise of replacing frequent injections of an expensive therapeutic protein or antibody with an infrequent or even one-time administration of a gene delivery vector, which would then provide continuous therapeutic protein production at the desired site. An appropriate system of gene expression will control and allow titration of protein levels, dosing to be adjusted as the disease evolves, and therapy to be initiated repeatedly or terminated at will. Regulation can be achieved by a physiological/pathological signal (e.g., glucose and hypoxia) or via dose-dependent ligand binding and activation of chimeric transcription factor proteins, which then interact with DNA elements incorporated into the vector and regulate therapeutic gene expression.

Much progress has been made on control systems, where gene expression is regulated pharmacologically by a small-molecule drug. Four major systems are known to date that have already been tested in animals: those regulated by the antiobiotic tetracycline (Tet), the insect steroid ecdysone or its analogs, the anti-progestin mifepristone (RU486), and chemical dimerizers such as the immunosuppressant rapamycin and its analogs. They all involve small-molecule-dependent recruitment of a transcriptional activation domain to a basal promoter driving the gene of interest, but they differ in the mechanism of recruitment. Such a pharmacological gene expression regulation system should meet the following criteria. Basal expression should be very low and inducible to high levels over a wide dose range. Induction should be a positive effect (adding rather than removing a drug) and use an orally active small molecule that has no untoward pharmacological effects in humans. The regulatory protein(s) should have no effects on endogenous gene expression and should be of human origin to minimize immunogenicity. It has been successfully used for the timing and dosing of circulating plasma levels of therapeutic proteins (such as IFNβ) expressed in the hind limb muscle of mice after i.m. delivery of their DNA in the form of AAV-1 or naked plasmid combined with electroporation.

Disease Targets for Gene Therapy

Ever since the first clinical attempt of gene transfer more than 17 years ago, numerous monogenic and complex (multigenic) diseases were targeted with a large variety of gene therapy strategies.

In 1989, Rosenberg et al. performed the first human gene therapy trial when they used a retrovirus to introduce the gene coding for resistance to neomycin into human tumor-infiltrating lymphocytes before infusing them into five patients with advanced melanoma. The first trials have been designed to establish feasibility and safety, to demonstrate the expression of therapeutic protein(s) *in vivo* by the genes transferred, and in some cases, to show therapeutic benefit.

As of January 31, 2004, there were 918 trials in 24 countries on record. The U.S. accounts for two thirds of these trials. Cancer is by far the most common disease indication, followed by inherited monogenic diseases and cardiovascular diseases. Viral vectors have been the most frequently used vehicles for transferring genes into human cells, with retroviruses and adenoviruses representing the vast majority. Over 100 distinct genes have been transferred.

FROM BENCH TO BEDSIDE: THE DEVELOPMENT OF AD5FGF-4 TO TREAT PATIENTS WITH RECURRENT ANGINA

A brief summary of the preclinical and early clinical development and manufacturing of the Ad5FGF-4 gene therapy product for the facilitation of angiogenesis in patients with chronic myocardial ischemia (recurrent angina) is provided below for the purpose of illustrating the complex processes involved in the many stages of preclinical and clinical development of an HGT product.

Preclinical Efficacy

Specific criteria need to be fulfilled for angiogenic gene therapy to be successful. The gene selected should code for a protein with proven angiogenic activity, the vector should provide high gene-transfer efficiency, the delivery technique should target the ischemic tissue, and the procedure should be safe, in both the short and the long term. In addition, appropriate current Good Manufacturing Practices (cGMP) need to be established. Preclinical and initial clinical studies indicate that angiogenic gene transfer with Ad5FGF-4, delivered by a single intracoronary injection, may meet these criteria.

Proof-of-concept study

Preclinical investigation of Ad5FGF-4 involved demonstration of myocardial angiogenesis in a porcine model of stress-induced myocardial ischemia. In this experimental model, an ameroid constrictor is placed around the proximal left circumflex coronary artery, leading to gradual closure of the artery over the following weeks. The subsequent development of collateral vessels allows normal myocardial function and blood perfusion at rest, but blood flow is insufficient to prevent ischemia during periods of increased oxygen demand. In the proof-of-concept studies, stress-induced (atrial pacing) left ventricular function and blood flow changes were evaluated by two-dimensional echocardiography approximately 35 days after ameroid placement. Ad5FGF-4 (10^{11} viral particle [v.p.] per animal) ($n = 6$) was then administered by intracoronary injection. Ventricular function and blood flow were reassessed 14 days later, and the animals were killed to quantify the presence of adenoviral DNA and FGF-4 mRNA and protein expression in the myocardium.

Polymerase chain reaction (P CR) and reverse-transcription–PCR (RT–PCR) analysis demonstrated the presence of Ad5 DNA and FGF-4 mRNA, respectively, in the injected pig hearts. Immunoblotting showed that pigs treated with Ad5FGF-4 expressed FGF-4 protein in heart tissue but not in other organs, such as the liver and eye. Contractile function, assessed as the degree of wall thickening of the ischemic region during atrial pacing, had improved significantly 2 weeks after FGF-4 gene transfer compared with preinjection. This functional improvement was associated with a normalization of regional blood flow during atrial pacing. Thus, this study provided experimental evidence that a single intracoronary injection of Ad5FGF-4 ameliorates deficits in myocardial blood flow and function in the setting of chronic myocardial ischemia in pigs. Follow-up studies in the same pig model showed that the effect of single Ad5FGF-4 injection lasted at least for 3 months, and that the effect was dose dependent.

Toxicology and Biodistribution

A Good Laboratory Practices (GLP) toxicology and biodistribution study was performed to determine the potential adverse effects of Ad5FGF-4 in healthy pigs after either intracoronary or left ventricular (systemic) administration (10^{12} v.p. left ventricular, 10^{10}–10^{12} v.p. intracoronary). Systemic biodistribution of the product was also assessed. This study found no significant test article-related toxicologic effects. PCR analysis for adenoviral DNA and RT–PCR analysis for the transgene (FGF-4) mRNA were performed to assess vector biodistribution. Adenoviral DNA was detected in 27 of 110 organs examined from animals injected intracoronary with 10^{12} v.p. Ad5FGF-4. Adenoviral DNA was detected in the lung, liver, spleen, and testis. Detectable adenoviral DNA typically decreased over time in most organs. The presence of viral DNA in the testis was observed at 5 days but not at 28 or 84 days. In no case in which adenoviral DNA was present in extracardiac sites was transgene expression detectable at the mRNA level after RT–PCR analysis. These results (along with cGMP) supported the submission of an investigational new drug (IND) application in 1998.

cGMP Manufacturing and Characterization of the Gene Therapy Vector

This section summarizes the various activities required in the course of cGMP manufacturing and testing of the Ad5FGF-4 product for the initiation and advancement of its clinical development and reaching a "well characterized product" status with the Regulatory Authorities.

Vector construction

Construction of the recombinant replication incompetent (E1/2 deleted) adenovirus serotype 5 (Ad5) expressing the human FGF-4 cDNA required three components: the FGF-4 transgene, a plasmid shuttle vector to carry the transgene as well as 5′ Ad5 sequences, and a second plasmid carrying the bulk of the Ad5 genome. The full-length cDNA for human FGF-4 (the "transgene") was isolated from a cDNA library, which was constructed from mRNA of Kaposi's sarcoma DNA transformed NIH3T3 cells. The cDNA that encodes the FGF-4 peptide is approximately 1.2 kB in size, and the FGF-4 protein has 206 amino acids, including a 33-amino-acid signal peptide at the N-terminus.

Plasmid pACCMVplpASR(-) (the "shuttle vector") contains the heterologous CMV promoter, a polylinker, and SV40 polyadenylation sequences flanked by partial human Ad5 sequences. The FGF-4 cDNA was subcloned, as an Eco R1 fragment, into this adenovirus shuttle vector at its single Eco R1 site. Plasmid pJM17 (the "*adenovirus plasmid*") contains the required Ad5 sequences except that the El region is disrupted by the insertion of pBR322 sequences. A unique feature of this plasmid is the presence of some nonviral sequences in the E3 region that become relevant for the viral vector identity testing. To generate the Ad5FGF-4 viral vector, plasmids pACSR/FGF-4 and pJM17 were co-transfected into HEK 293 cells using a calcium phosphate method. The cells were overlaid with nutrient agarose. Homologous recombination between the vectors created El-deleted, FGF-4 gene-containing vector genomes capable of replication in HEK 293 cells.

Master virus bank

Six clones were isolated from one round of virus plaque purification and were screened for protein expression. One clone was selected, amplified on HEK 293 cells, purified by cesium chloride (CsCl) ultracentrifugation, and used for preparation of a Master Virus Bank (MVB). A purified Ad5FGF-4 virus seed was propagated through three consecutive rounds of plaque purification. A final plaque was then expanded and purified by anion exchange chromatography, sterilized by filtration, and stored at –70°C. This virus stock was checked for sterility and absence of measurable replication competent adenovirus (RCA). An MVB was then created by one additional cycle of propagation in serum-free suspension culture of HEK 293 cells, and this virus was purified, aliquoted, and frozen. The MVB was tested and confirmed to be free of RCA as well as adventitious agents. The MVB was stored at –70°C.

Master cell bank and manufacturer's working cell bank

A scalable manufacturing process to meet clinical, as well as commercial, needs for recombinant adenovirus vector would only be attractive if it could be performed without using bovine serum in the culture medium. For these reasons, attachment and serum-dependent HEK 293 cells were first adapted to suspension culture by direct transfer into shake flasks in a modified William's essential medium containing 2% fetal bovine serum. The cultures were passaged continually for over 6 weeks in the same environment until the cells exhibited a consistent growth pattern of less than 48 hours of doubling time and greater than 90% viability. These suspension-adapted cells were subsequently adapted to serum-free medium by gradual weaning. Cells from this bank were thawed and expanded and then used to generate a Master Cell Bank (MCB). Culture identification as human cells, growth on soft agarose to assess potential tumorigenicity, and screening for adventitious agents were also performed (according to current cell-line testing guidelines). Starting from the MCB, a Manufacturer's Working Cell Bank (MWCB) was prepared and then similarly tested before routine use.

Manufacture of the bulk drug substance

The Ad5FGF-4 vectorwas manufactured under cGMP in a state-of-the-art, validated facility, following Biosafety Level 2 (BL2) practices. For the preparation of the Ad5FGF-4 drug substance, cells from the MWCB and virus from the MVB were employed. The virus was propagated in suspension cultures of HEK 293 cells using serum-free medium and the virus progeny was purified using a combination of anion exchange chromatography (AIEX) and ultra-filtration (UF). The purified bulk drug substance was stored at -70°C.

Drug substance (virus) purification

Medium components and extracellular (nonviral) contaminants were largely removed from adenoviral infected HEK 293 cells using three successive physiological buffer solution (PBS) washes and centrifugation of the cells at the time of harvest. The harvested cells were then frozen in a solution of PBS with 2% sucrose and stored at -70°C, until purification. The virus purification process was initiated with two additional cycles of freeze and thaw steps. After the final thaw, the ruptured cell suspension was centrifuged to remove cell debris. Virus purification was established with a protocol based on traditional protein purification techniques: column chromatography and ultrafiltration. Separation from nucleic acid contaminants was achieved by combining strategic peak collection and utilization of a tangential flow ultra-filtration step with a 100-kDa molecular-weight cutoff pore size membrane. Both of these purification procedures are readily and linearily scaled up and thus can support the large-scale production of Ad5FGF-4 for both clinical testings and commercial use.

Manufacture scale-up

The adenovirus harvest process consisted of three general steps: concentration, lysis, and clarification. In the small-scale process, the intact adenovirus-infected cells in culture medium were aliquoted and batch centrifuged to achieve a 30-fold concentration, and the supernatant was manually removed and replaced with a smaller volume of the freeze buffer. Although sufficing for harvest volumes of no more than 10 L, such a manual process would prove to be inadequate on a larger manufacturing scale. A successful harvest method was identified using continuous centrifugation in a Westfalia CSC-6 disk-stack device with a hydroheratic feed system (HHFS). Scale-up of the adenovirus harvest process using a continuous centrifuge with HHFS has been shown to efficiently separate and concentrate an infected cell pellet while allowing the relatively easy exchange of growth medium for freezing buffer without open, manual manipulation. This patented process step combined separation of the cell pellet from culture medium, medium/buffer exchange, cell concentration, and then cell lysis in a single-unit operation step. The resulting lysate could be clarified and the virus purified.

Analytical techniques and release specifications of bulk virus lots

The crude viral harvest was tested for adventitious agents as needed to comply with current regulatory guidelines. Purified virus was tested to confirm the absence of RCAs, residual host cell proteins and DNA, and endotoxin, and to quantify total and infectious vector particles and, thus, the infectivity ratio. Bulk virus lots were released after meeting specifications, which included <1 endotoxin unit/mL and infectivity ratios of $>2\%$ (infectious titer/total viral particles).

Chromatographic assays for the quantitation of intact viral particles

One main challenge in the development of the adenovirus purification process is the quantitation of intact viral particles in crude samples. Nonaggregated, purified viral samples were easily quantified by the reverse phase (RP)–high-performance liquid chromatography (HPLC) method. The RP–HPLC assay quantitates the individual structural proteins with UV absorbance at 214 nm as the basis for the measurement of the adenovirus concentration. Unfortunately this assay could not be used to calculate the yields of the purification steps because it could not reliably quantitate crude samples. To solve this problem, an anion exchange (AIEX)–HPLC procedure was developed using a trimethyl anion exchange (TMAE) resin. The TMAE- HPLC was suitable for the analysis of all in-process samples ranging from clarified cell harvest to the final formulated, purified recombinant adenovirus product.

Endpoint dilution (EPD) assay for infectivity

To determine infectivity, an end-point dilution assay was developed. The precision of this assay has a standard deviation of 0.2 when viral titers are expressed in $\log_{10}$.

Replication competent adenoviruses (RCA)

Recombination between the viral E1 gene carried by HEK 293 cells and the E1 deleted recombinant adenovirus can and does occur at low frequency to generate RCAs, essentially wild-type Ad5 lacking the FGF-4 transgene. A highly sensitive assay involving viral amplification and cytopathic effect (CPE) readout has been described. The limit of detection of this assay was one RCA in 3.2×10^{12} virus particles. Virus banks and bulk Ad5FGF-4 virus batches testing positive for RCA were not used in clinical studies.

Host cell protein detection by ELISA

Typically biotechnology products have been produced in cell lines not of human origin. In such cases, residual host cell proteins (HCPs) are perceived as a safety concern to the patient. In the case of Ad5FGF-4 produced in HEK 293 cells, it is expected that the patient may respond to viral proteins with an immune response, but it is less clear that human HCPs will be immunogenic or pose a serious safety concern. One approach to detection of such HCP is by enzyme-linked immunosorbent assay (ELISA) using a polyclonal antibody reagent such as the HEK 293 HCP detection kit offered by Cygnus Technologies. This ELISA was used to show a consistent, high HCP titer in crude cell lysates and to show that the diethyl-aminoethyl (DEAE) chromatography step is sufficient and reproducible to reduce HCPs to below the level of quantitation (20 ng/mL).

Residual DNA

Two methods were used to quantitate residual host cell (HEK 293) DNA in Ad5FGF-4 preparations. The first, using membrane hybridization of an oligonucleotide probe followed by chemiluminescent detection, was based on a procedure described by Walsh et al. Extracted samples were blotted onto a positively charged nylon membrane using a slot blot apparatus, the blot was then hybridized with a biotinylated oligonucleotide probe specific to the primate alpha-satellite sequence D17Z1, and the bound probe was detected with a streptavidin- alkaline phosphatase conjugate, followed by a chemiluminescent alkaline phosphatase substrate. The second method used TaqMan PCR quantitation of *Alu* repeat sequences in virus samples extracted using the Qiagen QIAAmp Viral RNA Mini Kit. In-process sample testing showed that the two methods gave similar results, both demonstrating a greater than 3 log reduction in the level of host cell DNA by the purification process, with final purified material containing less than 0.5-ng/mL DNA.

Product identity tests by PCR

The adenoviral backbone of the Ad5FGF-4 genome is derived from *dl*309, an Ad5 mutant, commonly used for the construction of E1-deleted adenoviral vectors. This mutant has a short stretch of foreign DNA inserted in place of a portion of the E3 region. PCR confirmation of the type of adenovirus backbone served as a test for product identity and purity. It was possible to confirm transgene orientation as well as differentiate the product digest pattern from those obtained from either wt Ad5, RCA, or vectors containing different transgenes.

Product potency tests

Two assays were developed that measure the potency of the FGF-4 protein. In the first case, a "one-step" growth promotion assay is conducted on normal, human retinal pigment epithelial cells (ARPE-19). The assay measures metabolic activity (Alamar blue dye metabolism) after infection of ARPE-19 cells with a serial dilution of the drug substance (Ad5FGF-4). The increase in metabolic activity correlated with FGF-4 protein production (determined by an FGF-4 ELISA), increased *de novo* DNA synthesis (measured by BrdU incorporation), and an increase in cell number.

The second assay measured the production of FGF-4 protein produced in and secreted by A549 cells after infection with different doses of Ad5FGF-4. An FGF-4 specific ELISA allowed quantitation of FGF-4 protein present in the cell culture medium. The FGF-4 produced was confirmed as biologically active by stimulating the growth of ARPE-19 cells.

DNA sequencing of the entire viral vector

The complete DNA sequence of the Ad5FGF-4 genome was determined using double-stranded DNA sequencing of Ad5FGF-4 DNA extracted from an MVB expansion. A total of 166 oligonucleotide primers were used to obtain overlapping readings from both strands of DNA. The observed sequence was compared with that predicted for Ad5FGF-4 by insertion of the FGF-4 transgene sequence into the wild-type Ad5 sequence, into which the *dl*309 specific mutations had been incorporated. The observed sequence matched the predicted 5′ 4.9 kB of vector sequence including the FGF-4 transgene. The sequence data distal to the transgene (3′ end) confirmed that the Ad5FGF-4 backbone was derived from the Ad5 mutant *dl*309.

Genome analysis

As a further safety precaution, and as a specific regulatory request, the DNA sequence of the FGF-4 transgene was analyzed for other possible open reading frames (ORFs) that might encode unexpected foreign proteins upon infection of target cells with the recombinant adenovirus. This analysis also included any reading frames that crossed the transgene/virus junctions and might therefore involve viral sequences. The genome analysis confirmed that only FGF-4 protein is made from the transgene carried in Ad5FGF-4.

The cGMP manufacturing and analytical process and the facility where it took place have been approved by both the U.S. Food and Drug Administration (FDA) and the European Regulatory Agencies. Based on the test data, the FDA qualified Ad5FGF-4 as a "well characterized product."

Clinical Studies

There are several goals of Ad5FGF-4 angiogenic gene therapy for patients with chronic myocardial ischemia. It should promote new collateral vessel formation in the heart. In turn, this should increase perfusion of ischemic regions, leading to improved myocardial oxygen delivery and left ventricular function. From the patient's perspective, the ultimate goal of treatment should be to reduce or ameliorate symptoms of angina, increase exercise capacity, improve quality of life, and decrease the long-term risk of acute coronary events (such as acute myocardial infarction).

The clinical development program was initiated in 1998 to determine whether the improvement in cardiac perfusion and function (without any product-related adverse effects) detected in pigs translates into a clinical therapeutic benefit in patients with chronic stable angina. Four clinical studies [Angiogenic

Gene Therapy (AGENT) phase 1/2 trial, AGENT 2 phase 2 trial, and AGENT 3 and 4 phase 2B/3 trials] have been initiated, and some (AGENT and AGENT-2) have been completed to date.

Phase 1/2 AGENT trial

The Angiogenic Gene Therapy Trial (AGENT) was the first ever randomized, double-blind, placebo-controlled (12 sites) U.S. clinical trial of angiogenic gene therapy for myocardial ischemia. The objectives of the AGENT trial were to evaluate the safety and anti-ischemic effects of five ascending doses of Ad5FGF•4 (3.2×10^8 to 3.2×10^{10} v.p.), randomizing in a ratio of 1 : 2 (placebo : active) in patients with chronic stable exertional angina, who had recurring angina despite optimal medical treatment and were not in need of immediate surgical revascularization.

A total of 79 patients with chronic stable angina were enrolled. Patients could exercise for ≥3 minutes in an exercise treadmill test (ETT) using the modified Balke protocol. The adenovirus vector was infused over 90 seconds through sub-selective catheters into all major patent coronary arteries and grafts, 40% into the right coronary distribution and 60% into the left coronary distribution. Repeat treadmill exercise tests were performed at 4 and 12 weeks posttreatment.

The increase from baseline in treadmill exercise duration at weeks 4 and 12 was greater among patients receiving 10^{10} v.p. Ad5FGF-4 than among those receiving placebo (the difference at week 4 was statistically significant). Analysis of the subgroup of patients with a baseline ETT time of <10 minutes showed the gene therapy produced a statistically significant increase in exercise capacity compared with placebo at 12 weeks (27% vs. 12%; $p = 0.01$).

Phase 2 AGENT-2 trial

AGENT 2 was designed to assess whether Ad5FGF-4 improved myocardial perfusion in patients with stable angina. It was also designed to further evaluate safety. Based on the results of the AGENT trial, a dose of 10^{10} v.p. was selected. The primary endpoint was the change in stress-related (adenosine-induced) reversible perfusion defect size (RPDS) as assessed by single-photon emission computed tomography (SPECT), 8 weeks after treatment. A total of 52 patients underwent double-blind randomization (35 to Ad5FGF-4, 17 to placebo). Total perfusion defect size (PDS) at baseline was 32% and RPDS was 20%.

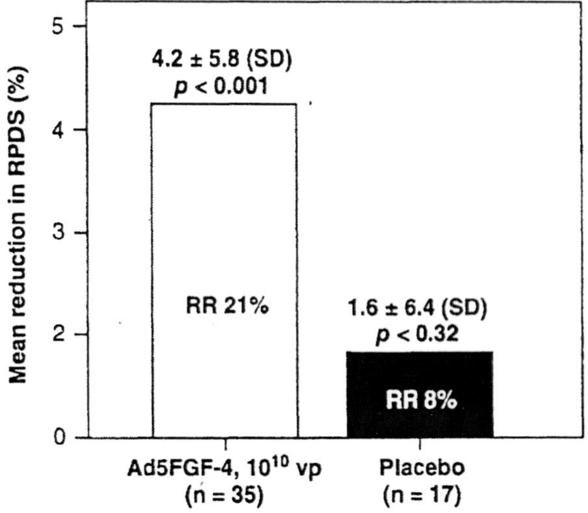

Fig. 16.2. AGENT-2 trial perfusion result.

The mean reduction in RPDS from baseline at 8 weeks posttreatment in the Ad5FGF-4 group was $4.2 \pm 5.6\%$ ($p < 0.001$), a 21% decrease from baseline, versus a reduction in the placebo group of only $1.6 \pm 5.4\%$ ($p = 0.32$), corresponding to a decrease of 8% from baseline. Similar results were observed for the change in total PDS from baseline at 8 weeks posttreatment: Ad5FGF-4 decreased total PDS by a mean of $4.6 \pm 5.6\%$ ($p < 0.001$) compared with a reduction of $2.4 \pm 6.5\%$ with placebo (p = NS). More of the patients who received the active product than those who received placebo reported complete resolution of angina (30% vs. 13%) and no nitroglycerin use (43% vs. 17%) at 8 weeks. In addition, the incidence of worsening/unstable angina and revascularation by coronary artery bypass grafting or angioplasty at 12 months was considerably lower in the Ad5FGF-4 group (6% and 6%, respectively) compared with those in the placebo group (24% and 16%, respectively).

Safety in AGENT and AGENT 2 trials

In the AGENT and AGENT-2 trials combined, a total of 131 patients (95 on Ad5FGF-4 and 36 on placebo) were treated and followed for 12 months. Overall, Ad5FGF-4 was well tolerated. There was no rise in cardiac enzymes, electrocardiographic change, or clinical evidence of myocarditis associated with the treatment.

Vector distribution after intracoronary administration was examined in the AGENT trial. Adenovirus could be detected by endpoint dilution infectivity assay in the pulmonary artery during intracoronary infusion and in peripheral venous blood 1 hour later. The frequency of positive samples increased with increasing doses of Ad5FGF-4. Virus was not detected in the urine collected over 6 hours after treatment. Neutralizing antibody titer to Ad5 increased in most patients, but no FGF-4 protein was detected in the circulation at any time. Semen samples (n = 8) were tested by PCR (8 weeks posttreatment) and found to be negative for Ad5FGF-4 DNA. Ad5FGF-4-related adverse effects included dose-related transient fever (n = 8) and transient increase in liver enzymes (n = 3). Overall, the safety profile was reassuring and consistent with safety data in other cardiovascular adenoviral gene therapy trials. There was no evidence of myocarditis, retinal neovascularization, or angioma formation.

The positive trend toward efficacy and the safety observed in these two trials were in good agreement with the preclinical safety and efficacy data obtained in pigs, and they provided the basis to progress the clinical development to larger, multinational phase 2b/3 trials (AGENT-3 and AGENT-4), the results of which will be reported in the future.

Lessons Learned from Past Failures

The remarkable clinical safety observed in most cardiovascular gene therapy trials to date is of no coincidence. Lessons learned from past failures at the manufacturing, preclinical efficacy and safety, and clinical development levels were all taken into account in the development of Ad5FGF-4. Failures were due primarily to two factors: safety issues and lack of clinical efficacy.

The tragic death of Jesse Gelsinger at the University of Pennsylvania treated with a very high dose (>10 e13 vp) of a first-generation adenoviral vector raised the issue of dose and innate immune response. We learned that side effects of Ad5 are dose dependent, which follow a so-called "elbow" shape (i.e., no effect up to a certain dose and severe effects at the next dose). Therefore we have tested the dose-response relationship of efficacy, biodistribution, side effects, and toxic effects very thoroughly in our preclinical models, and we chose the doses of10e9 and 10e10 vp (more than three orders of magnitude lower than the dose used in the "Gelsinger" case).

Another gene therapy clinical trial that led to serious side effects was the SCID trial in France, where several of the children treated developed leu kemia. These later were attributed to retrovirus integration at a site in the genome, which led to significant clonal expansion of the treated lymphocytes. Therefore, the choice of vector could be of great importance. In our product candidate, we intentionally avoided the use of integrating vectors (e.g., retrovirus, lentivirus, and AAV). As relatively short-term and transient gene expression is sufficient for therapeutic angiogenesis, we did not need to use these integrating vectors.

Both the "Gelsinger" case and the "SCID Trial" intensified regulatory scrutiny, which served the field very well. Small (mostly physician sponsored) trials using poorly characterized material are not allowed anymore. Both the FDA and the European Regulatory Agencies require well-controlled cGMP Manufacturing to be in place before clinical testing can start.

The recent failure of Hemofilia B trials due to lack of efficacy raised other important issues. All animal tests using the AAV.fIX product showed positive results from mouse to subhuman primates. The lack of efficacy in humans is now attributed (at least in part) to a memory T-cell mediated immune response against the AAV vector, which is absent in animals. However, no human-specific immune response to Ad5 vectors has been identified to date.

The progress of gene therapy in the past 17 years has been slower than was expected, which is due to several factors. Gene therapy is a pioneering new therapeutic modality based on complex biological systems occurring at the leading edge of biomedical knowledge. Incomplete knowledge of the genes involved in the pathomechanism of diseases constitutes a limit to generate clinically effective gene therapies, especially in complex diseases with mul tiple interacting genetic and environmental factors. Stringent and time-consuming safety studies are needed as is the establishment of new regulatory frameworks essential to control the applications of gene therapy and ensure safety to the patient and the population at large. High costs are involved in the R&D of gene therapy and complex issues of intellectual property and commercial rights need to be resolved.

Despite the early high exceptions and the subsequent setbacks, one has to recognize that this new therapeutic modality is still in its infancy. It will neither deliver medical "miracles" (as its early proponents predicted) nor will it "disappear" because of a few disappointing setbacks (as some of its recent antagonists predict). As with all new technologies, gene therapy has to run its course in its current "*development phase*" before it reaches "*maturation*," when its full potential will be exploited.

17

GENETIC MARKERS

Over the past decade, major research efforts have resulted in a wealth of sequence information for many genomes. In addition to the human genome, several other mammalian genomes have also been completely sequenced, providing a tremendous resource for biomedical researchers to examine gene sequences, their regulation, and their role in health and disease. However, although we commonly talk about "the genome" when we refer to the genome sequence, every individual of a species has a slightly different genome sequence. It is this variation in the genome sequence that accounts for phenotypic differences, and for different susceptibilities to a large number of diseases. In humans, if we knew which sequence differences predisposed individuals to common human disorders such as hypertension or Alzheimer's disease, we could develop preventive treatments that could prevent disease, despite the genetic risk. It is this vision that has driven researchers involved in the Human Genome Project over the past years. Likewise, if we understood the genetic variation in model organisms, such as rats or mice, responsible for disease susceptibility or variability in drug metabolism and efficacy, we could use this information to test novel drugs more efficiently and target specialized drugs toward individuals with specific genetic predispositions.

Although there has been significant progress in biomedical research to suggest that this vision may one day become reality, we do not yet have a good understanding of the genetic differences in the genome sequence, and how they influence the development of disease. One reason why progress has been slow is the fact that there are so many differences. The sequence of any two human genomes differs in at least three million bases. Most differences in mammalian genomes are single base pair differences in the DNA sequence, but others include length variation in repeated sequences and chromosomal rearrangements. This presents a tremendous challenge to geneticists and biomedical researchers: How do you distinguish between DNA sequence variation that has no functional consequences and the differences that affect gene function and possibly the well-being of the organism? After all, only about 5% of any mammalian genome encodes for genes, and only small portions of the remaining 95% have discernible functions. As a consequence, it is likely that most DNA sequence variation has no effect on the organism because it is located in these regions without (known) function.

To further identify the determinants of genetic disorders, different approaches have been used to zoom in on regions of the genome that contain the mutation(s) that are responsible for the genetic defect. Both commonly used approaches, family-based linkage studies and association analyses, require genetic markers, i.e., sequences that are variable between individuals and can be used to distinguish the DNA from different individuals. Even before the completion of the various genome sequencing projects, linkage analyses identified numerous loci in the genomes of both humans and model organisms that harbor genes involved in the development of a variety of common disorders. These studies used genetic polymorphisms, i.e., differences in the DNA sequence, to distinguish individuals with and without the disease and to identify regions shared by affected individuals. It is this initial use of DNA sequence variation as markers for genetic studies that this chapter will focus on. We will describe two types of genetic variation commonly used as markers in genetic studies, describe how they were discovered and can be interrogated by genotyping in large numbers of individuals, and will end by briefly describing the approaches of linkage and association studies that are aided by and rely on these genetic markers. Numerous review articles have summarized different aspects of this chapter, and we will focus primarily on the methodologies underlying the different genotyping approaches commonly used today in genetic laboratories.

Simple Sequence Length Polymorphisms (SSLPs)

Eukaryotic genomes contain interspersed repetitive sequence elements, many of which have no known function. Incredibly, these "nonfunctional" sequences comprise about 20% of the human genome. It is thought that these repetitive motifs were generated by transposons or retrotransposons that replicate and then "jump" to other locations to propagate their genome, in the form of either DNA (in the case of transposons) or RNA (in the case of retrotransposons). Some repetitive sequence elements are long, about 1000–5000 base pairs (bp) in length, and they are known as LINES (long interspersed elements), whereas others are shorter, about 200–500 bp, and are known as SINES (short interspersed elements). The Alu element, approximately 300 bp in length, is the most abundant SINE in the human genome and comprises about 3% of the human genome.

Another type of repetitive element consists of very short sequences (2 to 5 bp), arrayed in tandem. These sequences, called microsatellites, simple sequence length polymorphisms (SSLPs), simple sequence repeats (SSRs), or short tandem repeat polymorphisms (STRPs), tend to vary in unit size (from 5 to 30 units). The number of these tandem elements varies, and as a result, so does their length, making these sequences *polymorphic* (having different forms). The most abundant class of microsatellite repeat, is the dinucleotide repeat of cytosine and adenine, or (CA) · (GT) repeats. In the human genome, these dinucleotide repeat microsatellites occur every 30 to 60 kbp, corresponding to approximately 50,000 to 100,000 microsatellites in the 3 billion base pair human genome. Other common microsatellites include trinucleotide and tetranucleotide repeats (3 and 4 bp repeats, respectively).

The length of the microsatellite repeat is thought to be due to errors in DNA replication. During DNA replication, the polymerase machinery is thought to "slip," either eliminating or adding repeat units. The deletion or addition of a single repeat unit occurs most frequently (91%). The frequency of this type of mutation, on average, is 1.2×10^{-3} per microsatellite, translating to roughly 1 in 1000 meioses (as determined by examining how often a parent passes an expanded or contracted microsatellite repeat to his/her offspring). The range of mutation frequency for any given microsatellite is 0 to 8×10^{-3} and seems to occur more frequently in the male vs. the female germline.

With a few exceptions, microsatellites do not have functional consequences on clinical outcomes. They are most commonly found in intergenic or intronic portions of a eukaryotic genome. However, it is important to keep in mind that, although the microsatellite is repeated throughout the genome, there is a unique sequence flanking it, corresponding to the location within the genome in which it integrated. Therefore, this class of polymorphic repeat is ideal for an assay that can tag a specific genome location for use in genetic studies, which will be discussed in detail in this chapter.

Discovery

The microsatellite was first discovered in 1981 by Miesfeld et al. by screening a human gene clone library with a mouse 6-kbp (6 kilobase pair) ribosomal gene nontranscribed spacer probe (rDNA

NTS). They found this sequence was interspersed not only throughout the human and mouse genomes, but also in every other eukaryotic organism they studied—pigeon, frog, slime mold, and yeast. However, it was not identified in *Escherichia coli*. Therefore, the rDNA NTS has been conserved throughout all eukaryotes, but not down to prokaryotes. Miesfeld et al. then narrowed down the conserved element, which they called ECl (evolutionarily conserved), to a 251-bp fragment of the rDNA NTS that contained a tandem array of the (TG) · (CA) dinucleotide. However, the reason for its dramatic evolutionary conservation remained a mystery.

In 1989, two back-to-back manuscripts were published, by Weber and May and Litt and Luty, reporting the use of microsatellites as genetic markers; i.e., they could be used to identify inheritance patterns from parent to offspring. By cloning and sequencing several microsatellites, it was found that each tandem repeat was flanked by a unique genomic sequence, thereby providing the ability to identify an individual's "*genotype*" at a specific DNA location (locus) containing a microsatellite. By sequencing 59 of these microsatellites, Weber and May found that more than half of them contained repeats of 13 or greater dinucleotides, with the longest being 30 units in length. They went on to test 10 microsatellites for Mendelian inheritance. All microsatellites tested displayed expected Mendelian inheritance in three-generation families. Each band represents the length of the microsatellite fragment, separated according to its length by gel electrophoresis. Each parent, being diploid, has two alleles for the microsatellite, each having a different number of dinucleotide repeats. The mother and father each contribute one of these alleles to their offspring, with a 50% probability of a child inheriting either allele. The inheritance of each allele from their parents is shown in the children, in the expected Mendelian ratios.

The discovery of the microsatellite as a highly polymorphic genetic marker, and its ability to generate genotypes in a high-throughput manner, revolutionized genetic analyses of disease and greatly facilitated the mapping and sequencing of not only the human genome but also several model organisms, as discussed in the following sections.

Methods for Genotyping

The major advantage of genotyping using SSLPs over previously used genetic markers, e.g., restriction fragment length polymorphisms (RFLPs), is twofold. First, SSLPs are highly polymorphic, with alleles ranging anywhere from just a few to over 30 nucleotide repeat units. This greatly increases the likelihood that an individual will have alleles of differing sizes for any assayed SSLP, i.e., the marker is informative, and can be used across multiple families for genetic analyses. In fact, many tens of thousands of SSLP assays have been developed for organisms ranging from human to mouse, rat, dog, cat, cow, chicken, pig, fish, frog, fruit fly, corn, rice, poplar, and yeast.

Second, the relatively short stretch of DNA containing a microsatellite allows it to be readily assayed using the polymerase chain reaction (PCR). PCR is a chemical reaction that can exponentially amplify DNA fragments. In the case of SSLP assays, short oligonucleotide primers (~18–25 nucleotides in length) are generated that are complimentary to sequences flanking either side of the tandem repeat. The double-stranded genomic DNA is denatured (unraveled) by heating to 94°C, after which the reaction is cooled to approximately 55°C to 60°C. This temperature allows the oligonucleotide primers to anneal to the denatured genomic DNA. Finally the reaction is heated to 72°C, which allows a temperature stable polymerase, generally *Taq* polymerase isolated from a thermostable bacterium (*Thermus aquaticus*), to extend the oligonucleotide chain, using the complimentary genomic DNA strand as its template and the four dNTPs (dATP, dTTP, dCTP, and dGTP) as building blocks to extend the DNA fragment. This procedure is repeated multiple times, doubling the copy of the sequence contained between the primers with each cycle. Therefore, at the end of 30 cycles of consecutive denaturing, annealing, and extension, there are 2^{30} copies of the desired fragment, which is a sufficient amount of product for detection using radioactive isotopes or fluorescent dyes, as described below. Because PCR can be carried out in high-density microtiter plates (up to 1536 wells/plate) on commercial thermocyclers (machines that heat and cool the reaction samples required for PCR), genotyping of thousands of individuals can be performed in a single day.

Radioactive detection

Initially, PCR amplified product (amplicon) containing an SSLP, was most commonly detected using gel electrophoresis and a radioactively labeled nucleotide. This was done by either directly incorporating a radioactive tag in the PCR amplicon or by labeling the oligonucleotide primer. For direct incorporation, a radioactively tagged nucleotide, either ^{32}P or ^{35}S attached to the α position of one of the dNTPs (i.e., α^{32}P-dCTP or α^{35}S-dATP), is added to the PCR reaction. During each extension step of the reaction, labeled nucleotides are directly incorporated into the amplicon. An alternative approach used to detect the PCR amplicon is to label one primer used in PCR. In this approach, ^{32}P attached to the ã position of a dNTP (generally γ^{32}P-dATP or γ^{32}P-dCTP) is added to the 3´ end of one PCR primer, using T4 DNA kinase before the PCR reaction. During PCR, this labeled primer is annealed to the target sequence and extended, thereby labeling the PCR amplicon. The advantage of direct incorporation is that only a single step amplifies and labels the desired PCR fragment; however, this method can also lead to labeling of nonspecific PCR product, making results more difficult to interpret. End-labeling of the PCR primer can eliminate the detection of nonspecific product, but also it requires high levels of radioactivity and an extra experimental step. However, both approaches have been used extensively and successfully, and which approach is used depends on individual preference.

To detect the radio-labeled SSLP amplicon, one must be able to separate the labeled fragments, based on their length. With radioactively labeled amplicons, this is done using denaturing gel electrophoresis. Reaction samples are mixed with a loading buffer containing blue tracking dye and formamide, and then heated to 94°C to denature the product. The formamide keeps the product denatured. Samples are then loaded onto a standard denaturing polyacrylamide sequencing gel. As the fragments migrate through the gel, the smaller sized fragments (containing fewer tandem repeats) migrate more quickly, whereas the larger fragments move more slowly, separating the two alleles. The blue dye allows tracking of the migration so that the product does not travel off the end of the gel. The polyacrylamide gel is then transferred to a piece of paper, dried, and exposed to autoradiographic film for detection and genotype determination.

Fluorescence detection

The use of radioactivity has been largely supplanted by fluorescent dyes for genotyping, due to the obvious reduction of health hazards and a greater flexibility. As with radioactive labeling, the PCR amplification of the specific SSLP is largely the same, except that one dNTP is labeled with a fluorescent dye (fluorophore). Also, rather than detecting the electrophoresed product by autoradiography, the fluorescently labeled amplicon is detected as it passes a laser detector, either on a gel-based (e.g., an ABI 377 automated slab gel sequencer) or capillary-based DNA sequencer (e.g., an ABI 3700 or 3730 capillary sequencer). A major advantage of using fluorescent detection lies in the automation of genotype determination. As the labeled product passes by the laser detector, the signal is transferred to a computer algorithm that automatically converts the signal detection to a genotype. This greatly reduces manual genotype interpretation, reducing technical time and error as well as increasing overall genotyping throughput. Another important advantage of fluorescent genotyping lies in the ability to label different SSLP amplicons with different fluorophores. Up to three different fluorophores are commonly used, 6-FAM, HEX, and NED, each of which has a distinct excitation and emission profile. A fourth dye, ROX, is used to label a common internal size standard, allowing accurate determination of product size. The ability to distinguish multiple SSLP amplicons, each labeled with a different fluorophore, allows for simultaneous detection of multiple SSLPs in a single assay, increasing genotyping throughput.

This approach is also amenable to high-throughput robotic sample preparation, as it eliminates the precautions necessary for handling radioactivity.

Again, as with radioactive detection, the fluorescent tags can either be directly incorporated into the amplicon or added to the PCR primer. A disadvantage of the labeled primer is that each SSLP must be synthesized with the fluorescent tag attached, which greatly increases the cost of the primer. Oetting et al. devised a method to overcome this cost issue by combining unlabeled template-specific primers and a labeled, common M13 primer. By this method, one template-specific primer for each SSLP is synthesized with an 18-bp tail specific to the M13 phage on its 5′ end. This primer is combined with its template-specific mate, as well as a common M13 primer labeled with a particular fluorophore, and subject to PCR amplification. The amplification begins with the tailed primer incorporating into the template sequence in the initial cycles. In subsequent reactions, the incorporated sequence becomes the docking site for the M13 primer-dye conjugate. The single M13 tailed primer-dye conjugate is common for all SSLPs, greatly reducing the cost of genotyping.

Multiplex analysis

As discussed, using fluorescent detection of SSLPs greatly improves genotyping throughput because of the availability of multiple fluorophores and the ability to multiplex (determine genotypes of multiple SSLPs simultaneously). The amplicon size of SSLPs varies not only within a single SSLP but also from one SSLP to another, depending on the distance from the repeat the flanking primers are chosen. This allows for the ability to detect multiple SSLPs within a single sample on a gel or capillary, as again each SSLP migrates according to size. For example, the allele size range for one SSLP amplicon may be 120–140 bp, whereas another may range from 200 to 250 bp, and a third may range from 325 to 341 bp. Therefore, all three amplicons could be combined in a single reaction, as the laser can detect the size differences and their ranges are sufficiently different to differentiate the genotypes of the three SSLPs. Furthermore, because the fluorophores have distinct excitation/emission profiles, multiple fluorophores can also be combined in a single sample. Therefore, by combining amplicons of distinct sizes labeled with one fluorophore with those labeled with other fluorophores, one can genotype up to nine SSLPs in a single sample.

Two means of multiplexing are possible, either at the PCR or the electrophoresis steps. It is possible to combine PCR primers specific for multiple SSLPs in a single PCR reaction, whereby each SSLP is amplified simultaneously. The advantage of this approach is the reduction in PCR costs, as the overall reaction size is not modified. However, this approach requires up-front knowledge of the allele-size range of each SSLP in the samples being genotyped. Furthermore, some level of up-front optimization of the PCR reaction may be required so that each SSLP amplicon is generated with the same efficiency within the reaction. Once a set of two or three SSLPs are optimized for PCR multiplexing, these combinations are generally not modified. This approach is most efficient when the same set of SSLPs is used time and time again with varying DNA samples. The other multiplexing approach involves independent PCR amplification of each SSLP, followed by pooling of the amplicons before electrophoresis (gel or capillary). The advantage of this approach lies in the freedom to mix and match different marker sets. Marker sets may be slightly different depending on the population being genotyped. In some cases, the entire genome may be screened for initial linkage results. In other cases, an individual locus may be the focus of higher density mapping, for instance, to narrow a disease gene interval by identifying critical recombinant individuals. This assay allows the individual to mix and match markers from a characterized set to do these specific scans. By this approach, multiple pooled amplicons, regardless of primer sequence, have a high success rate. The use of fluorescent detection, combined with robotics and automated data analysis pipelines, facilitate highly automated, high-throughput genotyping platforms, resulting in thousands of genotypes per day at a relatively low cost.

Tools and Resources

To increase the efficiency of genotyping, major efforts have been made to generate a well-characterized and highly efficient marker set for genetic linkage analysis. One such effort was the Cooperative Human Linkage Center (CHLC). This National Institutes of Health (NIH) -funded project characterized thousands of di-, tri-, and tetranucleotide repeat polymorphisms to determine their informativeness (i.e., the number and frequency of SSLP alleles) and to array them according to their genetic position in the human genome (i.e., to develop high-quality genetic maps). Furthermore, the NIH went on to fund a centralized genotyping center, allowing investigators to submit research proposals for genome-wide linkage scans of their study populations. A European group, Genethon, also led a major effort to develop human SSLPs and generate high-density genetic maps for use in genetic linkage studies. These efforts have also reached the commercial arena, where companies such as DeCode will generate genotypes on a genome-wide or region-specific basis on a fee-for-service basis.

The discovery and use of microsatellites have revolutionized the ability to perform genome-wide genetic linkage studies, resulting in the positional cloning of many important genetic diseases ranging from mental retardation, glaucoma, heart defects, to neurological disease. They are particularly powerful for the localization and identification of single-gene disorders. Furthermore, the high-density genetic maps generated using microsatellite markers were instrumental to laying the groundwork for the eventual sequencing of not only the human genome, but also several other model organisms.

Single Nucleotide Polymorphisms (SNPs)

DNA is constantly modifying and mutating. During DNA replication, the duplication of the genetic material during cell divisions and inaccurate copying of the existing DNA leads to minor sequence changes in the copied version of the genome. Likewise, environmental influences such as mutagenic chemicals, ultraviolet (UV), or other radiation can also alter the DNA. On the basis of these constantly occurring changes in the DNA sequence of any organism, it becomes obvious that all individuals of a species are slightly different based on their DNA sequence. Most of these differences are single base changes in the DNA. Essentially one nucleotide in the sequence of one individual is replaced by a different nucleotide in another individual. These differences are called *single nucleotide polymorphisms* (SNPs). SNPs are the most common genome sequence variation. For the human genome, a comparison of two individuals reveals on average one SNP every 800 bases. As a consequence, two humans differ in their DNA sequence at over 3 million positions, or approximately 0.1%. Similarly, other mammalian species show significant sequence variation as well. In mice, one SNP can be found every 250 bases across the genome when 13 inbred (i.e., genetically identical) and two wild strains are compared. Inbred rat strains show a similar rate of SNPs. These sequence differences are responsible for all genetically caused differences between individuals, such as eye color, hair or coat color, or disease susceptibility. If we could unravel the DNA sequence of every human individual, we would be able to decipher all genetic mutations that cause the most common diseases such as diabetes, stroke, or Alzheimer's disease. Unfortunately, though, the cost of sequencing every patient far exceeds the available budgets for these studies. Therefore, scientists have focused on discovering the most important and most common SNPs in the human genome, and now use this subset of SNPs in the human genome to investigate the genetic causes of these disorders. Similar efforts are under way in other mammalian (and nonmammalian) species that serve as model organisms for specific diseases or traits in humans. Below we will describe and discuss the methods commonly used to discover SNPs, and the methodologies used to interrogate these SNPs in large numbers of individuals simultaneously by genotyping.

Discovery

Often, SNPs are discovered by sequencing the same genomic sequence in a number of unrelated samples. For this approach, a region of genomic DNA is amplified by PCR from different DNA samples. The resulting amplicons are resequenced using common sequencing technology. Approaches using gel-based resequencing and hybridization-based oligonucleotide array sequencing have successfully been used for large-scale SNP discovery efforts in the human and mouse genome as well as in other species. Analysis of the resulting sequences reveals base pair differences, or SNPs. Software tools have been developed to automate the SNP discovery from sequencing data, and these tools are routinely used today in a variety of organisms for SNP discovery. Although sequencing is commonly used for SNP discovery today, other indirect methods exist to uncover genomic sequences containing SNPs. Given the cost of sequencing, it may be desirable to preselect these DNA fragments for subsequent sequencing, and to eliminate DNA sequences that do not contain polymorphisms.

One of the first reported methodologies for SNP discovery was the PCR-based single-stranded conformational polymorphism method. In this approach, a region of DNA is amplified using PCR. The resulting amplicons are denatured, and they are allowed to re-anneal under conditions that favor the formation of single-stranded secondary structures. As the formation of secondary structures is sequence-dependent, any difference in the sequence of the PCR amplicon would lead to different folding. These differently folded products can be separated through non-denaturing polyacrylamide gel electrophoresis. Samples with different sequences will fold differently and, as a result, migrate differently in the gel, allowing for the detection of SNPs. This method has been used extensively for targeted screening of genes for potential disease-causing mutations in a variety of species. Recently, it has been adapted for capillary electrophoresis to facilitate large-scale screening.

Another approach to identify PCR amplicons that contain sequence variants uses denaturing high-performance liquid chromatography (DHPLC). In this approach, PCR amplicons are first denatured and then reannealed. In contrast to SSCP analysis, products are then allowed to form double-stranded duplexes. If the PCR product contains an SNP, this re-annealing process will generate homoduplexes (matching sequences reanneal) and heteroduplexes (strands containing the different two alleles of an SNP will anneal and form a single base pair mismatch). When these duplexes are separated on a liquid chromatography column under partially denaturing conditions (separation at temperatures close to the melting temperature of the duplex), the elution times of homo- and heteroduplexes will differ because the melting temperature of the heteroduplex will be slightly lower than the homoduplex due to the base pair mismatch in the sequence. The method and instrumentation has been automated, and it is commercially available. DHPLC has been used successfully for the identification of mutations in a large number of disease genes, and it has been adapted for the analysis of cancer samples and chromosomal abnormalities. Other modifications of the heteroduplex analysis exist, and they have been used by laboratories for a variety of studies. These include mobility analysis or enzymatic cleavage of heteroduplexes.

One additional methodology for SNP discovery should be mentioned because it is based on an entirely different experimental approach. In 1995, Faham and Cox described a method called mismatch repair detection (MRD) that used the bacterial mismatch repair system in *E. coli* to enrich for DNA fragments containing SNPs. The template for mismatch repair in *E. coli* is hemi-methylated double-stranded DNA (only one strand of the DNA is methylated), which is formed by mixing and annealing different single-stranded DNA samples grown in methylation-competent and -incompetent *E. coli* strains. The method has been developed into a high-throughput screening platform that can simultaneously analyze pooled PCR amplicons from large numbers of individuals. The method has been shown to enhance the discovery of rare SNPs that would be missed in pooled sequencing (or would require large numbers of individual samples to be sequenced).

In summary, several methods exist to identify SNPs in genomic DNA. Although some of them may be useful to enrich for SNP-containing PCR amplicons before traditional DNA sequencing, the commonly used approach of discovering SNPs from aligned sequence data from different individuals remains the "gold standard" and the basis of the majority of SNPs publicly available in databases.

Methods for Genotyping

Numerous methods have been developed and are being marketed for SNP genotyping, i.e., the specific determination of the nucleotide present at a polymorphic site in a genome. Theoretically, this information could be obtained by resequencing each and every sample using the same approach as for SNP discovery. However, this process is labor- and cost-intensive and provides significantly more information than is needed; i.e., it delineates the complete flanking sequence of the SNP, which, in most cases, will not differ between samples, and therefore is redundant. Instead, genotyping methods provide a cost-efficient alternative that can quickly generate genotype information on large numbers of samples. No attention is paid to the remainder of the genome sequence and its potential variation; the only information obtained is the nucleotide present in the sequence at the specific site of a known SNP. To develop methodologies for this genotyping procedure, the SNP in question, its possible nucleotides (alleles) that can be present at the site, and the sequence adjacent to the SNP need to be known. All methods discussed below use this information to obtain genotyping information for a large number of DNA samples. As outlined below, the different methods allow the analysis (genotyping) of individual SNPs in large numbers of samples, or varying numbers of SNPs for one sample at a time. All methods have been shown to result in reliable genotyping results with low error rates. The choice of the appropriate methodology primarily depends on the number of SNPs and the number of samples that need to be interrogated.

Essentially all genotyping approaches used to date fall into one of four categories: allele-specific hybridization, primer extension, oligonucleotide ligation, or invasive cleavage. We will first briefly describe the principles of each approach and then outline commercially available genotyping platforms based on these approaches for different study applications.

Allele-specific hybridization

Allele-specific hybridization distinguishes the allele present at an SNP using two different oligonucleotide probes. Each probe contains the SNP position in the middle and is complementary to one allele of the SNP. For hybridization to genomic DNA or PCR amplicons, conditions are chosen that allow the hybridization of the matching probe but not the mismatch probe. The successful hybrids between the target DNA and the oligonucleotide probes can be detected using a variety of approaches. Methods include the use of fluorescence resonance energy transfer (FRET) probes (e.g., in the 5′ exonuclease TaqMan assay), molecular beacon probes, or oligonucleotide arrays.

Primer extension

Primer extension uses the standard principle of PCR. Here, an oligonucleotide primer extends up to the SNP site. The assay then determines what nucleotide is incorporated into the extended PCR product by the polymerase. Often, the assay is performed in two steps. First, the genomic interval is amplified by PCR. The amplified product is subsequently mixed with another primer that anneals adjacent to the SNP site. Then individual dideoxynucleotides are added to the reaction. Upon incorporation of the matching nucleotide at the SNP site, the resulting extension product can no longer be extended further because it lacks a 3′-OH group required for nucleotide incorporation. Thus, the reaction essentially stops once the nucleotide has been incorporated.

Dideoxynucleotides are commercially available with different fluorescent tags; therefore, the resulting extension products can be examined using laser scanners to see which fluorophore has been incorporated. This method directly reveals the genotype of the template DNA. The method can be multiplexed and is commercially available (SNaPshot). Alternatively to the use of dideoxynucleotides, regular deoxynucleotides can be used sequentially in the extension reaction. Here, the primer is essentially extended as in a regular PCR reaction. The only difference is the sequential addition of one nucleotide at a time. This method is commercially available.

Oligonucleotide ligation

Similar to DNA polymerase, DNA ligase is a highly specific enzyme that repairs nicks in the DNA. Nicks are missing phosphodiester bonds in one of the two strands of the DNA molecule. DNA ligase detects and repairs these nicks, provided the nucleotides on both sides of the missing bond are complementary to the nucleotides in the intact DNA strand. Landergren et al. first described a novel approach for SNP genotyping that uses specific oligonucleotides that will hybridize to single-stranded DNA templates. One oligonucleotide will align with the sequence upstream of an SNP, including the actual nucleotide at the SNP site. A second oligonucleotide is complementary to the downstream template sequence, starting with the first nucleotide adjacent to the SNP. Although the latter oligonucleotide can be used to interrogate both alleles of the SNP, the first oligonucleotide is specific for one allele of the SNP, because it will end with the specific SNP nucleotide. Only the oligonucleotides perfectly matching the template sequence will be ligated by the ligase, whereas a mismatch will prevent the ligation of the alternate oligonucleotide. The method has been incorporated in a variety of commercial platforms such as the SNPlex platform or the Illumina GoldenGate technology, which is described below in more detail.

Invasive cleavage

The last SNP genotyping method we describe is invasive cleavage, which is commercially available as the Invader assay. This method depends on the ability of flap endonucleases to recognize specific three-dimensional structures that are formed when two overlapping oligonucleotides hybridize perfectly to a target DNA molecule. The overlap occurs at the SNP site, and only the oligonucleotide combination that is complementary to the SNP allele will be cleaved by the enzyme. The reaction is highly specific, and a mismatch to the target DNA will prohibit the enzymatic reaction. This methodology has been adapted for SNP genotyping assays, as described in more detail below.

Analysis of individual SNPs

Historically, investigators have used a variety of PCR-based methods to genotype individual SNPs. For all of these methods, the genomic sequence around the SNP was known and amplified using specific PCR primers that selectively amplified the genomic interval, including the SNP. SNPs that alter a restriction enzyme recognition site could then be genotyped by performing a restriction digest of the PCR product and by separating the resulting DNA segments by agarose gel electrophoresis. PCR products that contain the restriction enzyme recognition site will be cleaved into two products and will result in two bands of different size on the agarose gel. In contrast, PCR products from samples that contain an SNP in the recognition site will no longer be cleaved by the enzyme, and will result in a single band of larger molecular weight upon gel electrophoresis. Finally, PCR products from samples heterozygous for the SNP would result in a total of three bands, one band for the uncleaved product and two additional bands from the portion of the PCR product that can be cleaved. The method enjoys widespread use to this day because it is robust and uses basic molecular biology technology available to most laboratories. With the ever increasing number of commercially available restriction enzymes uncovered from various microbes, the repertoire of SNPs that can be genotyped by this approach has been steadily increasing.

Unfortunately, many SNPs do not lead to an alteration of a restriction enzyme recognition site in the genome sequence. For these SNPs, alternative approaches have been developed that use PCR and gel electrophoresis. In one approach, one initial PCR primer is designed so that it includes the polymorphic SNP site at its 3′ end. Two separate primers are used in two PCR reactions. One reaction includes the forward primer ending with one nucleotide present at the SNP, and the other reaction includes a primer ending with the alternative nucleotide. As the thermostable DNA polymerase used in PCR requires a perfect match of the primer at the 3′ end to attach additional nucleotides and amplify the DNA segment, the PCR reaction will only yield a PCR product when the forward primer perfectly matches the DNA template. Accordingly, the presence or absence of PCR product depending on the primer used indicates the genotype for the template DNA. Although this method works well for established assays, each assay needs to be optimized individually to ensure that both alleles of the SNP are successfully amplified when present. Furthermore, the design of the PCR primers may be difficult for some SNP sequences.

As an alternative to the allele-specific PCR and the restriction digest of PCR products (often called PCR–RFLP), several commercial platforms are available to genotype individual SNPs in large numbers of samples. In our discussion here, we will focus on three commonly used platforms: the 5′-exonuclease TaqMan assay, based on allele-specific hybridization; pyro sequencing, based on the primer extension principle; and the Invader assay, based on the invasive cleavage reaction of a flap endonuclease.

TaqMan assay

The TaqMan assay uses the 5′ exonuclease activity of Taq polymerase. Two FRET oligonucleotide probes complementary to the sequence around an SNP are hybridized to the target DNA. Each contains a different fluorescent dye that is quenched in the FRET probe. Each probe is specific for one of the two SNP alleles; i.e., it contains the complementary base to the SNP allele in the middle of the probe. The hybridization temperature is chosen such that only the matching probe hybridizes efficiently. After hybridization, a normal PCR extension reaction begins starting from an oligonucleotide primer annealed upstream of the FRET probe. The Taq polymerase extends the primer and, upon reaching the hybridized FRET probe, begins to remove it from the template DNA by cleaving one nucleotide at a time. The reaction is mediated by the specific 5′ exonuclease activity of the *Taq* polymerase. Once the entire oligonucleotide FRET probe has been cleaved, the fluorophore and the quencher molecule have been separated, and the energy transfer can no longer take place because the two molecules are no longer in close physical proximity. As a consequence, the fluorophore will now emit light upon excitation. As the two FRET probes contain different fluorophores depending on the allele, the resulting fluorescent color unambiguously determines the allele of the SNP in the target DNA.

TaqMan assays are commercially available for many SNPs and can be designed on demand by Applied Biosystems. The method requires a real-time PCR instrument or a fluorescent plate reader to measure the fluorescence of the two dyes at the end of the PCR reaction.

Pyrosequencing

Pyrosequencing has been described as a sequencing-by-synthesis method. In this approach, four different enzymes and specific substrates are used in a sequential reaction to produce light whenever a nucleotide complementary to the template DNA strand is incorporated. If the added nucleotide is not complementary to the base in the template DNA, no light is generated. The light-generating reaction is depended on the pyrophosphate that is released during the DNA polymerase reaction. If the added nucleotide forms a base pair, the DNA polymerase incorporates the nucleotide and pyrophosphate will be released. The released pyrophosphate will be converted to ATP by another enzyme (ATP sulfurylase). Luciferase then uses the ATP to generate a detectable light signal. The light intensity is proportional to the number of the ATP molecules, which in turn is proportional to the number of the incorporated nucleotides. After the completion of the reaction, the excess of each nucleotide is degraded by apyrase.

The reaction is repeated in the same order, with a different nucleotide added. If the added nucleotide does not form an incorporated base pair with DNA template, no light will be produced. The four nucleotides are added to the mixture in a defined order (e.g., ACGT), and thus, the sequence of the template DNA can be deduced by matching the nucleotide with the light signal generation.

Pyrosequencing provides rapid real-time determination of 20–30 nucleotides of target DNA sequence. With this technology, not only the SNP alleles but also the adjacent nucleotides are determined, providing greater confidence in the correct SNP detection. The reaction is automated and requires a dedicated instrument.

Invader assay

The Invader assay uses two oligonucleotide probes that are hybridized to target DNA containing an SNP site. The two oligonucleotides hybridize to the single-stranded target and form an overlapping invader structure at the site of the SNP. One oligonucleo-tide, the Invader oligo, is complementary to the target sequence 3´ of the polymorphic site, and it ends with a nonmatching base overlapping the SNP nucleotide. The second oligonucleotide, the allele-specific probe, contains the complementary base of the SNP allele, and extends to the sequence 5´ of the polymorphic site. This probe can also extend on its 5´ site with additional noncomplementary nucleotides. Once the two oligonucleotides anneal to the target DNA, they form a three-dimensional invader structure over the SNP site that can be recognized by a specific enzyme, cleavase, or flap endonuclease. The enzyme cleaves the probe 3´ of the base complementary to the polymorphic site (i.e., 3´ of the overlapping invader structure). If the probe is designed as a fluorescence resonance energy transfer (FRET) molecule containing a fluorophore at the 5´ end and an internal quencher molecule, the cleavage reaction will separate the fluorophore from the quencher and generate a fluorescent signal. If, in contrast, the probe oligonucleotide does not match the SNP allele present in the target DNA (i.e., the probe is complementary to the alternate SNP allele), then no overlapping invader structure is formed, and the probe is not cleaved. This distinction is highly specific, with only minimal unspecific cleavage of the mismatch probe.

Often, the Invader oligonucleotide is designed to permanently anneal to the target DNA at the assay temperature. In contrast, the probe oligonucleotide is designed to have a melting temperature close to the assay temperature. As a consequence, the probe constantly anneals and detaches. During the annealing, cleavase can cleave the oligonucleotide, the remnant detaches, and a new uncleaved oligonucleotide probe can reanneal to the same site. This design ensures the cleavage of a large number of probes, resulting in a strong signal even from small amounts of template DNA. Therefore, SNPs can be genotyped directly from genomic DNA using Invader assays, eliminating the need for additional PCR amplification. In addition to the FRET probes, other methods of detection (polarized light, mass spectrometry) have been used. However, the benefit of the fluorescence detection is the ability to read the assay after isothermic incubation in a standard fluorescence plate reader.

Multiplex analysis

Although the methods described above work well and reliably, they are not suited for genotyping multiple SNPs in large sets of samples. As each SNP has to be assayed individually, all SNPs have to be interrogated sequentially rather than in parallel. However, numerous other platforms exist that allow the genotyping of several SNPs at the same time. Here, we will discuss methods that allow up to 10 SNPs to be genotyped in one reaction. In addition, we will discuss high-throughput approaches in the next section.

Both methods described here are based on the primer extension reaction. In both platforms, oligonucleotide primers are designed that extend up to the nucleotide adjacent to the SNP site. The following primer extension reaction will use ddNTPs to incorporate the matching base for the SNP allele present in the target DNA. The resulting products are then separated and detected by different methods.

The first detection method, as implemented in the MassEXTEND platform from Sequenom, uses mass spectrometry to determine the accurate molecular weight of the resulting extension reaction product, using matrix-assisted laser desorption/ionization time-of-flight (MALDI–TOF) mass spectrometry. For this approach, the reaction products are mixed with a matrix and deposited on the surface of a metal plate. The matrix and the reaction products are hit with a pulse from a laser beam, resulting in the vaporization of a small number of DNA molecules from the reaction product. The vaporized molecules are transferred into a vacuum flight tube and charged with an electrical field pulse. This accelerates the resulting ions toward the detector at the end of the tube. The time between the application of the electrical field pulse and the collision of the ions with the detector is referred to as the time of flight. As the time it takes for the ion to pass through the flight tube to the detector is directly proportional to the mass of the ion (with larger molecules flying slower), this is a very precise measure of the molecular weight of the DNA products. The detectable mass differences are small, and the difference between an incorporated ddA and ddT of 9 mass units can be clearly distinguished. The assay allows further multiplexing even for reactions resulting in very similar mass for the products by adding noncomplementary tail sequences to the 5′ end of the primer, thus increasing the mass of the extension product.

Alternatively, the single base extension products can be analyzed using the SNaPShot technology from Applied Biosystems. In this approach, fluorescently labeled ddNTPs are used in the primer extension reaction, and the resulting extension products are separated and detected using commercially available capillary sequencers. Each ddNTP is labeled with a different fluorescent dye; thus, the different alleles of a SNP can be distinguished by the different color. Similar to the MassEXTEND approach, multiplexing can be improved by adding noncomplementary tail sequences to the primer. According to the manufacturer, 10-plex reactions can be performed with high accuracy.

High-throughput approaches

Currently, three high-throughput platforms for SNP genotyping are commercially available. All platforms allow the genotyping of large numbers of SNPs (1000–500,000) in a single experiment for one DNA sample. Although this significantly reduces the genotyping cost per SNP, it results in a tremendous cost for a project when 1000–2000 DNA samples need to be genotyped for thousands of SNPs. In addition, all approaches require specialized equipment and therefore are only of interest to laboratories that intend to perform large numbers of genotyping projects.

The first assay platform, developed by Illumina, combines allele-specific ligation with an extension reaction. The method, called the GoldenGate assay, uses the BeadArray technology, a method using fiberoptic substrates with randomly assembled arrays of beads.

In the assay, three oligonucleotides are designed for each SNP locus. Two oligos are specific to each allele of the SNP site, called the Allele-Specific Oligos (ASOs). A third oligo that hybridizes downstream from the SNP site is the Locus-Specific Oligo (LSO). All three oligonucleotide sequences are complementary to the target sequence and contain universal PCR primer sites. During the primer hybridization process, the assay oligonucleotides hybridize to the genomic DNA sample bound to paramagnetic particles. Hybridization occurs before any PCR amplification step; therefore, no amplification bias is introduced into the assay. Extension of the appropriate ASO and ligation of the extended product to the LSO joins information about the genotype present at the SNP site to a unique address sequence on the LSO. These joined, full-length products provide a template for PCR using universal PCR primers, two of which are fluorescently labeled. As a last step, the single-stranded, dye-labeled amplification products are hybridized to the complement bead type through their unique address sequences, and the labeled beads can be analyzed using arrayed optical fibers. Up to 1536 SNPs may be interrogated simultaneously in this manner using this Golden-Gate technology.

Similar degrees of multiplexing can be achieved using oligonucleotide array technology from Affymetrix. These arrays contain 25-mers that are synthesized directly on chip surfaces. In recent iterations, Affymetrix has developed arrays that allow the interrogation of 10,000, 100,000, or even 500,000 SNPs per reaction. The 500K array methodology uses an approach called whole-genome sampling analysis to selectively amplify regions of the genome containing SNPs, and subsequently interrogate the alleles present in the amplification products by hybridization to allele-specific oligonucleotides.

In the first step of the analysis, a single genomic DNA sample is digested with a restriction enzyme. After complete digestion, adaptors are ligated to the digestion products that allow the amplification of a subset of the fragments using a universal primer pair complementary to the adaptor sequence. Any SNP located in close proximity to the restriction site will be amplified by PCR and can be interrogated on the chip. The resolution is primarily driven by the restriction enzyme used. The more it cuts the genomic DNA, the more small amplification products can be obtained and hybridized to the chip. Accordingly, the different chips, (10K, 100K, 50 0K) use different enzymes in the initial step of the reaction, but subsequent steps are identical.

Although the assay allows the interrogation of a large number of SNPs simultaneously, the user has no influence on the composition of the chip, i.e., the SNPs that will be interrogated. The complete panel of 500,000 SNPs has been preselected during the design of the chip, primarily driven by the technical requirements of the restriction digest and amplification described above. However, a novel methodology developed by Parallele Biosciences uses the chip-based hybridization approach for the ultimate analysis, but it uses a different approach for the SNP interrogation. The approach, termed molecular inversion probe (MIP) technology, uses a long oligonucleotide that will hybridize with its end sequences in inverted fashion to the flanking sequences of an SNP. Using one dNTP in four different reactions, the SNP site can be filled in to form a circular padlock probe around the SNP site. The probe will only circularize when the dNTP added is complementary to the SNP allele present. The circular probe is resistant to DNAse digestion. Once the nonfilled probes have been digested using DNAse, the padlock probe is opened, using a cleavage site within the MIP to form a linear template for a PCR reaction using universal primers. The amplification product contains a unique tag sequence for each MIP that can be detected by hybridization to an Affymetrix TrueTag array. Assays can be designed and genotyped in parallel for up to 10,000 SNPs. This platform offers a new tool to design custom panels of SNPs for a specific study, rather than depend on a preselected set of SNPs on other Affymetrix chips.

Overall, all three approaches allow the efficient genotyping of large numbers of SNPs. All require specialized equipment, and although the cost of genotyping per SNP is low, the total cost of any genotyping project is high due to the large number of SNPs. These technologies are only suitable for large-scale studies, and they are best performed in collaboration with or support from institutional core facilities.

Linkage Disequilibrium and Haplotypes

Most SNPs in a genome probably arose from individual single mutation events at an early time during the history of the species hundreds of generations ago. From the time of each mutation event, the new allele (i.e., the new "mutant" nucleotide) is located on an individual chromosome that has specific alleles of other SNPs that arose previously on the same chromosome. This physical arrangement of SNP alleles along a chromosome is called a *haplotype*. Over multiple successive generations, recombination and novel mutation events will lead to a rearrangement or modification of this ancestral haplotype around the new SNP allele. As a consequence, the new allele only remains on the same portion of the ancestral haplotype with other SNP alleles that are on a short distance away; i.e., recombination events are less likely to separate the two alleles. This nonrandom arrangement of SNPs along the chromosome, i.e., the maintenance of a small segment of the ancestral haplotype, is called *linkage disequilibrium* (LD) or *allelic association*. This arrangement is used in disease association analyses that are based on the idea that it should be possible to identify the effect of any common disease-causing SNP allele by determining the ancient haplotype segment on which it is located. By using a sufficient number of SNP markers in a genetic study, any common variant, even if it was not assayed directly, should display significant LD with a neighboring marker SNP. This approach has been used successfully in human genetic studies to identify genes responsible for Mendelian disorders such as Hirschprung's Disease or cystic fibrosis.

The LD structure has been primarily studied in the human genome, although initial analyses have been performed for the mouse, rat, and dog genome as well. In the human genome, it has become clear over the past several years that the extent of LD and haplotypes in the human genome is not simply a function of distance between SNPs. Rather, the size of regions of significant LD is highly variable in different regions of the genome and reflects the complex history and interplay of recombination and mutation on different regions of the genome. If SNPs are not in LD, the alleles of the SNPs occur in seemingly random combination on individual chromosomes.

As a consequence, the alleles of neighboring SNPs, in the absence of LD between them, can form a large number of different haplotypes (2^n for n SNPs). In contrast, regions where neighboring SNPs are in significant LD, only a small number of resulting haplotypes is observed. These haplotypes are representative of the ancient haplotypes that have not been broken up by recombination. Therefore, an analysis of haplotype patterns would not only identify regions of significant LD between SNPs, but it would also identify those common (presumably ancient) haplotype patterns that represent the majority of chromosomes in that particular genomic interval. Knowledge of these common haplotypes would then permit the identification of "tag SNPs," individual representative non- redundant SNPs that would unambiguously differentiate all major haplotypes without analyzing all SNPs in that particular region.

To facilitate the selection of these tag SNPs, the International HapMap Consortium, a publicly funded effort by the National Institutes of Health, has analyzed the genome-wide LD structure comprehensively in four different human populations: A cohort of North Americans of Northern European descent, an African population, a cohort of Han Chinese, and Japanese individuals. In total, over 5.8 million SNPs have been genotyped in each of these populations, and the data of this effort are publicly available. It is the hope that selecting an informative subset of SNPs based on LD information from this study will provide a genome-wide coverage in whole genome disease association studies. Here, SNPs would be selected so that all other SNPs from the HapMap study not included in the representative set would be in LD with one or more of the selected SNPs. It has been estimated that this comprehensive coverage of the human genome will require around 500,000 SNPs across all chromosomes. Undoubtedly, commercial providers of genotyping platforms will offer high-throughput SNP panels based on the HapMap information in the near future.

Application for Genetic Analysis

As mentioned below, genotyping of SSLPs and SNPs is essential for the analysis of the genetic basis of common disorders. In the following section, we will briefly discuss the use of these polymorphisms in linkage and association analysis.

Linkage Analysis

A powerful means of identifying the location of genes causing disease is by genetic linkage mapping. During meiosis, when germ cells are being generated, homologous chromosomes can recombine, or cross over. As a result, offspring will have different combinations of parental alleles. We can use the percentage of recombinant offspring as a measure of physical distance, making a genetic linkage map. Linkage maps are based on probability. For instance, if two genes or loci are on different chromosomes, the probability of cosegregation of these loci is 50%. However, the closer loci are on the genome, the lower the probability of recombination between them. The measure of genetic distance is approximately the recombination frequency between loci. Although linkage is defined as <50% recombination, 47% recombination, for example, is not a reassuring or reliable measure of distance. Therefore, a genetic map needs many genetic markers to be reliable. Because of their relatively high abundance, their high informativeness, and their representation across all eukaryotes, SSLPs are the backbone of nearly every eukaryotic genetic map. To generate a genetic linkage map, large families, such as the three-generation families from The Foundation Jean Dausset-Centre d'Etude du Polymorphisme Humain (CEPH), are typically genotyped with hundreds or thousands of SSLPs. Analytical computer programs determine the frequency of recombination between parents and offspring, thus determining the distance between markers, and arrange the SSLPs according to their order and distance on each chromosome.

High-density genetic maps spanning the entire human genome have been generated by several groups and are commonly used for mapping disease genes and quantitative trait loci (QTL). Just as recombination determines the genetic distance between SSLPs, it also determines the distance between a disease gene and an SSLP. If a particular gene determines a specific phenotype or disease, then one can genotype families with SSLPs spanning the genome and identify cosegregation of an SSLP allele and a clinical phenotype. If recombination is significantly lower than expected between an SSLP allele and a clinical outcome, e.g., hemophilia, then the gene causing the disease is *linked* to that marker. Because the genome location of that marker is known, the location of that disease gene is also known. The first disease linked by the use of microsatellite genotyping was facioscapulohumeral muscular dystrophy in 1990. Since that time, thousands of loci have been mapped using this approach. Genetic linkage studies are most powerful when studying large, multigenerational families affected by a single gene (Mendelian) disease. However, linkage has proven more of a challenge with common complex diseases. Because multiple genes with relatively small effects are thought to be involved in common diseases such as hypertension or diabetes, combined with the fact that these diseases often affect older patients, it is often impossible to find large families with multiple generations. To address these issues, association studies offer the advantages of being able to study cases and controls or small families, which are much more readily ascertained. Furthermore, the large number of SNPs and high-throughput SNP genotyping technologies now makes genomewide association studies feasible, as discussed below.

Association Analysis

When it proves difficult to recruit a sufficient number of families for a genetic study, a popular alternative is an association study to elucidate the genetic basis of common diseases. In contrast to linkage studies where SSLP markers are used to identify a region of the genome that is inherited by affected offspring from affected parents, association studies aim to identify alleles that are found more often in individuals affected by a disease than in a control group. In the perfect association study, one would test the causal mutation for association with disease. However, in almost all cases, the causal mutation is unknown. As a consequence, association studies resort to indirect approaches relying on linkage disequilibrium (LD) between the causal mutation and another SNP that is being genotyped. If the SNP was associated with the disease, one would expect to find a higher frequency of the associated allele of the SNP in individuals affected by the disease (cases) when compared with a healthy control group.

Association studies can be performed in family-based cohorts. Numerous statistical approaches have been developed to test for association of SNP alleles with disease in small trios, nuclear, or even extended families. However, most association studies use unrelated patients in their analysis. In these cohorts. It is assumed that individuals are affected because they share a similar genetic susceptibility. However, as it is possible that some individuals may be affected for reasons other than genetic susceptibility (most common human disorders are also signifi- cantly influenced by environmental factors, e.g., lifestyle), it is imperative that a large number of patients is recruited for the study so that most individuals share the same genetic susceptibility genes and mutations. This cohort of affected individuals is then matched with a cohort of unaffected, healthy controls. Here, it is important that these control individuals match the patient cohort in the distribution of age, sex, ethnicity, and potential environmental factors that may influence the development of the disease.

Once the case and control cohorts have been collected, the DNA samples can be used for SNP genotyping. Depending on the scope of the study, samples are either genotyped for SNPs in candidate genes that were pre selected for the study or a genome-wide association analysis using a comprehensive SNP set across the entire genome will be performed. Published data to date primarily include candidate gene association analyses. A recent review by Newton-Cheh and Hirschhorn discusses in detail the important considerations for the design of these association studies and the potential problems that can be encountered. The number of SNPs to be analyzed would determine the best genotyping platform to be used in the study. Clearly, candidate gene SNPs can be genotyped with common approaches for individual SNP genotyping or moderate multiplexing platforms. However, genome-wide association studies will require high-throughput approaches.

Although the recent efforts to elucidate the LD structure of the human genome (HapMap Consortium) promise to facilitate the selection of informative subsets of SNPs for these types of association studies, it remains to be seen whether whole genome association studies will help uncover the genetic determinants for such common diseases as diabetes, asthma, or cardiovascular disorders. Clearly, candidate gene studies have yielded several well-replicated associations, but they account only for a small portion of the overall genetic susceptibility. Hopefully, comprehensive association studies of these disorders will help uncover additional genes responsible for the disease susceptibility. These discoveries would significantly advance our ability to predict, diagnose, and hopefully treat these disorders in affected individuals.

18

GENE EXPRESSION ANALYSIS

Pharmacogenomics combines genomics; investigations into the structure or function of very large numbers of genes undertaken in a simultaneous fashion, with the study of phenotypes and traits specifically related to drug responses. Gene expression analysis is an important and widely applied genomics tool. Gene expression analyses, either at the single gene level or by means of whole genome approaches, are integral to our understanding of how drugs work, whether they are effective, and whether a subset of the human population will either fail to benefit from a given drug or experience adverse affects from it. In this chapter, we focus primarily on three types of investigations that use gene expression technology to study pharmacogenomics. The first is the study of how human genetic variation affects the expression of genes, particularly genes relevant to drug response. The second topic is the use of gene expression analyses in the optimization of treatment, and the third type of investigation is the use of gene expression analyses in the discovery of pharmacologically important genes not previously implicated in drug response. In each case, we attempt to summarize the major types of techniques used for these investigations, and provide examples of both single gene (genetic) and multiple gene (genomic) experiments in these areas.

HUMAN GENETIC VARIATION AND GENE EXPRESSION

Genetic variation affects gene function in several ways. Nonsynonymous variants in translated regions cause amino acid changes that may alter protein function. Variants in exons or in introns may affect splicing, whilst those in the untranslated regions (UTRs) of genes can affect transcript stability. Finally, variants outside transcribed regions but within regulatory elements may affect the frequency of transcription of a gene and its level of expression, its tissue distribution, or its developmental or temporal expression. Given the ability of expression level changes to cause modest (and therefore developmentally viable) differences in phenotype without complete loss of gene function, differences in the expression levels of genes may be among the most important types of variation for common complex genetic diseases. Indeed, promoter variants have been shown to influence complex traits such as blood pressure and susceptibility to diseases such as rheumatoid arthritis.

Genetic variants that affect gene regulation may include either single-nucleotide polymorphisms (SNPs) or insertions or deletions ("indels"). The SNPs that affect gene regulation are sometimes referred to as regulatory SNPs or "rSNPs." Inclusion of such variants in genetic association studies will be important for the assessment of candidate genes with regard to pharmacologically relevant phenotypes and other complex genetic disorders. Studies of the effect of genetic variation on gene expression have lagged behind studies of variants that alter protein structure or function. This is due in part to the more straightforward interpretation of the effects of many nonsynonymous changes and a lack of effective assays for detecting genetically determined gene expression differences, particularly in the normal chromosomal context of each gene. Furthermore, we lack a full understanding of the sequence elements necessary for the expression and regulation of individual genes or groups of genes. In addition, it is known that sequence elements such as enhancers may be found at relatively large distances (of the order of 100 kb) from the transcriptional start of a gene, making it difficult to define precisely the genomic region containing important regulatory elements. For these and other reasons, variants in the regulatory regions of human genes have been more difficult to study and are now the subject of considerable attention, a key aspect of which is the development of high-throughput assays for the effects of specific genetic variants on gene expression.

Effect of Individual Sequence Variants and Haplotypes on Gene Expression and Phenotype

Inter-individual sequence-based variation in gene expression is now considered to be a major cause of phenotypic variation. Pharmacogenetic examples of such effects include, variation in the number of repeats in the promoter region of the thiopurine methyltransferase (TPMT) gene, which have been shown to affect gene expression in vitro. Sensitivity to thiopurine drugs such as immunosuppressants and cytotoxic compounds is affected by the inter-individual genetic variation in this gene. Alternate splicing also has clear functional effects on genes, many of which express isoforms with distinct functions. CYP4F3, for example, hydroxylates the pro-inflammatory molecule leukotriene B4. Alternate splicing of CYP4F3 alters the substrate specificity, tissue distribution, and function of this enzyme. Examples of genetic variants that affect splicing are a SNP in codon 242 of the cyclin D1 gene that affects the age of onset of hereditary nonpolyposis colon cancer and a VNTR (variable number of tandem repeats) polymorphism that prevents multiple alternate splicing of the cystathione beta-synthase gene.

A particularly well-characterized example of genetic variation affecting gene function, expression, and phenotype is the β2-adrenergic receptor gene (ADRB2). ADRB2 is a G protein coupled receptor for catecholamines (epinephrine and norepinephrine), and a major drug target for the treatment of heart failure and asthma. The functional or phenotypic consequences of several common individual ADRB2 variants are well characterized including a Gly16 variant that is associated with increased agonist-promoted down-regulation of the receptor and nocturnal asthma; a Glu27 variant markedly associated with obesity; and an Ile164 variant that decreases the coupling, binding, and sequestration of substrate. Ile164, Gly16, and the Gly16/Gln27 combinations are also associated with depressed exercise performance in patients with heart failure. In vitro expression studies using allele-specific constructs of ADRB2 or employing a reporter gene have shown that a Cys19 variant in the leader peptide of the gene increases expression at the level of protein without affecting mRNA levels.

A seminal paper by Drysdale et al. used 13 SNPs at ADRB2 to characterize 12 common haplotypes that differ in frequency between ethnic groups. They then correlated gene and protein expression, as well as in vivo response to albuterol, a β2-adrenergic receptor agonist, with haplotype pairs for a series of individuals, and found that both gene expression and response to the drug were significantly related to specific ADRB2 haplotype pairs. Importantly, ADRB2 haplotype pairs were predictive of drug response, whereas individual SNP variants were not, showing that unique interactions of multiple SNPs within a haplotype can affect biological and therapeutic phenotypes. If this observation holds true for many other human genes, haplotype analysis will be critical for pharmacogenetics, and pharmacogenomics.

Cross-Species Conservation: Indirect Evidence of Regulatory Elements

Cross-species comparison of genomic sequence, or comparative genomics, has become a widely used technique for the identification of evolutionarily and presumably functionally important DNA sequence elements. These computational methods use a variety of algorithms, strategies, and programs to align and compare sequences to identify conserved elements. Analyses such as phylogenetic footprinting and phylogenetic shadowing have been used to computationally identify the binding specificities of transcription factors. DNA sequence variants located within conserved or other computationally identified sequences are candidates for rSNPs.

In Vitro Functional Characterization of SNPs

Functional assessment of individual non-coding SNPs can be done by a variety of methods, including gel-shift assays, DNA footprinting, and allele-specific promoter constructs with reporter gene assays. Although these in vitro assays are valuable methods of assessing the effects of different genetic variants on gene expression, they have several major limitations. One is the difficulty of assessing the consequences of variation in regulatory elements located at a distance from the gene of interest. These methods also do not assess the effects of regulatory sequence variation within the gene's normal chromosomal context in the presence of other genetic and epigenetic effects within a mammalian genome. To overcome these limitations, two methods of assessing variants in their normal chromosomal/chromatin context have been developed. One measures allele-specific transcript abundance; the other assays allele-specific binding of polymerase II, which is a reflection of the frequency of gene transcription.

Assays of Allele-Specific Transcript Abundance

An effective and elegantly uncomplicated method for directly assessing allele-specific transcript abundance within a normal chromosomal context has been used by several groups to examine allele-specific expression in human samples. Cowles et al. have used this method to examine such variation between mouse strains. These groups use SNPs in the transcribed regions of genes as tools to measure allele-specific expression levels of genes of interest, or expression "*allelic imbalance*". Here, we will use the term "*expression allelic imbalance* (EAI)" to avoid confusion with tumor allelic imbalance; the latter is generally used to describe events such as loss of heterozygosity in cancers. Allele-specific differences in gene expression are likely due to the presence of either allele-specific cis-acting factors physically linked to the transcribed "*indicator*" SNP, or caused by epigenetic factors such as imprinting. The method does not generally discriminate between imbalances caused by unequal allele-specific transcription, allele-specific splicing, or differential transcript stability.

In this EAI method, single base extension (SBE) genotyping assays are used with either fluorescently labeled or acycloprime-labeled terminator nucleotides in assays using cDNA. Hudson and co-workers validate each assay using genomic DNA, for which robust assays give the expected 50:50 allele ratio in heterozygous individuals. When cDNA from heterozygous lymphoblastoid cell lines from unrelated CEPH (Centre d'Etude du Polymorphisme Humain) individuals was used, however, they found that 23 of 129 inflammation-related genes (18%) deviated from the expected equimolar ratio in one or more individuals tested. The frequency of EAI in different genes varied from 6% to 50% of the informative unrelated individuals tested. Kinzler and co-workers observed EAI in 6 of 13 genes tested, with 3–30% of individuals displaying EAI in different genes. Bray et al. find that roughly half (7 of 15) of genes tested in human brain cDNA show EAI. The Hudson group also demonstrated EAI in heterogeneous nuclear RNA (hnRNA) of three out of three genes tested, demonstrating that the imbalance originated at the level of transcription and, for these three genes at least, was not due to allelic differences in transcript stability.

A group led by Lee and Buetow describes an efficient approach to EAI analysis that uses Affymetrix HuSNP chips to assay for both sample genotype and allele-specific expression level. Of 602 informative (heterozygous) genes expressed in kidney or liver, 54% were found to show EAI in at least one of seven individuals tested. A subset of genes showing EAI was also tested for segregation of the EAI phenotype in CEPH pedigrees. Several genes showed transmission patterns of EAI that were compatible with Mendelian inheritance, one with incomplete penetrance of the EAI phenotype. BTN3A2, a gene for which EAI was consistently associated with a particular allele in different families, showed co-segregation of the EAI effect with a 15-kb haplotype composed of nine SNPs in three pedigrees as well as in unrelated individuals. The indicator SNPs in BTN3A2 are likely to be in linkage disequilibrium with the rSNP underlying its EAI. Other genes displayed apparently random expression of either one allele or the other in different individuals; this random monoallelic expression that may result from imprinting or other epigenetic phenomena.

Interestingly, most EAIs were bidirectional, with increased expression of a specific allele in some samples, but increased expression of the other allele in other samples. Pastinen et al. noted that this could be explained by allelic heterogeneity of cis-acting regulatory variants, epigenetic effects, or incomplete linkage disequilibrium between the indicator SNP and the rSNP underlying the EAI. They point out that the indicator SNPs chosen are on average 34 kb downstream of the start of transcription, a distance that is greater than the average size (20 kb) of a linkage disequilibrium block.

Several laboratory groups have used EAI assays to demonstrate that allele-specific expression is a widespread and heterogeneous phenomenon, and is therefore likely to have a key role in complex genetic disease. Experimental strategies such as those described above can be adapted for the high-throughput systematic discovery of the effects of rSNPs in whole genomes. Though the method does not identify the causative rSNPs per se, it can provide an invaluable snapshot of the effect of genetic variation on gene expression in the genome. If comprehensively applied across many genes in different tissues, this would be of particular value for genes of pharmacogenetic significance.

HaploChIP: Allele-Specific Protein–DNA Interactions Identify Putative rSNPs

Knight et al. have developed a novel technique based on chromatin immunoprecipitation (ChIP) that detects the allele-specific biases in the "*loading*" of phosphorylated RNA polymerase II (Pol II) onto promoter sequences. It is known that transcription begins when Pol II is phosphorylated on specific serine residues and is released from the initiation complex to begin transcript synthesis. ChIP involves the treatment of cells to cross-link proteins to DNA, followed by fragmentation of the chromatin by sonication. Protein–DNA complexes are then immunoprecipitated with antibodies that recognize DNA binding proteins. In the case of HaploChIP, an antibody specific for particular phosphorylated serine residues of Pol II is used to isolate Pol II-bound DNA fragments. The DNA–protein cross-links are then reversed and the protein digested away. The relative abundance of different alleles of the promoter region of a specific gene in the Pol II-bound DNA fraction is then measured using PCR with primers flanking a nearby SNP followed by primer extension genotyping and detection by quantitative MALDI-TOF mass spectrometry. Knight et al. used their technique to demonstrate haplotype-specific loading of Pol II at the lymphotoxin alpha (LTA) gene.

The HaploChIP approach does not require the presence of an indicator SNP in a transcribed region; SNPs in chromatin outside transcribed regions can be used to demonstrate and measure allele- or haplotype-specific loading of PolII, a surrogate measure for gene transcription. This method allows the high-throughput identification of allele-specific transcription for genes that lack transcribed SNPs, but does not determine the particular SNP or SNPs responsible for the allele- or haplotype-specific effect.

Neither EAI nor HaploChIP determine which SNP is causing an effect on gene expression; additional techniques are required for this. As noted by Hudson, such variants may be targets for manipulation of expression levels to restore full gene function.

Gene Expression Profiles as Quantitative Traits (eQTLs)

The experimental approaches described above, though amenable to high- throughput analyses, require a gene-by-gene assessment of expression levels. Another powerful approach marries large-scale microarray-based expression profiling to genome-wide linkage analysis. The method, first termed "*genetical genomics*" by Jansen and Nap, is referred to as "*expression quantitative trait locus*" (eQTL) analysis by Friend and co-workers who describe its application to the genome-wide genetic analyses of gene expression levels in maize, mouse, and man.

An example of the eQTL approach would be analysis of a series of F2 progeny of a cross between two inbred strains of mice. The genomes of each of these F2 mice would be a patchwork of blocks of sequence derived from one parental inbred strain or the other. In classical quantitative trait locus (QTL) analysis, genetic linkage analysis is applied to traits such as weight or size that vary quantitatively between mice of such an F2 series, to identify genomic loci that are responsible for that quantitative trait. In eQTL analysis, the quantitative traits used are the gene expression levels from gene expression profiles of the F2 mice. These F2 mice are subject to microsatellite-based genome scanning to provide the genetic data for linkage analysis. If a gene expression chip representing, for example, 10,000 genes was used, this would provide 10,000 quantitative traits to analyze for linkage using the genome scan data, i.e., genome-wide linkage analysis of 10,000 phenotypes!

Schadt et al. analyzed 23,574 profiled genes and found that 7861 (33%) were differentially expressed in the livers of the parental (C57BL/6J and DBA/2J) mouse strains or their F2 progeny. The eQTL mapping revealed 2123 genes with LOD scores (log of the odds in favor of linkage) greater than 4.3, and 965 genes with LOD scores greater than 7.0. eQTL hotspots, where multiple eQTLs clustered in a clearly non-random way, were observed on several mouse chromosomes. Such hotspots are likely to represent loci that affect the expression of multiple genes, or clusters of genes for which expression is under genetic control.

An observation that the expression of many genes was linked to more than one eQTL locus, and that some were linked to three loci, demonstrated that gene expression is a complex trait. Schadt et al. note that the Nnmt drug metabolism gene was known to differ in expression between the DBA and B6 parental mouse strains and they also observed a corresponding eQTL (LOD score 15.3) at the position of the Nnmt gene. Perhaps most interesting of all was that while many genes' expression levels map to an eQTL corresponding to the position of that gene, others identified eQTLs elsewhere in the genome that are likely to correspond to trans-acting genetic factors influencing gene expression.

Schadt et al. also performed initial eQTL analyses using gene expression profiles from the immortalized lymphocytes of members of four CEPH pedigrees. Almost one-third of the differentially expressed genes that were analyzed in this way showed inheritance of their EAI. Given that only 16 "normal" individuals were studied, it is remarkable that genetic effects could be detected in such a high proportion of genes. This result underscores the importance of genetic effects on gene expression in the determination of human phenotypes such as susceptibility to complex diseases and drug responses.

The eQTL analyses in humans, either based on linkage studies of pedigrees or on association studies in case/control groups, are likely to be valuable for those pharmacologically relevant genes that are expressed in accessible tissues such as lymphocytes. For tissues such as liver, which is the site of many steps in the metabolism of various drugs, studies in model organisms like mice will be particularly fruitful for pharmacogenomics research.

Early examples of pharmacogenetics represent Mendelian or near-Mendelian traits. A true picture of pharmacogenomics will be multifactorial and will more closely resemble complex genetic disease. As for other complex phenotypes, studies of drug responses will benefit from new genomic methodologies and resources such as inexpensive genotyping methods and the HapMap project. New assays for gene regulatory processes such as EAI and particularly new genome-wide methods for relating expression levels to phenotypes, such as eQTL analyses, will be critical for an understanding of the genetic basis of drug response and other medically important phenotypes.

Gene Expression Analysis for Tailoring and Optimizing Drug Treatment

Gene expression analysis has broad applications in pharmacogenomics including molecular profiling of patients for optimizing drug treatment, selection of target genes, and pathways for drug development and toxicological profiling of novel drugs (e.g., determination of the activation patterns of drug-metabolizing enzymes).

Molecular profiling of tumors and tissues to assess the optimal treatment strategy and to adjust drug dosage prior to drug administration is advantageous, and is available for some therapeutic compounds. Implementation of such measures is expected to lead to a new era of individualized molecular medicine. Patients in general, and cancer patients in particular, can be profiled by gene expression analysis using advanced high throughput technologies. In particular, advances in DNA microarray technology, high throughput DNA sequencing, and proteomic assays accelerate the generation of high quality patient profiles at ever-decreasing costs. The combination of these methods with sophisticated bioinformatics tools for data analysis has enhanced the basis of drug discovery (identifying targets genes and pathways) and molecular patient profiling (identification of drug responders and non-responders).

It is widely hoped that the broad implementation of DNA microarray technology will revolutionize future pharmacologic investigations. Monitoring gene expression profiles may provide insights into (a) the molecular fingerprints of different diseases including cancer, diseases of the central nervous system, and the cardiovascular system, (b) therapeutic treatments, (c) environmental agents, (d) avoiding toxicity and achieving personalized treatment, and (e) methods of achieving the ultimate goal of preventing these diseases altogether.

High-Throughput Gene Expression Analysis

DNA microarrays are often used to analyze genome-wide changes in gene expression patterns. Either cDNA microarrays or oligonucleotide-based gene chips can be used for gene expression analysis. A cDNA microarray contains a large number of cDNA fragments physically spotted onto glass slides or nylon membranes. Alternatively, oligonucleotides corresponding to known genes or ESTs can be synthesized in situ on a miniature matrix using a photolithographic process to produce oligonucleotide-based microarrays. Oligonucleotide-based DNA chips can also be used to screen individuals for DNA mutations and polymorphisms by analyzing variations in genomic DNA.

The traditional gene-by-gene approach to assess gene expression induced by pharmaceutical compounds includes Northern blotting of mRNAs, reverse-transcription-coupled polymerase chain reaction (RT-PCR) of mRNAs, Western blotting of proteins, and various enzymatic assays. These techniques, however, allow evaluation of only a few to tens or at most hundreds of genes/gene products per study. With the advent of DNA microarray technology, expression of thousands or tens of thousands of genes can be queried simultaneously, including various drug metabolizing enzyme (DME) genes and a battery of genes that may be relevant pharmacologically (as potential therapeutic targets) or toxicologically (leading to undesirable or toxic effects of the drugs) to drug response in humans. Microarray data have also been used recently to analyze gene expression changes in response to environmental toxins, chemotherapeutic agents, and cytokines. The use of DNA microarrays to interrogate the gene expression patterns of cells exposed to pharmacologic small molecules and environmental toxins may yield insights into the mechanisms of drug- or chemical-induced toxicity and carcinogenesis.

An important use of microarray-based gene expression analysis is the sub-classification of cancers. Two methods are currently used: supervised and unsupervised analyses. A supervised analysis first defines sample subcategories and then searches for genes that are differentially expressed between these two groups. Unsupervised analysis (or clustering) of expression data identifies gene expression "*clusters*" in phenotypically uncharacterized samples that are significantly related in terms of their expression profiles. Samples that share expression profile features might be expected to share phenotypic features, treatment outcome for example, that can be clearly defined pathologically.

Expanding our knowledge of basic biological processes and developing a detailed understanding of the signaling pathways that participate in the development of disease has led to opportunities for diagnostic and therapeutic intervention. Validation of drug targets within patient groups is critical, and for a successful clinical application it is also critical to determine whether the putative target can be identified as present or absent in a consistent, practical, and inexpensive manner.

Molecular Profiling of Cancers

Examples of specialized molecular therapeutics that have been developed from discoveries made using expression profiling experiments include chimeric human/murine antibodies for the treatment of various cancers. Rituximab, an anti-CD20 antibody in use since 1997, was the first chimeric monoclonal antibody to receive FDA approval for treatment of CD20-positive Non-Hodgkin lymphomas. Cells from most Non-Hodgkin lymphomas express this antigen on their surface. Shortly thereafter Trastuzumab, which targets the human epidermal growth factor receptor 2 (HER2) was approved for breast cancer treatment; it is now part of the clinical management of metastatic disease. Further examples of monoclonal antibodies in clinical use include Cetuximab, which targets the epidermal growth-factor receptor (EGFR) and Bavacizumab, which reacts with vascular endothelial growth factor (VEGF). Both have been approved for treatment of metastatic colorectal cancer and are in clinical testing for use with other types of tumors.

From a pharmacological viewpoint these molecular therapies change the "one drug fits all" approach that was applied previously. As with a plethora of classical therapeutics, where the actual drug targets and the mode of action are not entirely understood, these new-generation therapeutics are only effective when the target protein is present in the malignant tissue. The specific investigation of one gene product does not require the sophistication of complex microarray analysis. Specific assays or small- customized arrays, consisting of tens rather than thousands of genes or customized real-time quantitative PCR platforms represent realistic alternatives for clinical use.

Examples of diagnostic tests in clinical use in cancer therapy include evaluation of HER2 and EGFR expression levels. The HER2 diagnostic tests marketed by Dako and Abbott Laboratories detect overproduction of HER2 protein and gene amplification, respectively. Dako also markets an FDA approved test kit, EGFR-pharmDx that identifies EGFR-positive tumors and thus helps determine whether a patient can benefit from Cetuximab therapy. These single gene expression-based diagnostic tools are among the first steps towards applied pharmacogenetics/genomics and individualized medicine. Future challenges for pharmacogenomics in clinical settings will be the transformation from single-protein diagnostics to detection of multiple biomarkers and, if necessary, the integration of whole genome analysis.

High-density microarrays allow the parallel investigation of all transcripts in a given cellular system. This global gene expression analysis will advance drug-associated gene and pathway discovery, functional characterization of genes, and tumor sub-classification. Although molecular testing has been increasingly used in clinical practice, the precise diagnosis, and prognosis of most human cancers still relies heavily on descriptive histopathological data. Identification of robust molecular markers associated with distinctive morphological parameters will assist in diagnostic and prognostic assessment. In the past several years, DNA microarray technology has been widely used in the context of cancer research, resulting in a deluge of new information that can be used to identify molecular alterations common to all tumors of a specific type as well as signatory profiles unique to a subcategory of cancers. Expression-profiling studies have been performed in almost every major type of cancer.

Although many of these studies were initially designed for cancer classification, a large proportion of the published data contains information that can be used to identify cancer-specific markers. Rhodes et al. demonstrated a successful model for performing meta-analysis of independent microarray datasets. Analysis of four prostate cancer gene expression data sets revealed striking similarities, despite the different sample preparation methods and array platforms used. Results from this and other studies have generated a number of promising cancer specific markers that will probably out-perform other prostate cancer markers previously identified. Based on existing well-illustrated examples such as AMACR (a-methylacyl-coA racemase), which is commonly up-regulated in prostate cancer specimens, the complete molecular distinction between normal and cancer cells can be surprisingly easy to achieve, if a combination of a few robust markers is used.

Tumor Classification

Sub-classification of tumors originating from a specific tissue holds much promise for accurate cancer diagnosis and individualized treatment. Expression profiles unique to each subtype of cancer can be used for development of subtype specific therapies and for monitoring their therapeutic efficacy. Although advanced cytogenetics and molecular analysis tools have been used in subclassification of some cancers (e.g., acute leukemia), molecular classification based solely on gene expression has proven to be a viable alternative and may provide further information regarding the disease state. Proof of this principle was first illustrated by Golub et al. in a study involving samples from 72 acute leukemia patients. Supervised learning methods based on known identities of acute myelogenous leukemia (AML) and acute lymphocytic leukemia (ALL) generated a profile that was successfully used to classify a new group of samples into the correct category. This study established the feasibility of expression-based tumor classification.

Genetic microarray analysis was also extensively studied to classify and predict prognosis in a series of hematological malignancies. Some of the earliest clinical studies that used gene array analysis studied acute leukemia, a disease for which one has access to essentially pure tumor cell populations. An important initial question was whether expression arrays could be used diagnostically to distinguish AML from ALL. Using unsupervised learning based solely on gene expression, 36 of 38 AML and ALL patients were correctly assigned, demonstrating that microarrays can be used to classify acute leukemias without prior clinical knowledge. Using supervised learning, 50 genes were identified that were differentially expressed between AML and ALL. Profiling of these genes in unknown leukemia samples classified 29 of 34 samples correctly. Gene expression signatures have also been defined for prognostic subgroups of diffuse large B-cell lymphoma (DLBCL) that show statistically significant differences in overall survival. The sub-classification into germinal center B-like DLBCL (GC-DLBCL) and activated B-like DLBCL involved gene expression patterns of approximately 3000 genes identifying each group. Although the entire patient group showed an overall 52% survival at 5 years, 76% of GC B-like DLBCL patients were alive after 5 years in contrast to only 16% of activated B-like DLBCL patients, suggesting that these two subgroups represent distinct disease entities. Germinal center B-like DLBCL has a more favorable response to standard therapies, whereas activated B-like DLBCL is less responsive to them. More aggressive and/or investigational treatment approaches may be justified for the latter group. This DLBCL subgroup classification resulted from the development of a custom microarray-based prognostic tool, the LymphoChip capable of identifying these two distinct subgroups of DLBCL.

Rituximab, which targets the B cell surface protein CD20, is therapeutically useful for treating follicular lymphoma (FL). A recent study has examined the expression of more than 20,000 genes in tumor samples from patients who received rituximab for treatment of FL in order to identify differentially regulated genes in responding and non-responding patients. Based on their expression profiles, the tumors fell into two groups, one clustered with normal lymphoid tissues from spleen and tonsil, and the other with more malignant samples. Rituximab non-responders were found in the normal lymphoid tissue group, whereas rituximab responders were mainly found in the more malignant group.

Other hematological malignancies have also been studied using DNA microarrays, particularly with respect to prognosis, including chronic lymphocytic leukemia, mantle cell and marginal zone lymphoma, and multiple myeloma. All these studies used high-density microarrays in class prediction experiments to identify diagnostic markers and to improve the characterization of and therapeutic strategies for these malignancies.

A key clinical classification of breast cancer tumors is estrogen receptor (ER) expression. The more ERs are present on tumor cells, the more likely an anti-estrogen therapy such as tamoxifen can be successfully applied. Classification of each tumor is important, as only about 60% of breast cancers are ER-positive. Initial studies set out to demonstrate that breast cancers with distinct pathological features could be separated by microarrays. Several groups demonstrated that supervised data analysis could be used to distinguish ER-positive from ER-negative tumors. Surprisingly, these studies also demonstrated that the gene expression profiles of ER-positive and ER-negative breast cancers differ both qualitatively and quantitatively in expression of a large number of genes.

The fact that ER-positive and ER-negative tumors are different at the level of gene expression suggests that these molecular subtypes are entirely different disease entities that may have arisen from distinct precursor cell types. Furthermore, only a few of the genes that discriminate between ER-positive and ER-negative tumors appear to be part of the ER signaling pathway, adding further weight to the concept of distinct lineages for ER-positive and ER-negative tumors. In a landmark study, van't Veer et al. performed gene expression microarray analysis on 78 sporadic lymphnode-negative tumors arising in women under the age of 55 years.

Microarray analysis of these primary tumors identified a list of 70 discriminatory genes whose expression patterns, in an internal validation, identified a group of patients who had not developed metastases at 5 years from diagnosis. A method such as this that can identify patients at very low risk of developing metastases allows chemotherapy to be targeted only to those women who are likely to benefit from it.

If accurate determination of chemosensitivity were predictable by gene expression analysis, the overall number of patients receiving cytotoxic treatment unnecessarily would decrease, and the overall survival benefit derived per patient treated would increase accordingly. Large increases in the absolute survival of patients diagnosed with breast cancer, however, will require the development of novel therapeutic agents.

Microarray-based gene expression profiling for gene and pathway discovery, functional classification of genes, and new tumor sub-classifications have also been applied to various other malignancies including lung, bladder and prostate cancer, and cutaneous melanoma.

Identification of Drug Targets and Toxicological Profiles by Gene Expression Analysis

In addition to molecular profiling of diseases to identify drug responders/ non-responders and to classify sub-groups within a given disease, large scale gene expression analysis is also broadly used to determine the effects of drugs on target cells or tissues. It is well known that genes control drug effects, but there is increasing evidence that drugs also affect gene function. Accordingly, microarray analysis can be used to monitor gene expression changes that directly reflect the cellular response to drug exposure. This kind of information is valuable in several ways: (a) altered gene expression patterns of drug-metabolizing enzymes highlight specific drug response pathways, (b) the single genes or whole signaling pathways activated represent potential novel drug targets, and (c) toxicological information, especially induction of apoptosis, stress response genes, and multi drug-resistance genes (toxicogenomics), can be assessed with genome-wide gene expression analyses.

Gene Expression Analysis of Drug-Treated Cells

Rae et al. used microarrays to measure the effects of rifampin, an antibacterial agent, on the mRNA expression of drug-metabolizing enzymes in human hepatocytes. They showed increases of cytochromes P450 CYPC9, CYP2C8, and CYP3A4 but not of CYP2C18, CYP2E1, or CYP2C9. This cytochrome P450 expression pattern resembles the specific drug metabolizing enzyme profile for rifampin.

To investigate the toxicological profile and to identify novel downstream mediators of tumor cell response, two recent studies investigated MCF-7 breast cancer cells that were treated with different chemotherapeutic agents. Maxwell et al. used DNA microarrays to identify genes that are transcriptionally activated in MCF-7 cells by 5-fluorouracil (5-FU) treatment. They found specific genes that were consistently up-regulated in the treated group (spermine/spermidine acetyl transferase, annexin II, thymosin-β-10, chaperonin-10, and MAT-8). As the major limitation to the clinical use of 5-FU is acquired or inherent resistance, these identified genes may prove valuable in overcoming these limitations.

Kudoh et al. used DNA microarrays to monitor the expression profile of human MCF-7 cells that were either transiently treated with doxorubicin or selected for doxorubicin resistance. They identified a subset of genes (microsomal epoxide hydrolase 1,26S proteasome regulatory subunit 4, and XRCC1) that were constitutively over-expressed in both the short-term treated and resistant groups and may therefore be functionally relevant for drug resistance. Identification of drug-target genes and the underlying signaling pathways using advanced gene expression technologies can indeed facilitate the development of new therapeutic strategies to improve the efficacy, safety, and tolerance of novel or existing drugs.

In the field of toxicogenomics (i.e., the study of how genomes respond to environmental stressors or toxins) large-scale gene expression analysis of toxin-treated cells and animals has demonstrated its highly accurate capacity to recognize the toxic potential of novel drug candidates, resulting in an increase in the efficiency, quality, and safety of drug selection in drug development pipelines.

Gunther et al. used human primary neurons treated with multiple classes of antidepressant drugs, antipsychotic drugs, and opioid receptor agonists to generate DNA microarray gene expression data representative of these classes of treatment. They investigated whether gene expression profiles from these drug treatments could be used to construct statistical models capable of predicting drug efficacy. They showed that supervised classification schemes could be used to accurately predict the functional category of members of each of these drug classes, based on analysis of the drug-induced gene expression profile.

Gene Expression Analysis of Combination Therapy

Recently, Cheok et al. examined the gene expression profile of a combination therapy. They examined the DNA microarray-based gene expression profile of childhood acute lymphoblastic leukemia bone marrow cells 24 hr after the randomized initiation of patient treatment with mercaptopurine (a purine antagonist), methotrexate (a dihydrofolate reductase inhibitor), or a combination of these two agents. This study addressed two important questions: (a) do mercaptopurine and methotrexate elicit similar changes in gene expression, as they both affect purine metabolism in similar ways, and (b) does the combination of mercaptopurine and methotrexate treatment result in gene expression changes that simply reflect the sum of the two parts? Interestingly, the effects of mercaptopurine and methotrexate when given as single agents were largely non-overlapping. Only 14% of the genes regulated by either mercaptopurine or methotrexate alone were similarly regulated by the combination therapy. These data support a model in which the combination does not simply function as a sum of the component parts. Whether this combination treatment represents synergistic action impinging on a single molecular pathway, or modulation of independent pathways that subsequently converge remains to be determined.

Reverse Pharmacogenomics Approach

A new twist in the use of gene expression as a drug discovery tool was reported by Stegmaier et al., who devised a new screening strategy for identifying compounds that force the myeloid differentiation of AML cells. Their approach is based on the observation that all-trans retinoic acid produces clinical remissions by inducing differentiation of acute promyelocytic leukemias harboring a mutated retinoic acid receptor alpha. They developed a surrogate marker approach that uses post-treatment gene expression signatures in AML cell lines as the read-out for screening the ability of candidate compounds to induce differentiation of AML cells. This "*reverse pharmacogenomics*" strategy inverts the classical model of assessing therapeutic agents by first defining the drug-induced pattern of gene expression that is the therapeutic goal, and then screening compounds that can induce this endpoint. In some ways, this can be viewed as a modern, mechanistically insightful reimplementation of classical pharmacology, using a whole-cell response to drive drug discovery. The ultimate tests would be in vivo experiments illustrating that compounds identified by this approach actually induce AML differentiation in preclinical models, and clinical trials. Gene expression analysis is an important genomic tool that has wide applications in pharmacogenomics. Successes to date include the subclassification of many types of tumors to optimize treatment or prognosis, as well as the use of drug-induced expression profiles in target discovery and toxicity studies. New techniques that enhance our understanding of how human genetic variation affects gene expression contributes to drug response will be important in predicting individual responses to drugs, both for efficacy and for the prediction of adverse events.

19

POSITIONAL CLONING

Advances in recombinant DNA technologies and the sequence data provided by the human genome project have provided an unprecedented opportunity to characterize the molecular pathophysiology of disease. It is now evident that the majority of human diseases arise as a result of the interplay between environmental factors and genetic background. Genetic and environmental interactions play an essential role not only in disease predisposition, but also in the modulation of disease characteristics (such as age at onset and expression of various subphenotypes), therapeutic responsiveness, and outcome. Recently, the elucidation of these complex interactions has been greatly facilitated by the completion of the human genome project and publication of the full genome sequence, currently estimated to encompass about 22,000 protein coding genes.

The major challenge now facing medical science is to exploit this genetic information so as to identify the sets of genes responsible for specific illnesses and thereby unravel the molecular processes coupling such genetic determinants to expression and persistence of disease. Such knowledge will allow for definition of molecular biomarkers for use in diagnosis and prediction of disease risk, prognosis and drug responsiveness, and will thereby enable "*individualized*" medical care wherein both diagnosis and therapy are predicated on the individual's profile of susceptibility gene variants. Thus, definition of the full complement of susceptibility alleles involved in common diseases will pave the way for earlier, more precise diagnosis and for developing the pharmacogenomic knowledge required to optimize drug therapy.

In view of the extraordinary potential for disease gene identification to improve health care delivery, a major thrust of human genetics research has been directed at developing technologies, which accelerate the disease gene discovery process. For many single-gene diseases, knowledge of the pathophysiology has been sufficient to allow for direct screening of newly cloned genes as possible disease gene candidates. This "*candidate gene*" approach, which builds upon understanding of the disease pathophysiology and a given gene/protein function, has, for example, been used to characterize the molecular basis for phenylketonuria, β-thalassemia, and many other single-gene disorders. For the majority of human diseases, however, information on etiopathogenesis is insufficient to render candidate gene testing feasible. This situation is true for most single-gene diseases and for virtually all of the common human diseases having a significant genetic or inherited component.

These latter conditions are referred to as "*complex genetic*" diseases, conditions which collectively account for the majority of the healthcare burden in developed countries and which include, for example, atherosclerotic cardiovascular disease, rheumatoid arthritis, and diabetes. Discovery of genes involved in complex genetic diseases is further confounded by many other issues such as lack of knowledge of mode of inheritance (dominant, recessive, multifactorial, etc.), incomplete penetrance, genetic and allelic heterogeneity, and the fact that many disease-associated genetic variants are likely to occur commonly in the general (healthy) population. Additionally, until relatively recently, most of the genome had remained uncharacterized. For these and other reasons, most of the initial work on disease gene identification utilized an alternative gene discovery approach, "*positional cloning*," wherein disease genes are isolated based on their chromosomal localization.

Positional cloning, a strategy allowing disease gene discovery despite lack of knowledge of disease pathophysiology or mode of inheritance, has proven extraordinarily successful to gene discovery in single-gene disease and, more recently, also in relation to uncovering genes involved in complex genetic disease. While the steps involved in positional cloning and candidate gene analysis are initially distinct, positional cloning approaches lead ultimately to the identification of sets of candidate genes at specific locations in the genome. Thus, these two methodologies converge and the challenge becomes identifying which one of a (generally small) number of "good candidate" genes represents the gene responsible for the disease under study. In this chapter, these technologies and challenges are described and illustrated using the specific example of the inflammatory bowel disease, Crohn's disease.

Candidate Gene Approaches

Detailed understanding of disease pathogenesis provides a knowledge framework for predicting the genes likely contributing to disease susceptibility. The relevance of such "candidate" genes to a specific disease can be directly established by demonstrating that the disease state is associated with variants (alleles) of the gene(s) in question. Candidate gene analysis involves investigation of fully characterized genes encoding putative disease-relevant products (e.g., tumor suppressor genes in cancer, cytokines in inflammatory disease, etc.).

Alternatively, candidate gene analysis may require the isolation of a gene encoding a protein that seems likely to be related to disease, for example by using oligonucleotide-based probes or antibodies to screen cDNA or expression libraries. This latter strategy was used, for example, to isolate the factor VIII gene involved in Haemophilia A, the globin genes involved in thalassemia and sickle cell anemia and one of the genes responsible for Fanconi anemia. However, as the specific pathophysiological processes and proteins underlying the majority of human diseases are unknown, this approach has limited scope for application.

As gene cloning has progressed and the human genome has been increasingly well characterized, candidate gene investigation has largely shifted from the direct cloning approach to the screening of already-identified genes for their potential relevance to disease. Although this approach involves some degree of "educated" guessing, with candidates being selected on the premise of relevance to disease etiology, the candidate gene strategy has proven successful in many instances. Identification of the genetic defect underlying Marfan's syndrome, for example, was based on the realization that a newly cloned gene encoded a protein, fibrillin, with functional properties potentially relevant to the cellular defects found in Marfan's patients.

Genes encoding the human leukocyte antigens (HLA) have also been investigated as candidate susceptibility genes for a broad spectrum of diseases, including autoimmune and other immunological disorders such as asthma, inflammatory bowel disease, multiple sclerosis, type 1 diabetes mellitus (T1D), and psoriasis. Indeed, certain variants of the HLA genes have been shown to contribute to a significant proportion of the genetic risk for T1D, rheumatoid arthritis, and inflammatory bowel disease. As the functions of the full complement of human genes become increasingly well characterized, opportunities for disease gene identification by candidate gene analysis will continue to grow and likely permit discovery of many important disease susceptibility genes.

Positional Cloning

In contrast to the candidate gene approach, positional cloning involves disease gene identification in the absence of assumptions as to the functional properties of the relevant genes. Thus, at least in its initial stages, this approach does not require prior knowledge of the disease pathophysiology. The first and most well known example of disease gene discovery by positional cloning was the identification of the gene (CFTR) responsible for cystic fibrosis, a discovery involving the use of physical and genetic mapping methods to "home in" on the chromosome 7 region harboring the gene mutation underlying this disease.

The basic strategy used in positional cloning involves definition of chromosomal region(s) containing the genes of interest and the subsequent analysis of the genes within such regions for disease-associated mutations. This approach involves screening the >3 billion bases of the haploid human genome for as minor a change as a single-base alteration, a magnitude of task that can be likened to the challenge associated with finding a specific individual person on this planet with no prior knowledge as to his/her address. However, despite the enormity of the challenge, many genes associated with single-gene disorders have been identified by positional cloning. These successes have validated positional cloning as a valuable strategy for disease gene isolation and have provided incentive for the field to progress toward the search for genes underlying the chronic multifactorial disorders constituting the bulk of human disease.

Clinical Materials

Regardless of the approach taken, disease gene identification generally involves a series of discrete steps, the earliest and often rate limiting of which is the ascertainment and clinical characterization of affected individuals. The importance of patient collection cannot be overstated, as the quality of the phenotypic data collected in the population under study has immense impact on the results and interpretation of the data obtained from genetic analysis. In contrast to candidate gene association analysis, positional cloning involves the analysis of families as well as affected individuals. Multigenerational pedigrees including multiple affected individuals such as affected relative pairs and affected sib pairs, as well as parents and ideally, grandparents, are most useful for such studies, but are often difficult to obtain, particularly for diseases where age of onset is late in life. Other unaffected relatives may also be included in order to "link" affected individuals in the pedigree.

Genetic material, usually genomic DNA extracted from a peripheral blood sample, is collected from the affected and unaffected study participants and clinical records obtained and reviewed so as to ensure the affectation status of all subjects. In more sophisticated studies, the affectation status may be denoted as "unknown," if a subject is young enough to be pre-symptomatic for a late-onset disease. The importance of establishing stringent diagnostic criteria for the phenotype of interest is crucial as the failure to do so may obfuscate subsequently obtained linkage data. These clinical data should, in turn, be formatted and stored in databases in a fashion that facilitates easy retrieval and flexible queries, so as to enable multivariate analyses, stratification of the population based on various demographic/clinical characteristics and definition of subpopulations treated with and/or responding to specific medications.

Family-based Linkage Analysis

Following completion of family collection, genotyping studies can be initiated so as to enable linkage-based disease gene localization. Linkage refers to the cosegregation of loci in close proximity on the same chromosome. By contrast, loci which map to different chromosomes or far apart on the same chromosome segregate independently due to meiotic recombination and therefore show no linkage. The greater the (physical) distance between two loci, the higher the likelihood that these loci will be separated by recombination events, and thus show a greater interlocus recombination fraction. By contrast, loci mapping close to each other are unlikely to be separated by recombination and are referred to as "linked." Importantly, "linkage" implies a physical relationship between genetic loci and needs to be distinguished from the concept of "association," the latter of which refers to the coincident presence of a specific genetic variant and a given disease, but which does not necessarily imply physical proximity between the disease gene and the marker locus. A number of different approaches to determining linkage between disease and DNA markers are commonly used, including both parametric and non-parametric approaches.

Genetic Markers for Linkage or Association Analysis

In recognition of the potential for linkage to localize and ultimately reveal novel disease susceptibility genes, enormous effort has been directed at identifying genetic markers that are sufficiently polymorphic and/or sufficiently frequent in the genome to be of value in linkage studies. Older marker typing technologies such as restriction fragment length polymorphism (RFLPs) and variable number of tandem repeats (VNTR) marker testing have since given way to the two most frequently used genotyping tools: short tandem repeats (STRs), also commonly called "*microsatellites*," and single-nucleotide polymorphisms (SNPs). The SNPs also form the basis of newer mapping approaches such as haplotype-tag mapping, a strategy underpinning the international haplotype mapping effort directed at delineating all haplotype "blocks" across the genome and sets of SNPs representative of each block.

The STRs represent regions of the genome containing stretches of tandem repeats of about two to seven nucleotides in length and occur frequently throughout the genome. The STRs are generally highly polymorphic and can be detected by PCR amplification using primer pairs corresponding to conserved STR flanking sequences. Detection is typically via size-separation on fluorescent capillary or slab gel DNA sequencers and automated software is used to obtain genotype "calls," i.e. to identify the different sized alleles from either chromosome of an individual DNA sample. The vast majority of genome-wide scans for disease susceptibility loci use STR-based approaches, although SNP-based approaches are now becoming feasible and are gaining in popularity. Most STR-based scans involve the use of approximately 300 di-, tri-, or tetranucleotide repeat markers spaced at about 10-cM intervals, so as to provide coverage of the approximately 3300 cM genome. Standardized primer sets for such genomewide scans are readily available from commercial vendors.

While STR markers have proven highly useful for disease gene mapping, the level of resolution provided by these markers is sufficient only for regional localizations of genes involved in complex disease (i.e. refinement to, at best, perhaps 1 cM, or roughly 1 million base pairs of DNA). Typically, such regions are defined through family-based linkage analysis, although linkage disequilibrium (LD) mapping using STRs can also be very successful in many regions of the genome. Indeed, our own search for inflammatory bowel disease susceptibility genes involved an initial standard STR-based genome-wide linkage scan approach, followed by LD mapping with microsatellite STRs to refine the Crohn's disease-associated IBD5 locus to a small region of chromosome 5q31. Regions of this magnitude in size are expected to contain multiple genes, perhaps even dozens in some particularly gene-rich areas of the genome.

In this context, SNPs, the most common form of genetic variation, are useful for refining regions and identifying specific disease-associated genes. The SNPs represent sites in which single-base pair variation occurs from person-to-person and in which the least frequent allele has a population frequency of 1% or greater. In contrast to STRs, SNPs occur at an average frequency of about 1 per 1000 bp and are generally mutationally stable, facilitating LD mapping strategies which rely upon co-segregation of ancestral alleles that are in close physical proximity to each other. Many SNPs occur within genes, and accordingly, some will represent the genetic lesions of interest (e.g. a missense or nonsense mutation in a coding region). By contrast, the utility of SNPs is reduced by their biallelic nature, meaning that heterozygosity cannot be greater than 50% and thus more SNPs than STRs are required to provide adequate information for disease gene discovery. Estimates of the numbers of SNPs required for genome-wide genetic association studies have been as high as 0.5–1.0 million, and even a recent estimate suggests that no fewer than 200,000 SNPs may be required to achieve this goal.

This problem has been addressed in part with the development of microarray-based SNP genotyping approaches incorporating greater than 100,000 SNPs per array, or through other very high-throughput genotyping platforms such as the Illumina BeadArray system. New approaches such as single-molecule sequencing using nanoscale fluidics may also further optimize such studies. These and other technologies, coupled to robotic systems for sample and liquid handling, should render high-throughput SNP genotyping increasingly feasible and, in conjunction with worldwide efforts to identify and validate all common SNP variants in the human genome, enable the scale of whole-genome association studies to be ramped up to the level required for disease gene mapping in complex genetic diseases.

Use of Families for Positional Cloning

In conjunction with polymorphic markers spanning the genome, family collections represent a cornerstone of gene mapping studies. The choice of family structures to be used in positional cloning is very much influenced by the disease under study. For example, large pedigrees including multiple affected individuals are particularly relevant to the mapping of single-gene disorders in which the pattern of inheritance is known and parametric linkage methods (those including parameters specifying mode of inheritance, penetrance, etc.) thus easily applied. By contrast, in instances in which the mode of inheritance is unknown, as is the case for most complex genetic diseases, a more widely used family structure is the affected sibling pair (ASP), which can be studied by non-parametric methods that assess sharing of chromosomal regions by the affected individuals.

The ASP analysis is predicated upon the fact that siblings are expected to share 0, 1, or 2 parental alleles at frequencies of 0.25, 0.5, and 0.25, respectively, if the alleles segregate at random. In contrast, siblings affected by a given disease would predictably share the chromosomal region containing the disease relevant loci (and thus polymorphic alleles located within such a region) at frequencies greater than would be seen under the null hypothesis of random chance segregation. The ASP analysis has proven very valuable in the search for complex disease gene loci and remains the state of the art in this regard. However, there are drawbacks to this approach, including, for example, the fact that sib pairs share many chromosomal segments by chance alone. Thus, in order to avoid false-positive results, a large number of ASPs must be examined.

Once genotypes have been derived from genome-wide scans, the data can be analyzed so as to determine whether any markers cosegregate with the disease/phenotype. Segregation of alleles is evaluated using linkage analysis and is generally quantitated using a lod (logarithm of odds) score (Z), which depicts the likelihood of linkage vs. the null hypothesis of no linkage (i.e., random segregation between marker and disease phenotype). For single-gene disorders and two-point linkage analysis, a lod score of 3.0 is considered definitive evidence of linkage; under these conditions, linkage is rejected if $Z < -2.0$ while values between −2.0 and +3.0 are considered inconclusive. However, these standards do not hold in the context of multiple testing in genome-wide scans, wherein the simultaneous analysis of >300 rather than one or two individual loci markedly increases the chance for false-positive results. Accordingly, for linkage analysis in which genome-wide scans are used to identify single-gene disease loci, the accepted threshold for significance is a lod score of 3.3 or greater. For complex genetic diseases, defining the level of significance in a genome-wide study is crucial to establishing which disease linked marker loci represent real disease susceptibility loci. The difficulties inherent to this issue arise in part from the incorporation of multiple test markers. While it is generally agreed that genome-wide scans require a threshold p value more stringent than required for two-point analysis, controversy has existed as to the level of this value.

A set of criteria for interpreting linkage data have been proposed by Lander and Kruglyak and these have been widely accepted, but the correct thresholds of significance for use in such studies remains controversial. Based on the 1995 criteria set out by Lander and Kruglyak, a lod score of 3.6 ($p < 2 \times 10^{-5}$) can be considered as the threshold for significant linkage, a lod score of >2.2 ($p < 7 \times 10^{-4}$) can be considered suggestive of linkage in ASP analyses, and replication of previously reported significant linkage data requires a $p < 0.01$. These guidelines are likely to be revisited in the near future in view of the increasing complexity and density of genotype data derived from genome-wide scans, particularly those based on tens to hundreds of thousands of SNPs.

As evidenced by the extensive variation in the linkage data derived from independent groups working on the same complex genetic disorder, linkage analysis in multifactorial disease is not straightforward, independent genome-wide screens typically revealing overlapping, but non-identical, sets of loci contributing to a specific disease. One solution to resolving such discrepancies involves the meta-analysis of data from multiple genome screens, a strategy which may identify the most consistently linked loci and thereby redirect research efforts towards discovery of disease genes most likely to be relevant in many different populations.

While some of the disparities between linkage data may reflect easily correctable errors such as misread gels, switched samples, incorrect scoring of family relationships or misdiagnosis/misclassification of phenotype, other key contributing factors such as incomplete penetrance and genetic heterogeneity are difficult to address. An additional problem is the relatively low resolution of STR-based marker scans, and the consequent necessity for analysis of very large numbers of families so as to delineate a target region amenable to gene identification (i.e., <2 cM). Most commonly, linkage data emanating from STR marker scans has revealed target regions that are far too large (e.g., 10-40 Mb) to attempt disease gene isolation. Accordingly, genome-wide scanning needs to be complemented by additional mapping strategies, which enable refinement of regions of interest to sizes amenable to physical mapping and candidate gene analysis.

One other confounding factor in the use of high-throughput genotype data for disease gene mapping is the possibility of undetected genotype errors in large datasets. While Mendelian (inheritance) errors can be identified readily, genotype errors that yield data consistent with Mendelian inheritance can significantly interfere with downstream genetic analyses, for example, through the introduction of spurious "*double recombination*" events or through the elimination of *bonafide* "real" recombinations. Even in the highest-quality datasets, problems such as missing genotypes, sample mix-up, or miscalled genotypes can introduce significant biases that can be difficult to detect and which can reduce ability to localize disease genes with the accuracy required for such studies.

Reffinement to Chromosomal Localizations

The disease gene localizations provided by STR marker-based genome-wide scans are usually broad, and thus regions of interest identified in this manner need to be refined using additional genetic strategies. One commonly used approach involves screening for associations between the disease locus and markers in the candidate region. To this end, additional microsatellite markers that increase the density of coverage (e.g., from 10 to 1 cM resolution) are placed across the region so as to search for disease-associated LD. The term LD is applied in instances in which association occurs in the presence of linkage, as opposed to situations in which association is found without linkage (e.g., in candidate gene analysis, or, spuriously, as a result of other factors such as population stratification). In the presence of LD, the cosegregation of two or more alleles across many generations and the consequent transmission of a "*haplotype*" of alleles arranged along a single chromosome can be demonstrated. The use of LD mapping in disease gene localization is predicated upon the notion that disease gene alleles segregate in association with a set of flanking alleles that comprise an ancestral haplotype derived from a founder individual who originally introduced the disease gene allele into the population under study. Thus, affected individuals may share a set of contiguous alleles within a chromosomal region that comprise a disease-associated haplotype encompassing the disease-related allele. Regions of LD are generally much smaller than "linked" regions and thus LD mapping can facilitate refinement of candidate regions elucidated from linkage data.

Additionally, the increasing definition of comprehensive maps of "blocks" of LD in the human genome should allow for LD mapping with SNPs "*tagging*" specific haplotypes and should therefore markedly reduce the numbers of SNPs required for LD mapping studies. Thus, for example, one analysis of such haplotype-tagging SNPs revealed the information provided by 122 genotyped SNPs to be completely reproduced by analysis of 34 SNPs, a 3.6-fold reduction in genotyping effort. Similarly, we have shown that any one of 11 SNPs within a 250 region on chromosome 5q31 serves to tag a Crohn's disease-associated haplotype at this locus. Thus, while complex haplotype structures are likely to be the rule rather than the exception in most regions of the genome, the identification of haplotype blocks, a major goal of the international HapMap consortium, should greatly reduce the number of SNPs required for both genome wide and refinement mapping efforts.

The transmission disequilibrium test (TDT) is a non-parametric test that is commonly used to identify association in the presence of linkage (i.e., LD) in datasets derived from "trio" families, (two parents and their affected child). This family-based association test involves comparison of the number of times a specific allele is transmitted to an affected offspring versus the number of times that allele is not transmitted, the expectation being that a marker allele in LD with the disease gene variant will be disproportionately transmitted to affected progeny. As TDT is typically carried out by analysis of trio families including a single affected individual, it is usually possible to ascertain many more families for TDT than for affected sib pair analysis.

To accommodate parent inavailability, variant approaches to TDT, incorporating, for example, affected/unaffected sib pairs in the absence of parental samples and extended family structures, have also been developed and can be combined with traditional TDT to increase power in datasets lacking some of the parental information. Although the TDT circumvents some of the major problems inherent to case-control association approaches (most notably, population stratification), under some circumstances, the latter strategy may have greater statistical power to detect disease associations with similar sized sample sets. Thus, the choice of study design and methodologies for association analyses is most often influenced by the presence or absence of suitable family structures in the sample set.

Case-control Genetic Association Studies

The increasing feasibility of candidate gene-based disease gene identification has engendered enormous interest in case-control genetic association studies, wherein relevance of a specific gene to a disease/phenotype is examined by comparing affected individuals and matched controls with respect to frequencies of particular allelic variants of the gene of interest. Such case-control studies involve the analysis of putative susceptibility (positively associated) or protective (negatively associated) alleles. This methodology has many advantages over traditional linkage analysis for disease gene discovery. Such advantages include, for example, lack of requirement for parental DNA samples, which may be very difficult or impossible to obtain in the context of late-onset diseases. Both family based and case-control association methods also involve the analysis of gene variants (polymorphisms) which may not only exhibit LD with the gene defect of interest, but which may actually represent the disease-relevant defect per se.

To render possible LD mapping in the context of a case-control design, statistical methods such as the expectation-maximization (EM) algorithm have been developed to enable definition of haplotypes (arrangements of alleles along a single chromosome) associated with disease susceptibility. One major consideration, however, which needs to be factored into any genetic case-control study, is the ethnic constitution of the cases versus the controls. Because of the potential for allele frequencies to vary significantly between different ethnic populations independent of differences related to disease susceptibility, divergence in the ethnic representation in cases compared to controls creates a significant potential for spurious false positive results. This problem, referred to as population stratification, together with inadequate sample size and incomplete or inaccurately derived assignment of phenotype, may account for the high rate of failure in replicating case-control genetic association data in independent studies.

To address these problems, standard guidelines identifying criteria required for rigorous case-control genetic association studies have been derived and include: large sample sizes (on the order of 1000 unrelated cases and at least as many controls); a requirement for low p values, appropriately corrected for multiple testing, and correspondingly high odds ratios for susceptibility; inclusion of a replication study performed on an independently ascertained population; and "biological sense" for the demonstrated association—that is, the disease-associated allele(s) should affect the gene product in a physiologically meaningful way. The last of these criteria, however, is often difficult to fulfill and even under circumstances in which all these criteria are met, some genetic association data still prove non-reproducible. Nevertheless, with the increasing availability of high-density SNP maps, better technologies for automated high-throughput SNP genotyping, international haplotype mapping (HapMap) data and higher quality DNA sequence data for most of the human genome, the quality of genetic association data is continually improving and this study design is almost certain to become the most practical and rapid approach to disease gene discovery, particularly for identifying genes relevant to late-onset diseases.

The potential for SNP-based genome-wide association studies to identify susceptibility genes in complex diseases have been investigated by assessing the extent of LD between known disease susceptibility genes and specific SNP markers flanking these genes. Data from one such analysis, for example, involving the *APOE* gene implicated in late-onset Alzheimer disease, revealed that of 10 SNPs lying within the 800kb flanking the gene, only three SNPs located 10, 12–30, and 440 kb, respectively, from APOE showed significant LD with APOE and strong association with Alzheimer disease.

By contrast, other SNPs located as little as 60–80kb from the gene showed no evidence of LD or disease association. LD has also been reported between a number of other genes and STR markers mapping up to 400kb from the genes of interest, although more typically, LD between disease genes and associated SNPs is in the range of 60 kb, at least for European Caucasian populations (59). The size of LD blocks across the genome is, however, highly variable, some regions of LD on chromosome 22, for example, spanning >700kb. Moreover, extent of LD across specific chromosomal segments is likely to vary between different ethnic groups, a point which needs to be considered in selecting haplotype-tagging SNPs for association studies.

These considerations illustrate the complexity inherent to SNP-based candidate gene analysis dependent on marker-disease LD and further highlight the need to analyze many SNPs in or near a gene of interest and to assess the impact of suspected disease-causing variants on the function and/or expression of the relevant gene product. The SNPs for such studies can be selected and prioritized based on their physical location near or within genes of interest, presence within a specific haplotype block, and/or by computational approaches enabling functional impact of SNP variants to be predicted and analysis thereby focused on putative deleterious SNPs.

Utility of Isolated Populations

Isolated populations have been used successfully to identify a number of complex disease loci, including for example, putative susceptibility loci for types 1 and 2 diabetes mellitus, multiple sclerosis, hyperlipidemia, and Hirschsprung's disease. In such populations, inbreeding and genetic isolation alters disease allele frequencies and often reduces genetic heterogeneity substantively compared with that found in outbred populations. Because affected individuals are more likely to share functional alleles identical by descent in this setting than in more admixed populations, the number of alleles contributing to a complex trait is likely to be lower and recessive genetic effects on phenotypes are more easily identified. Data from association studies have in fact directly shown the detection of small genetic effects on a quantitative trait to be enhanced in consanguineous populations. Similarly, inbreeding coefficients of approximately 0.01 have been shown to be associated with increased power in detecting the effect of a candidate gene.

In addition to consanguinity, isolated societies often contain large, multigenerational families with multiple affected individuals, a pedigree structure that greatly facilitates linkage analysis. In founder populations of recent origin, the extent of LD across a genetic interval may be larger than in older populations and therefore associations between polymorphic markers and a disease trait can be detected over greater genetic distances. This phenomenon may, however, represent a double-edged sword, potentially diminishing the extent to which genetics can be used to refine intervals of interest to sizes amenable to candidate gene analysis. In this latter situation, examination of a more outbred population may allow tighter refinement of the relevant interval, provided that the disease association seen in the inbred cohort is also present in the outbred population. Finally, population isolates may also have common traditions, lifestyles, and/or environmental exposures, which also contribute to overall lessening of the confounding effects of background environmental heterogeneity that may mask genetic effects in outbred populations.

Despite these advantages, there are a number of caveats to the interpretation of genetic data garnered from inbred populations. For example, distinguishing a disease-causing allele (which might be comparatively common in an inbred population) from a rare polymorphism unique to the population may be difficult in a population isolate. Consanguinity may also increase the type 1 error rate in sibling pair linkage analysis, leading to false positive linkage results. Finally, alleles identified as disease causative variants in such populations may be rare alleles that are not relevant to disease etiology in more admixed populations and the practical clinical utility of such data may therefore be limited to the isolated population studied.

Genome Sequence

The strategy of positional cloning, in which a disease gene is identified by virtue of its position within the genome rather than by functional characterization, has been used in the mapping and identification of many disease loci. However, with the completion of the human genome project, there has been a radical change in positional cloning technologies, the need for laborious physical mapping techniques such as radiation hybrid mapping, ordered library contigs, and pulsed-field gel electrophoresis mapping having been essentially abrogated by availability of the full genome sequence. Nevertheless, such resources are still of value in filling remaining sequence gaps and in understanding the biology of duplicated regions of the genome, which may not be correctly detected or assembled in genome sequence databases. The success of candidate gene identification by inspection of the genome sequence within a small region of linkage or LD is very much dependent on the accuracy and resolution of both genome sequence data and the precise positioning of both genetic markers and candidate genes. While the quality of human DNA sequence data in both public and private databases continues to improve, at the current time, not all genes are accurately represented or correctly predicted, and examination of multiple DNA sequence databases and gene prediction algorithms is still warranted.

Genetic maps provide critical tools for positioning disease gene loci ascertained from genome-wide or regional refinement linkage data within the framework of the sequenced genome. Integrating physical and genetic maps was, for many years, a laborious process and ambiguity as to the physical positions of some STRs often hampered efforts to identify disease genes. However, the physical positions of the markers used in contemporary genetic maps are now well established in relation to the genome sequence and the possibility to positionally clone disease genes has thus been greatly enhanced. A wide variety of genetic maps, including those derived by CEPH/Genethon and the Marshfield Clinic, are currently available and serve as the start-point for gene mapping studies. Nevertheless, it seems likely that in the near future, comprehensive SNP maps based on standardized panels of haplotype tagging SNPs will supplant these STR-based maps as the template for disease gene mapping projects.

Once the full complement of genes within a region of interest has been elucidated, the potential relevance of each gene to disease can then be explored. Identification of the sought after gene may be facilitated by prior knowledge of the gene product functions or expression patterns in tissues relevant to disease pathology. Our group's identification of *SLC22A4* and *SLC22A5* as Crohn's disease susceptibility genes, for example, was greatly facilitated by our data revealing these genes to be expressed in tissues relevant to intestinal inflammation, i.e., in cells of the colonic epithelium and in T cells and macrophages infiltrating colonic tissue. Based on such biological data, genes of interest can be prioritized for further investigation and studied by direct sequence analysis or other mutation detection methods (e.g., denaturing high-performance liquid chromatography or DHPLC) to identify disease-associated variants. As the genetic lesions responsible for complex genetic disease are likely to be more subtle (i.e., SNPs) than those found in single-gene disease, and will not be entirely correlated with the presence or absence of disease, verification of a candidate gene as etiologically relevant to this class of genetic disease will generally require some functional data linking the gene defect to the clinical phenotype.

Computational Algorithms and Database Mining

At the time of this writing, genome sequence for 9 of the 24 human chromosomes has been fully completed and the remainder will soon be available. These sequence data have dramatically changed the positional cloning process, substantively improving capacity to integrate genetic mapping with DNA sequence data and allowing for the application of computational methods to identify, within regions of interest, candidate genes, SNPs with potential pathological consequences, and other sequence properties of possible relevance to disease pathophysiology, such as transcriptional regulatory regions. Analysis of selected chromosomal regions for candidate genes has traditionally involved such strategies as exon trapping, CpG island identification, and isolation of cDNA clones representing genes within the region of interest. While such approaches may still be required to identify all of the genes within a given region, the need to involve these labor intensive strategies is progressively diminishing as new computational approaches and databases are used to prioritize and inform "wet lab"experimentation.

A number of programs incorporating algorithms for gene or exon prediction have been developed and output from many such programs is already available for the public builds of the genome sequence. The algorithms incorporated in such programs have varying sensitivities and specificities for exon/gene identification and a robust analysis would therefore require use of several such programs. Regions of interest can also be scanned for transcription start sites, potential splice sites, polyadenylation signals, CpG islands, transcription factor binding sites, and other indicators of coding sequence. In addition, sequences of interest can be compared by automated software methods to a database of expressed sequence tags (ESTs) in order to identify previously known transcribed sequences that correspond to genes in the region. The ESTs that occur in clusters, align to genomic sequence, are predicted by exon/gene prediction algorithms, and exhibit intron–exon structure are highly likely to represent fragments of *bonafide* genes, which will thus warrant further investigation.

Informatics is also key to many other aspects of positional cloning, such as, the mining of cumulative SNP databases. Novel computational approaches have been developed, for example, to assist in the identification of SNP variants with likely functional impact, such strategies incorporating epidemiological and evolutionary approaches and utilizing multiple sequence alignment comparisons of known or suspected functional domains. While some SNPs introduce easily predictable changes in protein function (e.g., a change of a conserved residue in an enzyme's catalytic site), others have more subtle effects, altering, for example, important non-coding regulatory regions or mRNA stability or engendering amino acid substitutions that appear conservative but have functional impact. In silico approaches to the identification of such functional variants are also emerging and include, for example, comparisons of comparable sites in genomes from different species and prediction of likely functional relevance based on the average rate of conservation between these species.

In addition to improvements in database mining strategies, increased sophistication in statistical methodologies for disease gene mapping is also a major factor in accelerating disease gene discovery research. Among the many difficult issues emerging from the trend to case-control study designs, a particularly important problem has been the analysis of non-phased genotype data (i.e., data in which the arrangement of alleles in haplotypes on individual chromosomes is unknown) in which haplotypes that may contribute to disease susceptibility cannot be explicitly determined. This problem has, however, been resolved to some extent through the development of algorithms such as the EM algorithm, a method now widely used to reconstruct haplotype frequency distributions from unphased genotype data. Association of specific haplotypes with disease susceptibility can then be determined using a likelihood ratio test based on the haplotype frequencies in cases as compared with controls. We have previously utilized EM analysis to show that a 250kb haplotype block delineated by 11 SNPs in strong LD contains a two SNP haplotype involving variants in the *SLC22A4* and *SLC22A5* genes, respectively, with genetic, functional and histopathological links to Crohn's disease. Identification of the *SLC22A4/SLC22A5* haplotype, which demonstrated the role of these genes in susceptibility to Crohn's disease, was made possible by use of these recently developed statistical methods.

Discovery of the genetic variants underlying the most prevalent and devastating human diseases is one of the most significant goals of the human genome project. As exemplified by the identification of *SLC22A4* and *SLC22A5* gene variants as susceptibility factors for Crohn's disease, highly integrated approaches to gene discovery can yield new knowledge of disease mechanisms, potential drug targets, and diagnostic tools. Ultimately, many such discoveries will lead to new insights into the mechanism of drug actions and toxicity and to the personalization of therapies based on the underlying genetic lesions specific to an individual's disease. While significant issues such as genetic heterogeneity, late onset of disease, and incomplete penetrance complicate disease gene isolation in complex, multifactorial disease, novel statistical, computational, and bioinformatic approaches, coupled to tremendous increases in throughput of genotyping technologies, have markedly accelerated the pace at which the genome can be screened and mined. In particular, the generation of genome-wide SNP microarrays and other very high throughput SNP genotyping technologies has brought genome-scale SNP association studies into the realm of possibility, from the standpoints of both cost and practicality.

To fully capitalize on the wealth of current and future disease gene discoveries, an acceleration in the pace at which such discoveries are translated to the clinic will also be required. Although DNA-based diagnostic products are now routinely used in many settings (e.g., mutation panels for diagnosis/risk prediction in Cystic Fibrosis, breast cancer, or cardiovascular disease), many attendant problems associated with the application of genetic data to the clinic remain unresolved. These include, for example, complex ethical, sociological, and legal issues that require continuous and proactive attention and management and the many problems inherent to communicating and even interpreting complex genetic data.

Despite these caveats, disease gene discovery has many potential immediate benefits, including, for example, the definition of disease-specific targets for pharmacological intervention and the possibility to personalize medical treatments so as to reduce risk and enhance efficacy. Disease gene discovery also opens the door to large-scale population studies directed at definition of the environmental-gene interactions which underlie disease, and for meta-analytical studies integrating data from multiple groups and thereby identifying the gene–gene interactions contributing to disease. These data, in turn, will inform and direct biological experimentation to elucidate underlying disease mechanisms. Such knowledge is anticipated to provide further novel drug targets, new molecular markers that can be used to stratify patient populations so as to predict severity, prognosis, and drug responsiveness, as well as basic knowledge of disease etiology of potential use in risk reduction. Ultimately, knowledge of the complete complement of genes which cause and modulate the common diseases afflicting humankind will shift the paradigm of medical care to "*individualized*" care, wherein disease risk can be identified and mitigated in healthy individuals and treatment for those affected by disease can be tailored so as to minimize toxicity and optimize efficacy of selected therapies. The era of genomic medicine is well underway, and the challenge in the early part of the 21st century will be to delineate the genetic basis of all human disease and to translate this extraordinary achievement to radical improvements in the quality of health care delivery.

20

RNAi in Drug Development

RNA interference (RNAi) is a phenomenon comprising the ability of double-stranded RNA (dsRNA) molecules to stimulate eukaryotic gene suppression in a sequence-specific manner. This article will first outline the essential molecular biological principles of RNAi and then focus on RNAi's practical applications. It will explain how dsRNAs can be delivered to or expressed inside mammalian cells, and what considerations are usually taken into account when choosing various RNAi approaches. In addition, the discussion describes how RNAi can be applied in the drug target discovery and validation process, and what potentials RNAi hold as a therapeutic modality.

RNAi phenomenon was first described, yet not properly understood, in the early 1990s, when instead of overexpression of transgenes responsible for pigmentation in plants, researchers observed "*cosuppression*" of the transgenes and their corresponding transcripts. It was later demonstrated in the nematodes *Caenorhabditis elegans* that dsRNA was causing the knockdown of homologous genes. Unfortunately, similar experiments using long dsRNAs in mammalian cells were unsuccessful. Introduction of long dsRNA into mammalian cells induced interferons and other stress-response genes, confounding the interpretation of data. In 2001, however, it was discovered that the effector molecules in the RNAi pathway were actually short dsRNA by-products (called short-interfering RNAs or siRNAs), generated by the cleavage of the long dsRNAs. This landmark discovery opened the door for use of RNAi in mammalian cells. Chemically synthesized siRNAs were then shown to effectively inactivate mRNA transcripts in many types of mammalian cells, suggesting a broadly conserved pathway for gene regulation. These findings marked a new chapter in the RNAi field, with its now widespread use in the biological community. By monitoring the phenotypes of RNAi-mediated gene knockdowns, it becomes easier to define the roles of corresponding proteins inside cells. This property of RNAi makes it an indispensable drug target discovery and validation tool. Furthermore, the unique nature of RNAi compounds makes them potential candidates for becoming drugs themselves. Indeed, by delivering RNAi compounds inside diseased cells and tissues and knocking down the genes that cause the problem, it is in principle possible to cure the illness.

RNAi Biology

RNAi Pathway

The natural role of RNAi has been theorized to be primarily cellular surveillance. RNAi functions as an antiviral and antitransposon system in diverse organisms. Indeed, animal and plant viral proteins, which inactivate the RNAi pathway at different steps, have been identified. Conversely, disruption of RNAi can lead to mobilization of transposable elements in the nematode *C. elegans*.

RNAi is initiated by trigger molecules usually dsRNAs. These can be formed during viral replication, from transcription antisense to an inserted gene or from aberrant "foreign" RNA structures detected in the cell. The first step in the RNAi pathway is the processing of these dsRNAs by a cytoplasmic RNase III enzyme. Appropriately named Dicer, the enzyme cuts the trigger into a series of ~22 bp siRNAs. This step produces multiple effector molecules from the original trigger dsRNA, in proportion to its size.

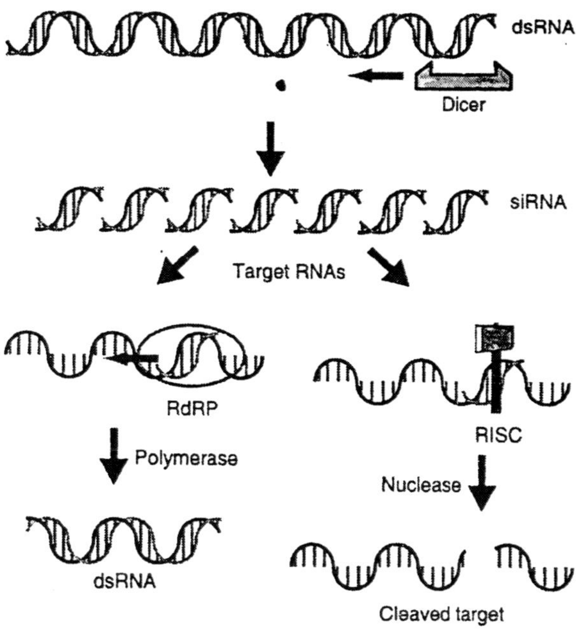

Fig. 20.1. The RNAi mechanisms.

In plants and nematodes, an additional amplification step involves the use of RNA-dependent RNA Polymerase (RdRP). The siRNAs can act as primers for RdRP to produce additional dsRNA using the homologous RNA as a template. Amplification may lead to two additional phenomena in these organisms—transitive and systemic RNAi. Transitive RNAi occurs when the original trigger molecule complements only one part of a target message. RdRP can extend siRNA primers binding this region of the target into more distal, usually 5′ regions. The dsRNA that results is then processed into new siRNAs, including those from regions not part of the original trigger. Systemic RNAi describes the spread of RNAi-mediated silencing from one cell or tissue in the organism to another. For example, in *C. elegans*, injection of dsRNA into the gut can trigger silencing in many other cell types, including germ cells. Silencing occurs in the injected animal's offspring and can last for several generations. Systemic RNAi requires RdRP-mediated amplification to produce sufficient trigger for silencing throughout the organism. In addition, it requires a system for transport of the silencing signal across cell membranes.

While they serve as primers for RdRP in some organisms, the primary function of siRNAs is as the RNA guide in the RNA-induced silencing complex (RISC). One strand of each small RNA duplex is "*loaded*" into RISC by a complex including Dicer and the RNA-binding protein R2D2. The other strand is rapidly degraded. Selection of a strand for loading is biased by the relative thermodynamic stability of the duplex ends: the more stable end tends to be bound by R2D2; the strand with its 3′ terminus at this end enters RISC. This RISC-incorporated "*guide strand*" is then used by RISC to identify complementary sites in target RNAs, which are cleaved within the base-paired region.

Various components of RISC have been identified in different organisms, but the key constituent, the nuclease or "Slicer," is an Argonaute protein. Argonautes share two motifs: the PAZ domain, which binds to the 3′ end of the siRNA guide strand, and the catalytic Piwi domain, which structurally resembles an RNase H.

MicroRNAs

MicroRNAs (miRNAs) are a diverse class of endogenous RNAs that regulate complementary targets through components and mechanisms overlapping with the RNAi pathway. The first miRNAs, lin-4 and let-7, were discovered by forward genetics in *C. elegans*. Later, attempts to clone siRNAs from cell lysates led to the discovery of hundreds of endogenous approximately 21–25 nt miRNA sequences in mammals, flies, and worms.

Analysis of genome sequences has revealed that miRNAs are derived from hairpin precursors (pre-miRNAs). Many of these are thought to be expressed from RNA polymerase II (Pol II) promoters, with the miRNA sequences lying within the introns of protein-coding genes and in both introns and exons of non-coding RNAs. The pre-miRNAs are processed from the transcripts in which they reside by the nuclear RNase III Drosha and the predicted dsRNA-binding protein DGCR8/Pasha. Transport to the cytoplasm is mediated by exportin-5, which also traffics some tRNAs out of the nucleus. In the cytoplasm the pre-miRNAs, which are partially double-stranded, are cleaved by Dicer to produce a short-lived duplex. In a manner analogous, if not identical to RISC loading of siRNAs, one strand of this duplex enters RISC or a RISC-like complex containing Argonaute. Like siRNAs, miRNAs complement the mRNAs whose expression they regulate. Many plant miRNAs and at least one animal miRNA complement their targets nearly perfectly and cleave them through an RNAi-like mechanism. Others carry multiple mismatches to their targets and regulate them by inhibiting translation.

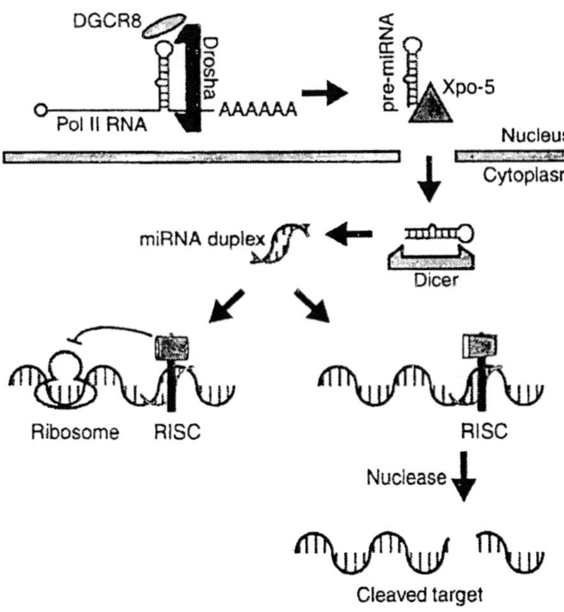

Fig. 20.2. The microRNA (miRNA) pathway.

Because miRNAs need not perfectly complement the transcripts they influence, miRNA target prediction can be difficult. There may be thousands of genes regulated by miRNAs through both strong and subtle interactions, and miRNAs themselves are often expressed in a regulated, cell-type specific manner. Relatively few biological functions for miRNAs have been identified, but the growing list includes differentiation and development, cell death and proliferation, aging, and fat metabolism.

RNAi Technological Aspects

RNAi with Synthetic Effector Molecules

The key challenges to achieving efficient gene silencing with RNAi compounds are delivery, potency, duration of activity, and specificity. Efficient delivery of RNAi molecules to cells is critical to achieving gene silencing in cell cultures (in vitro) and in whole organisms (in vivo). Commercial cationic lipid reagents are the mostly widely used method for delivering siRNA molecules into cultured mammalian cells. Optimal transfection conditions must be determined empirically for each cell type. Complexes of cationic lipid reagent and negatively charged nucleic acid molecules, termed "*lipoplexes*," are internalized most likely through adsorptive and fluid-phase endocytosis. Most lipid formulations also contain a helper lipid component such as dioleoylphos-phatidylethanolamine (DOPE) to facilitate release from the endosomal compartment by promoting vesicle membrane destabilization. Once internalized and released from the endosomal compartment, siRNAs can interact with cytoplasmic RISC to trigger silencing of homologous gene targets. Failure to achieve high levels of gene silencing in cultured mammalian cells is often because of poor uptake or inefficient release of siRNAs within the cytosol.

The use of fluorescently labeled siRNA molecules allows for visual monitoring of cellular uptake of dsRNA following lipid-mediated transfection, and is a good general indicator of transfection efficiency. Uptake is often optimized by altering the ratio of siRNA to lipid transfection reagent, thereby adjusting the charge ratio between nucleic acid and cationic carrier. An increase in the concentration of siRNA and/or lipid often results in higher transfection efficiency, but, in some cases, may also increase cellular toxicity. Optimal transfection conditions should incorporate a balance between transfection efficiency and toxicity. The amount of targeted siRNA that gives good inhibition of gene expression can usually be titrated down to reach the lowest effective level, to further minimize toxicity and potential off-targeting effects. For example, early RNAi experiments in mammalian cells used high concentrations of siRNA (often 100 nM or higher). Toxicity and off-target effects become very real risks at such high levels. Today, with better design rules, siRNAs can be identified, which are highly effective at much lower concentrations (2 nM or lower) with equal or better activity to their historical counterparts.

Most adherent cell types can be efficiently transfected with lipid reagents. Even notoriously hard to transfect cells such as neurons, certain primary cells, and embryonic stem cells can be successfully transfected under optimized conditions with the appropriate reagents, presumably because siRNAs only need to be delivered to the cytoplasm (unlike DNA plasmids that must enter the nucleus for expression). For reasons that are not yet clear, suspension cells tend to be refractory to lipid-based transfection and typically require electroporation or viral-based methods for delivery of siRNA. While electroporation efficiently delivers naked siRNA directly to the cytosol for access to RISC, thereby bypassing the endosomal compartment, the extensive cell death that results and large amounts of siRNA required are prohibitive for broader-range applications.

Once delivered to the cytosol, the silencing effect of siRNA molecules can be maximal as early as 18-hr post-transfection, while typically lasting two to four days in rapidly dividing cultured mammalian cells. Loss of activity is attributable to dilution through cell division and degradation by intracellular exo- and endonuclease activity. Chemical modifications to siRNAs can extend silencing activity for up to a week or more, presumably by conferring stabilization against nuclease activity. Furthermore, it appears that the more active the target site is, the longer the knockdown effect tends to last in the cell.

The discovery that siRNAs could be delivered exogenously to mammalian cultured cells to achieve targeted gene silencing opened the possibility for RNAi experiments to be performed on a wide scale in mammalian systems. The earliest RNAi studies utilized chemically synthesized siRNAs designed according to rules that specified siRNAs to be 19-mer dsRNA duplexes (sense and antisense complementary strands) with 3′ 2-nt deoxythymidine overhangs and 100% homology (anti-sense strand) to the target mRNA. Alternative, low-cost methods for generating siRNAs include digestion of long dsRNA (prepared using in vitro transcription) by purified Dicer enzyme prior to delivery into cells. In a few cases, where induction of the interferon (antiviral) response is not an issue, such as with mammalian oocytes and embryonic stem cells or fly cells, long dsRNA has been introduced directly into cells to serve as a substrate for endogenous Dicer activity. While each of these methods can lead to targeted gene silencing, the use of multiple sequences such as with pooled synthetic siRNAs or Dicer-generated siRNAs is generally reserved for high- throughput phenotypic screening assays (HTS), where identified "hits" can be followed up more rigorously with individual siRNAs to verify a given phenotype and rule out potential artifacts or off-target effects.

Sequencing of the human genome opened the possibility that short dsRNA sequences could be designed to silence virtually any gene in the entire genome. However, similar to past experience with antisense oligonucleotide design, it was immediately recognized that not all siRNA sequences were effective at triggering gene silencing. Identification of sequences with activity against a particular gene target has typically required screening through several (five or more) sequences to identify one or two with good activity (≥70% inhibition of gene expression). Recently, the labor and expense of screening has been significantly reduced by the development of algorithms that incorporate extensive basic local alignment search tool (BLAST) searching, sequence effects, thermodynamic properties, and other criteria to successfully select sequences with high activity and specificity. Recent research revealed that the efficiency of RNAi is determined largely by directional incorporation and unwinding of siRNAs in the RISC. The most thermodynamically unstable end (and therefore most easily unwound) of a given siRNA is preferentially incorporated into RISC, thereby determining whether the sense or the antisense strand is utilized as the guide strand to trigger silencing. Other studies have determined that some changes in siRNA structure can be tolerated without significant loss in activity, such as elimination of 3′ overhangs, changes in overall length, or addition of mismatches or chemical modifications to certain regions. Overall, a 15-mer central region containing the cleavage domain and largely intolerant of mismatches is thought to be essential for RISC activity. Similarly, the 5′ end of the antisense strand, where unwinding initiates, is sensitive to modification and does not tolerate mismatches with the target sequence. With advanced in silico design programs, it is now possible to routinely identify highly potent sequences that are active at low picomolar levels and that inhibit gene expression by 90% or greater. However, a subset of sequences remains that conform to design rules, but display poor activity against the target gene. A better understanding of the regulation of expression of these gene targets, along with further insight into how the base composition and structure of siRNAs function within RISC to trigger mRNA degradation, may lead to the design of highly specific and potent dsRNAs against the vast majority of targets.

Chemical modifications in RNAi compounds can also improve specificity of gene knock-downs by reducing the possibility of two undesired events: (i) off-target effects related to sense strand activity and (ii) activation of cellular stress response pathways. The ability of unmodified siRNA to stimulate off-target effects, i.e., knockdown of transcripts not intentionally targeted for destruction, was first reported in early 2003 using whole-genome expression profiling. Such non-specific effects can, in part, be attributed to the potential role of the siRNAs' sense strand. By chemically modifying the RNAi duplexes, however, it is possible to secure the exclusive activity of the antisense strand. Activation of cellular stress response pathways is yet another problem associated with certain unmodified RNAi compounds. The nature of such stimulatory effects, while not entirely understood, appears to be sequence specific, and chemical modifications in the RNAi duplexes can alleviate the problem. Indeed, siRNA sequences that have been shown to induce stress responses can become non-stress inducing by the addition of chemical modifications, without a loss in knockdown activity. Overall, the use of chemical modifications, contemporary design algorithms, pretested compounds, and appropriate experimental procedures can dramatically reduce the risk of the artifactual events associated with RNAi knock-downs and improve the quality and interpretation of the achieved results.

The use of exogenously delivered siRNAs to trigger gene silencing in vitro is advantageous, because the method is relatively simple, is cost-effective, and can be used to rapidly screen multiple gene targets. A primary drawback is that gene targets with particularly long protein half-lives will invariably be difficult to silence at the protein level. In such cases, stable long-term silencing driven by RNAi effector molecules expressed endogenously may be required.

RNAi with Endogenously Expressed Effector Molecules

To produce stable and long-lasting knockdown, viral vectors have been developed to efficiently express siRNAs or short hairpin RNAs (shRNAs) in a wide variety of mammalian cells. Expression vectors include standard plasmids as well as those made from adenoviruses, adeno-associated viruses (AAVs), onco-retroviruses, and lentiviruses. The viral expression systems have the added benefit of being able to deliver siRNA, shRNA, or miRNA expression cassettes efficiently into cell types that are otherwise difficult to transfect via common transfection or electroporation protocols.

The design of shRNAs most commonly features a 19–21 bp duplex that is joined by a 4–9nt loop sequence. The transcript is typically expressed by an RNA polymerase III (polIII) promoter, usually U6 or H1. PolIII promoters are ideal for this application for several reasons:

1. They can be designed to start and stop transcription at specific locations to create the requisite shRNA.
2. Their natural role in the cell is transcription of short, non-coding RNAs.
3. They are typically highly and constitutively expressed in most mammalian cell types.

Following transcription, the nascent transcript is transported out of the nucleus and into the cytoplasm where it is converted to an siRNA by Dicer.

An alternative vector-driven RNAi tool is patterned after the endogenously expressed miRNAs. Engineered miRNA transcripts can be driven by polII promoters and therefore have the potential to be expressed in a tissue- or temporal-specific manner. As with shRNAs, miRNA-based constructs can be delivered to cells via viral vectors. The miRNAs are designed to perfectly match their targets so that the mechanism of gene silencing is mRNA cleavage, making the resulting gene silencing as robust as that seen with shRNAs and siRNAs.

RNAi Applications

Gene Function Analysis in Cultured Cells

Since the discovery that RNAi can be induced in mammalian cells, considerable effort has gone into harnessing this mechanism and developing it into tools for genetic analysis. RNAi allows researchers to use a "*reverse genetics*" approach, determining the function of a gene by virtue of its disruption. Moreover, the tools of RNAi can be easily scaled up for use in high-throughput assessments, for instance, with attempts to decipher complex biochemical pathways. As described above, there are many ways that RNAi can be utilized to generate targeted gene knockdowns. The approach used is dictated by the nature of the questions asked, the organism or cell culture system, and the phenotypic readout.

With the large amount of genomic sequence information available, it has become possible to design and undertake a systematic genome-wide functional screen to examine the biological roles of tens of thousands of genes. Using the method of reverse transfection, it has been demonstrated that cultured cells can take up nucleic acid/lipid complexes that have been previously deposited on a plate. The coupling of RNAi and reverse transfection has made it possible to perform high-throughput "*loss of function*" assessment in mammalian cells. To illustrate the feasibility of this approach, prototype microarrays were assembled and used to cotransfect luciferase-directed siRNAs along with a luciferase reporter construct, yielding a robust knockdown of the reporter protein in a number of cell lines. To further validate the method, RNAi reverse transfection was used to target endogenous transcripts involved in cytokinesis and proteasome-mediated proteolysis in cultured mammalian cells.

While RNAi has obvious utility in reverse genetics, it also has tremendous potential in its use for discovering genes by forward genetics. Forward genetics is the strategy of identifying novel cellular components as a result of their induced mutant phenotype. By administering RNAi reagents to cells, isolating cell populations with novel phenotypes, and identifying the responsible silenced genes, rapid insight can be gained into complex physiological cellular processes.

In one study, a retroviral library of more than 23,000 shRNAs targeting nearly 8000 genes and a human fibroblast cell line with a temperature-sensitive block in p53-dependent proliferation were used in a forward genetic strategy to identify genes involved in the cancer- relevant p53 signaling pathway. Under conditions that would normally result in blocked cell growth, clones resistant to p53- and p19ARF-dependent proliferation arrest were selected. Genomic DNA from such clones was then pooled, and PCR amplified to generate shRNA inserts. By hybridizing the amplification products against a master shRNA array, vectors that conferred resistance to p53- and p19ARF-dependent proliferation arrest were identified. Amongst these were modulators of the p53 pathway, including p53 itself and five novel genes.

In another example, two conceptually similar strategies, called siRNA production by enzymatic engineering of DNA (SPEED) and enzymatic production of RNAi libraries from cDNA (EPRIL), recruited a series of enzymatic and cloning steps to convert a population of normalized double stranded cDNAs into shRNA expression libraries. The key advantages of these approaches include low cost of library production and high flexibility with the starting material (i.e., mRNA from diverse sources can be used). In addition, no knowledge of individual expressed sequences is required. SPEED- and EPRIL-generated shRNA libraries are expected to be useful for high-throughput whole-genome forward genetics screens. Among the powerful assets afforded by RNAi is the ability to discriminate amongst gene family members, even those that share a high degree of identity at the amino acid and nucleotide level. For example, using an shRNA collection directed against the family of deubiquinating enzymes, the tumor suppressor CYLD (encoded by the familial cylindromatosis susceptibility gene) was identified as a suppressor of NF-κB activation. This finding led to a therapeutic strategy to treat individuals suffering cylindromatosis.

Drug Target Validation In Vivo and RNAi Therapeutics

The term "*drug target validation*" continues to evolve within the research and development community. To some, the definition suggests that a target is validated when it is shown, in vitro, to be critically involved in a disease process such that modulation of this target is likely to have a therapeutic effect. Others may not consider a target to be truly validated until being proven to be effective in animal or human trials. The use of RNAi in vivo is still in its infancy and recent proofs of concept experiments are generating a great deal of excitement. However, as standard siRNAs are, by their nature, just two annealed strands of RNA, they are extremely sensitive to degradation by naturally occurring ribonucleases. One significant advance was the development of chemically modified siRNAs to increase plasma stability. Covalent chemical modifications have been widely used to stabilize and prolong activity of antisense oligonucleotides. Drawing from the expertise gained in the antisense field, siRNAs have been synthesized with a variety of chemical modifications without a loss of knockdown function. Synthetic RNAi molecules can be injected directly at the site of desired action, for example, into a solid tumor, the eye, limb joints, or the brain. Current data indicate that these direct delivery methods are enhanced by the combination of the siRNA with a lipid or other formulation. For many therapeutic applications, this may become the method of choice, because this approach would be expected to have less systemic side effects and requires much less material than a whole-body delivery.

Synthetic RNAi can also be administered systemically, with or without specific tissue targeting. Early efforts for RNAi delivery have focused on the direct administration of synthetic siRNAs. The first of these, termed "*hydrodynamic delivery*," is achieved when siRNA, i.e., suspended in roughly 1 ml of saline solution, is rapidly administered to the mouse via tail vein injection. The resulting high venous pressures force siRNA primarily into the cells of the mouse liver, kidney, and lung. In a study where the TNFR family member fas was targeted, 80–90% of fas mRNA was silenced in the 90% of the hepatocytes, which internalized the siRNA. The silencing was robust for up to 10 days. In other studies conducted in vivo, gene silencing was achieved by injecting smaller volumes of siRNAs packaged in cationic liposomes and administered without high venous pressure. As in the previous study, silencing was primarily seen in highly perfused tissues such as the lung, liver, and spleen. A more directed approach for delivering siRNAs was demonstrated with an siRNA modified by conjugating a cholesterol moiety to the 3′ end of the sense strand. Again, lower amounts of siRNA were required in the absence of high venous and organ pressure. This strategy was successful in targeting mouse *apoB* mRNA in the liver and jejunum as a regimen of reducing total serum cholesterol.

A number of other molecular modifications have also been shown to improve cell and tissue delivery of siRNAs. These modifications include conjugating siRNAs to membrane-targeted peptides such as monoclonal antibodies and then formulating into liposomes to encapsulate them. An alternative approach using peptide-targeted nanoparticles proved successful by assembling polyethyleneimine, polyethylene glycol and an Arg-Gly-Asp (RGD) peptide with the siRNA. This encapsulated siRNA was targeted to a tumor's neovasculature by virtue of the surface integrins that bind RGD. Both tumor growth and tumor angiogenesis were inhibited by an siRNA targeting vascular endothelial growth factor receptor-2 (VEGF-R2). Other formulations include other targeting proteins incorporated into "pegylated" immunoliposomes (PILs). These have been shown to direct gene silencing in a number of tissues, including brain. As compared to hydrodynamic delivery, these tissue-targeting strategies demonstrate some success in delivering siRNAs into an in vivo model using methods that more approach clinically acceptable routes of administration. For many in vivo applications, target gene knock-down must persist for an extended period of time (i.e., weeks, months, or even permanently). Further, if the target gene is essential, inducible knockdown methods are desirable. The best approach for extended or inducible gene knockdown is with DNA vector-based RNAi. This can be accomplished by transcription of an shRNA or miRNA designed to target the gene of interest. The use of recombinant viral vectors to deliver RNAi expression cassettes in vivo (via retroviruses and lentiviruses) has been reported to produce a stable and robust knockdown. Lentivirus has also been successful both ex vivo, targeting p53 in $CD34^+$ hematopoetic precursor cells, and in vivo, targeting transgene expression in the mouse brain. In another example, AAV was shown to efficiently deliver shRNA expression cassettes against mutant ataxin-1 into the brains of a spinocerebellar ataxia type 1 mouse model.

For the production of transgenic animals, lentiviral vectors that express shRNAs have been used This approach has been utilized mostly in mice, but can be applied to other organisms that are not amenable to traditional, homologous recombination-based gene knockout approaches. Embryonic stem cells or eight-cell embryos that are transduced with shRNA-expressing lentiviruses can generate animals in which gene expression is permanently knocked down in all cells and tissues. Moreover, because RNAi sequences may vary in their extent of silencing, it is possible to produce mice with graded degrees of silencing. This may be important in evaluating genes that are known to be linked to disease. Producing an RNAi mouse only requires the insertion of a single shRNA cassette; so "knockdown" mice can be generated in a fraction of the time that is required to produce a "knockout" mouse via traditional methods. RNAi technology has a short yet very prolific history. In less than four years since the first demonstration that RNAi compounds can work in mammalian cells, the technique has found its way into virtually every relevant academic and industrial institution in the world. One of the reasons for such success most likely stems from the desperate need to assign functions to the numerous genes identified during the human genome project. RNAi technology has become a tool to fulfill such need by finally enabling reverse genetics in mammalian cells. Another reason for enhanced interest in RNAi is its promise to become a new and powerful therapeutic modality. The potential of quick development of a drug based on simple information about the primary sequence of the target gene has always been a dream of drug developers.

The role of RNAi as a gene functional analysis and, hence, as a drug target discovery and validation tool has been at least partially utilized. Numerous projects have been reported, which successfully utilized RNAi to define novel functions to various genes. The key challenges for the future here are combining RNAi with the high-throughput screening and high-content phenotypic approaches, utilizing the most relevant disease cell systems (e.g., primary cell culture), and developing versatile and reliable in vivo approaches. Even more attractive, yet more difficult to achieve, therapeutic potentials for RNAi are being explored very aggressively by many industrial and academic groups. At this point, the key challenge is in developing reliable and physiological cell type and tissue-specific delivery protocols. If this task is accomplished, the potential for the RNAi will be truly astounding.

21

Recombinant DNA Technology

The biopharmaceutical sector is largely based upon the application of techniques of molecular biology and genetic engineering for the manipulation and production of therapeutic macromolecules. The majority of approved biopharmaceuticals are proteins produced in engineered cell lines by recombinant means. Examples include the production of insulin in recombinant *E. coli* and recombinant *S. cerevisiae*, as well as the production of EPO in an engineered (Chinese hamster ovary) animal cell line.

Terms such as '*molecular biology*', '*genetic engineering*' and 'recombinant DNA (rDNA) technology' are sometimes used interchangeably and often mean slightly different things to different people. Molecular biology, in its broadest sense, describes the study of biology at a molecular level, but focuses in particular upon the structure, function and interaction/relationship between DNA, RNA and proteins. Genetic engineering, on the other hand, describes the process of manipulating genes (outside of a cell's/organism's normal reproductive process). It generally involves the isolation, manipulation and subsequent reintroduction of stretches of DNA into cells and is usually undertaken in order to confer on the recipient cell the ability to produce a specific protein, such as a biopharmaceutical. 'rDNA technology' is a term used interchangeably with '*genetic engineering*'. rDNA is a piece of DNA artificially created *in vitro* which contains DNA (natural or synthetic) obtained from two or more sources. When developing a new protein biopharmaceutical, one of the earliest actions undertaken entails identifying and isolating the gene (or complementary DNA (cDNA)) coding for the target protein, the generation of an appropriate piece of rDNA containing the protein's coding sequence and the introduction of this rDNA into an appropriate host cell such that the target protein is made in large quantities by that engineered cell. This chapter aims to provide an introductory overview of the approaches and techniques used to isolate the target gene, generate an rDNA sequence and introduce it into an appropriate producer cell. Before we look at these techniques, however, we will briefly review the basic biology and structure of nucleic acids.

Nucleic acids: Function and Structure

Nucleic acids represent a prominent category of biomolecule present in living cells. The term incorporates both DNA and RNA. DNA represents the repository of genetic information (the genome) of most life forms. RNA replaces DNA as the repository of genetic information in some viruses. In most life forms, however, RNA plays a role in mediating the conversion of genetic information stored in specific DNA sequences (genes) into polypeptides. There are three subcategories of RNA, each playing a different role in the conversion of gene sequences into the amino acid sequence of polypeptides. Messenger RNA (mRNA) carries the genetic coding information from the gene to the ribosome, where the polypeptide is actually synthesized. Ribosomal RNA (rRNA), along with a number of proteins,

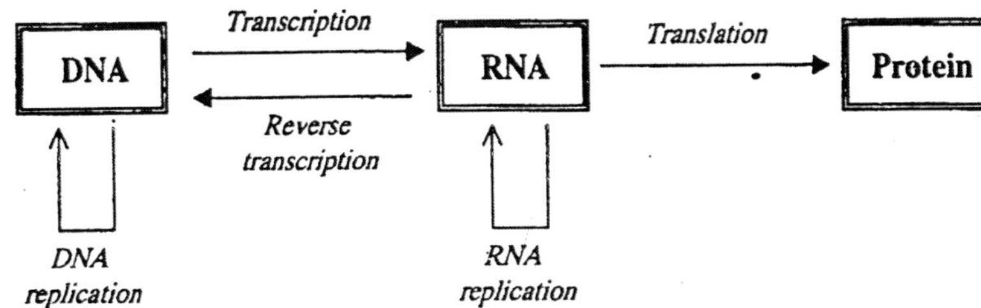

Fig. 21.1. Schematic representation of the so-called central dogma of molecular biology.

forms the ribosome itself, and transfer RNA (tRNA) functions as an adaptor molecule, transferring a specific amino acid to a growing polypeptide chain on the ribosomal site of polypeptide synthesis. Therefore, nucleic acids, between them all, mediate the flow of genetic information via the processes of replication, transcription and translation as outlined in what has become known as the central dogma of molecular biology.

Structurally, nucleic acids are polymers in which the basic recurring monomer is a nucleotide (i.e. nucleic acids are polynucleotides). Nucleotides themselves consist of three components: a phosphate group, a pentose (five-carbon sugar) and a nitrogenous-containing cyclic structure known as a base. The nucleotide sugar associated with RNA is ribose, whereas that found in DNA is deoxyribose. In total, five different bases are found in nucleic acids. They are categorized as either purines (adenine and guanine, or A and G, found in both RNA and DNA) or pyrimidines (cytosine, thymine and uracil, or C, T and U). Cytosine is found in both RNA and DNA, whereas thymine is unique to DNA and uracil is unique to RNA.

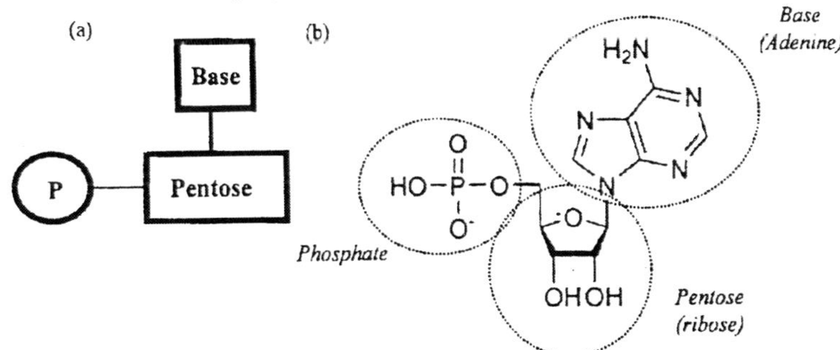

Fig. 21.2. (a) The basic structure of a nucleotide. (b) The actual chemical structure of one representative nucleotide.

The DNA or RNA polymer consists of a chain of nucleotides of specific base sequence, linked via phosphodiester bonds. RNA is a single-stranded polynucleotide, although RNA molecules tend to adopt higher order three-dimensional shapes. DNA, on the other hand, is a double-stranded molecule that assumes a double helical structure. The two polynucleotide strands face each other in an antiparallel manner, with the hydrophilic sugar and phosphate residues facing outwards, towards the surrounding aqueous-based environment, and the more hydrophobic bases point inwards. The base sequence of each chain displays complementarity. Wherever thymine is found in one chain, adenine is found positioned opposite it in the other. Wherever guanine is found in one chain, cytosine is found positioned opposite it in the second chain. Complementarity provides an obvious mechanism to ensure the fidelity of DNA replication and to underline transcription. The double helical DNA structure is stabilized by (a) hydrogen bonding between complementary opposite bases (two hydrogen bonds between A and T, three hydrogen bonds between G and C) and (b) by hydrophobic stacking interactions between the planar, largely hydrophobic bases effectively stacked above each other along the length of each strand.

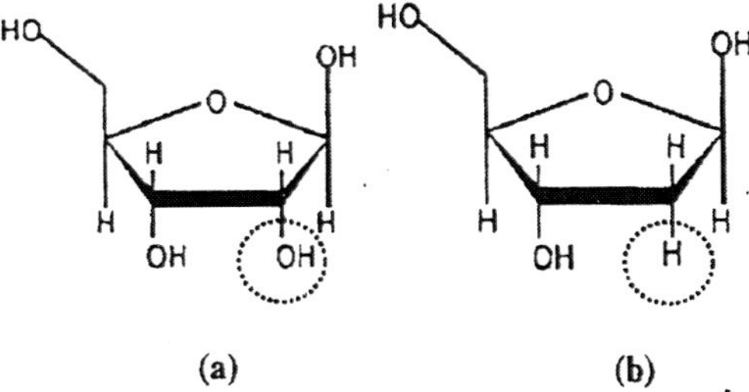

Fig. 21.3. Chemical structure of (a) ribose and (b) 2′-deoxyribose, the nucleotide pentoases found in RNA and DNA respectively.

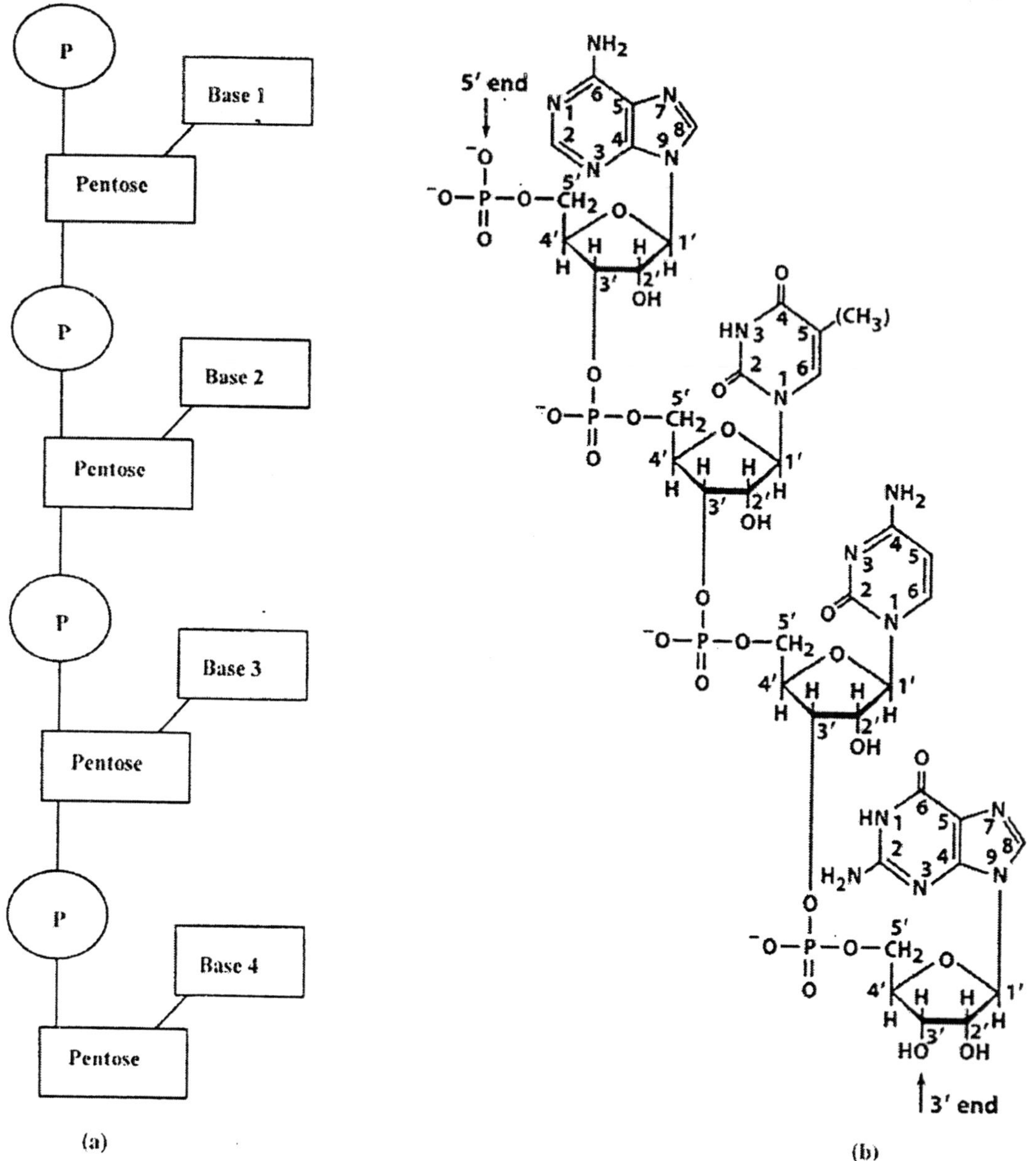

Fig. 21.4. The basic polynucleotide structure as shown in (a) outline form and (b) in chemical detail. The 5′ end of the chain is defined by lacking a nucleotide attached to the first sugar's carbon number 5; the 3′ end lack a nucleotide attached to the carbon number 3 of the last sugar in the backbone.

Genome and Gene Organization

The genome refers to the entire hereditary information present in an organism. As discussed earlier, this is usually encoded by double-stranded DNA (the genome of most plant viruses and some animal and bacterial viruses is RNA based). DNA-based genomes are largely or exclusively organized into chromosomes, each chromosome being a single DNA molecule housing multiple genes, as well as non-coding sequences. Bacteria normally harbour a single, circular chromosome that tends to be tethered to the bacterial plasma membrane and tends to have few if any closely associated proteins. Many bacteria also contain extra-chromosomal DNA in the form of plasmids, as will be discussed later. Eukaryotes (plants, animals and yeasts) posses multiple linear chromosomes contained within a cell nucleus, and these chromosomes are normally closely associated with proteins termed histones (the protein–DNA complex is termed chromatin). Eukaryotes also invariably possess DNA sequences within mitochondria and in chloroplasts in plants. The (usually circular) DNA molecules are much shorter than chromosomal DNA, are often present in multiple copy number and tend to house genes coding for proteins required within these organelles. Human mitochondrial DNA, for example, is 6600 base pairs (6.6 kbp) in length and houses 37 genes. Such DNA molecules are believed to be vestiges of chromosomes from ancient bacteria that gained entry into early eukaryotic cells.

Table 21.1 The number of chromosomes found in selected species/ cells, along with their predicted/ estimated (approximate) number of genes

Cell/species	*No. chromosomes*	*No. genes*
E. coli	1	4400
S. cerevisiae	16	6200
Fern	1200	13600
Fruit fly	18	13000
Mouse	40	30000–35000
Rat	42	23000
Dog	78	19300
Human	46	30000–35000

The genomes of different species are organized into different numbers of chromosomes. Chromosomes present in all cells contain both coding regions (i.e. genes, which are stretches of DNA that encode the specific amino acid sequence of a particular polypeptide or the exact nucleotide sequence of a tRNA or rRNA) and non-coding regions. Coding regions, as we will subsequently see, often represent only a small fraction of total genome sequences.

In close association with gene sequences are regulatory elements, i.e. stretches or regions of DNA that mark the beginning or end of a gene or a series of related genes or which regulate the level of gene expression. A characteristic regulatory sequence upstream (i.e. on the 5' side) of a gene is termed the promoter region (P), which RNA polymerases (the enzymes responsible for transcribing the gene into RNA) identify and bind. Immediately adjacent to this is a characteristic sequence that represents the starting point for transcription (T_C). Immediately downstream of the gene is a transcriptional termination site (t_C). The intervening sequence, of course, represents the precise stretch of DNA that is copied into RNA and is often called the *transcriptional unit*.

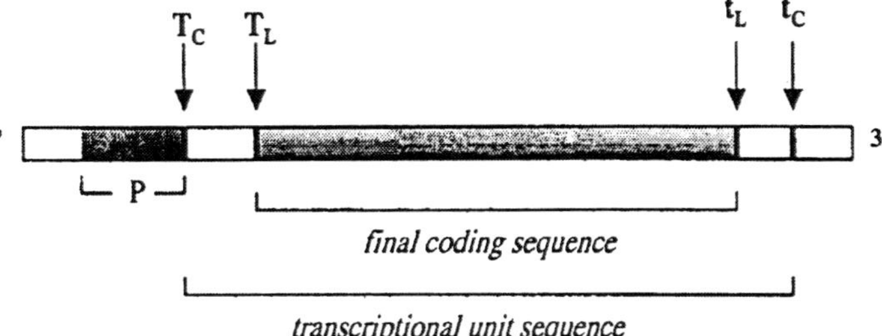

Fig. 21.5. Generalized gene organization within the genome.

The gene sequence will often contain start and stop signals or sequences (T_L and t_L) that ultimately dictate the precise stretch of transcriptional unit actually translated into polypeptide. Other regulatory regions controlling gene expression can also be present, either upstream and/or downstream of the gene itself. In addition to genes and their associated regulatory sequences, DNA molecules also invariably

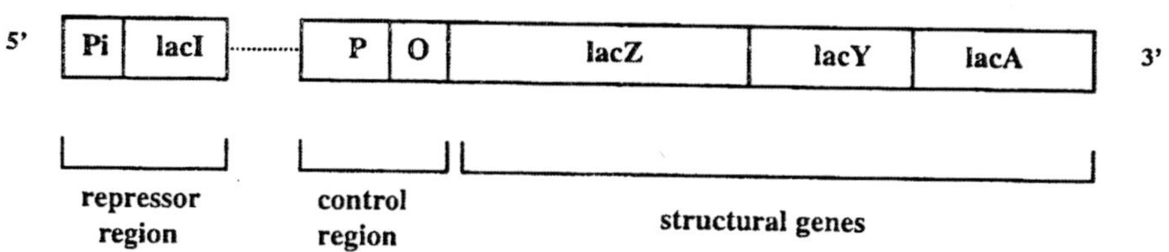

Fig. 21.6. The lac operon houses three structural genes: lacZ, lacY and lacA.

house additional non-coding sequences in the form of various kinds of repeat sequences. For example, genes account for only some 30 per cent of the total human genome sequence. The detail and arrangement of gene structure is also normally different in prokaryotes and eukaryotes. In prokaryotes, genes of related function are often clustered together in operons, which are usually under the control of a single promoter/ regulatory region.

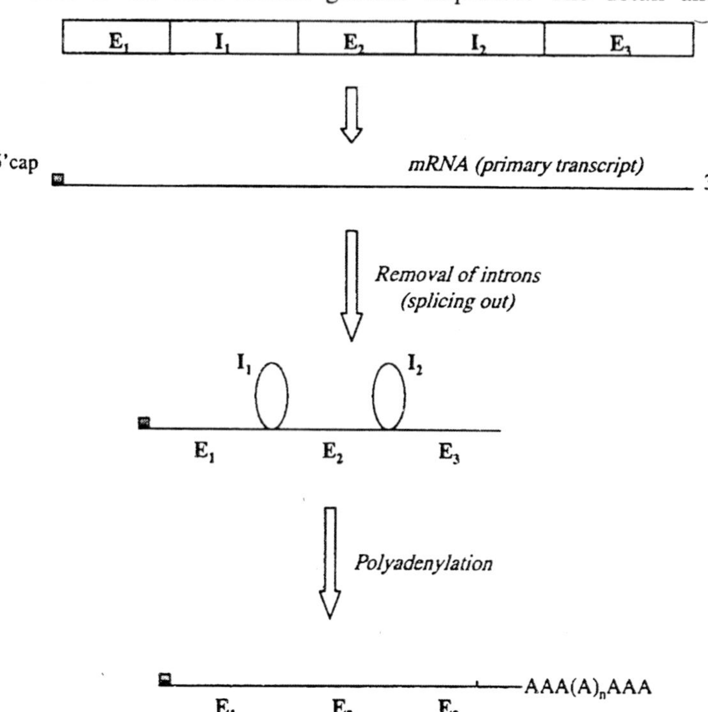

Fig. 21.7. Overview of the transcription of eukaryote genes and subsequent mRNA editing.

Transcribed operon mRNA thus usually contains coding sequence information for several polypeptides, and such mRNA is termed polycistronic. Although common in prokaryotes, the presence of polycistronic operons is infrequent in lower eukaryotes and essentially absent from higher eukaryotes, where virtually all protein-encoding genes are transcribed separately. Eukaryotic genes, however, usually contain coding sequences (exons) that are interrupted by non-coding intervening sequences (introns), and in many cases exons represent a minor proportion of the entire gene length. For example, of the 30 per cent of the human genome believed to be taken up by genes, an estimated 28.5 per cent is accounted for by introns with only some 1.5 per cent being accounted for by exons. mRNA transcripts in eukaryotes undergo substantial editing. The introns are enzymatically removed from (spliced out of) the primary transcript, and further characteristic modifications include the addition of a cap at the mRNA's 5' end and the addition of a polyadenine nucleotide tail (poly A tail) at the molecule's 3' terminus.

Nucleic Acid purification

A prerequisite step to any rDNA work is the initial isolation of DNA or RNA from the source material (which can be microbial, plant, animal or viral). Numerous methodologies have been developed to achieve nucleic acid purification, and some of these methodologies have been adapted for use in a variety of commercially available purification kits. Although details vary, the general approach adopted entails initial liberation of the nucleic acid by disruption of any cell wall present (or viral capsid) and of the cellular plasma membrane, followed by selective precipitation and often chromatography. In the context of plants and some microorganisms, initial disruption of the cell wall may require application of physical or other vigorous disruptive influences. This can potentially complicate DNA purification, particularly as it can cause physical shearing (fragmentation) of the extremely long DNA chromosome. The gentlest method of cell lysis usually involves incubation with cell-wall-degrading enzymes, and the addition of detergent will solubilize the plasma membrane.

Following cellular disruption, initial purification steps normally entail solvent-based extraction/ precipitation. For example, shaking in the presence of phenol (or a mixture of phenol and chloroform), followed by standing or centrifugation (to achieve phase separation) results in extraction of the (now denatured) proteins into the phenol phase and/or accumulation at the interphase, with nucleic acids remaining in the upper, aqueous phase. Further purification may be achieved by selective precipitation of the nucleic acids using ethanol or isopropanol as precipitant. If DNA is required, then the RNA present may now be removed by the addition of the enzyme ribonuclease, which selectively degrades RNA. On the other hand, if (eukaryotic) mRNA is required, then affinity-based purification may be undertaken using an oligo(dT) column. Nucleic acids absorb UV light maximally at 260 nm (compared with 280 nm in the case of proteins); thus, absorbance at 260 nm can be used to quantify the amount of nucleic acid present and to follow the purification protocol. The ratio of absorbance at 260 nm versus 280 nm can also be used to determine how contaminated the nucleic acid preparation is with protein. The ratio $A_{260}/A_{280} \approx 1.8$ for pure DNA and 2.0 for pure RNA preparations; lower ratios usually indicate the presence of contaminant protein. DNA can also be detected and quantified by the addition of the chemical ethidium bromide. Ethidium bromide molecules intercalate (bind) in between DNA bases and fluoresce when illuminated with UV light.

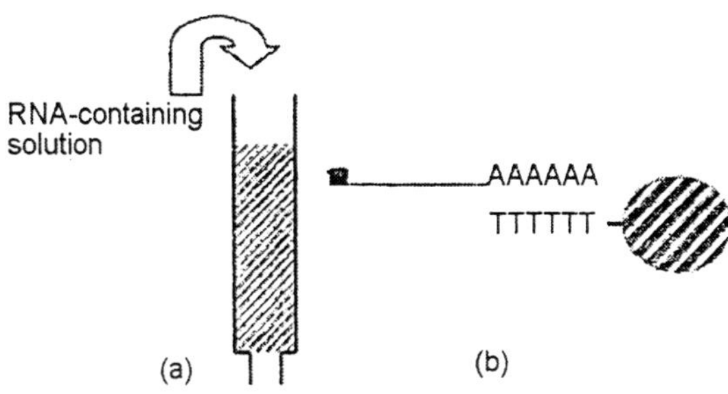

Fig. 21.8. Affinity-based purification of mRNA.

Nucleic Acid Sequencing

The determination of the exact base sequence present in a stretch of nucleic acid (particularly in DNA) underpins much of modern molecular biology. Sequencing plays a central role in rDNA cloning experiments, as well as in determining genome data. Two approaches have been developed to sequence DNA: the Maxam–Gilbert chemical sequencing method and the Sanger–Coulson enzymatic sequencing method. Both involve the ultimate generation of a full set of fragments of the DNA strand to be sequenced. The methodologies employed ensure that the identity of the final (3') base in each fragment is known. The fragments are then separated on the basis of their size by electrophoresis and, because the identity of the end base in each fragment is already known, the full sequence can simply be read from the ladder of fragments generated. Full details of sequencing methodologies are outside the scope of this book, but they are included in all core molecular biology and biochemistry student textbooks. RNA is sequenced by an enzyme-based method somewhat similar to the enzyme-based DNA method.

Recombinant Production of Therapeutic Proteins

The evaluation of any protein as a potential biopharmaceutical and its subsequent routine medical use are dependent upon the availability of sufficient quantities of the target protein. In most instances this is best achieved via production by recombinant means (i.e. via genetic engineering). In addition to facilitating the production of any protein in substantial quantities, recombinant-based production can have a number of additional advantages over direct extraction from a naturally producing source. Production of any protein via rDNA technology entails the initial identification and isolation of a DNA sequence coding for the target protein. This sequence can be direct genomic DNA, but mRNA coding

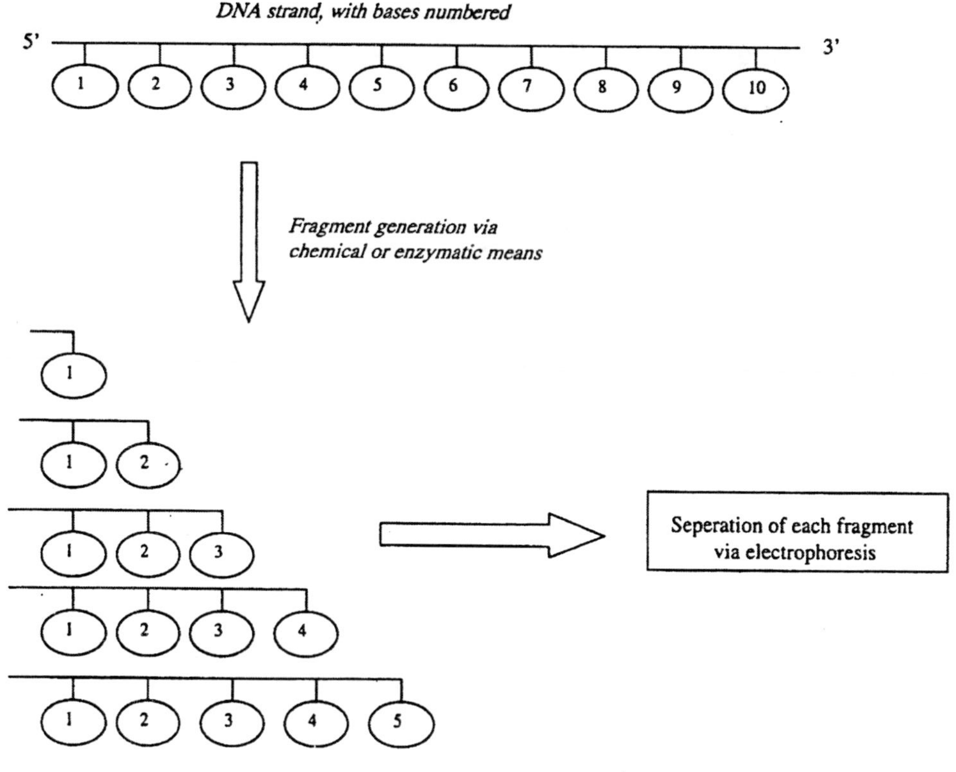

Fig. 21.9. A simplified overview of the approaches adopted to both chemical and enzyme-based DNA sequencing.

for the protein of interest can also act as a starting point. In the latter approach, the mRNA is enzymatically 'reverse transcribed' into cDNA. If the target therapeutic protein is eukaryotic (which is invariably the case) then the genomic DNA will contain both coding (exon) and non-coding (intron) sequences, whereas the cDNA will be a reflection of the exons only.

The desired gene/cDNA is normally amplified, sequenced and then introduced into an expression vector that facilitates its introduction and expression (transcription and translation) in an appropriate producer cell type. All recombinant therapeutic proteins approved to date are produced in *E. coli*, *S. cerevisiae* or in animal cell lines (mainly CHO or BHK cells). The general characteristics of these various producer cells and their advantages and disadvantages, along with factors taken into account when choosing one for biopharmaceutical production, are points considered elsewhere. In the remainder of this chapter we will review the basic molecular biology techniques that underpin the isolation, identification, cloning and expression of a target protein-encoding gene sequence. We will first overview the classical approach to cloning, which entails the generation of genomic libraries as described immediately below. We will then consider an alternative approach that has now come to the fore, and which is based upon the polymerase chain reaction (PCR) technique.

Classical Gene Cloning and Identification

The basic approach to cloning a segment of DNA entails:

1. Initial enzyme-based fragmentation of intact genomic DNA (usually chromosomes isolated) so that it is broken down into manageable fragment sizes for further manipulation. Ideally all/most fragments will contain one gene.

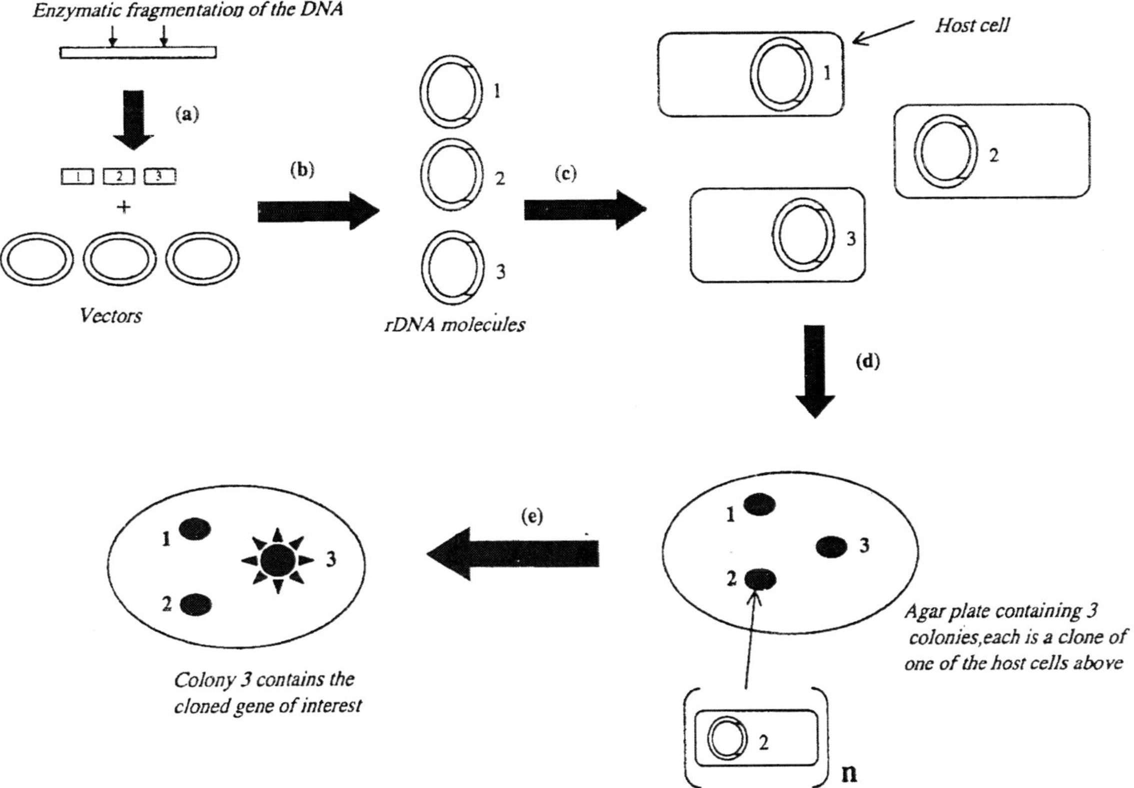

Fig. 21.10. A basic overview of the DNA cloning process.

2. Integration of the various fragments generated into cloning vectors, which are themselves small DNA molecules capable of self-replication. Typically, these are plasmids or viral DNAs and the composite or engineered DNA molecules generated are called rDNA.
3. Introduction of the vectors housing the DNA fragments into host cells.
4. Growing these cells on agar plates.
5. Screening/identification of the host cell colonies containing the rDNA molecules (i.e. screening the 'library' of clones generated) in order to identify the specific colony containing the target DNA fragment, i.e. the target gene.

We will now look at each of these stages separately. The initial fragmentation of genomic DNA is undertaken using enzymes known as restriction endonucleases (REs). Some 800 different REs have been identified thus far. These enzymes recognize, bind and cut DNA sequences which exhibit a defined base sequence. These sequences normally exhibit a twofold symmetry around a specific point and are usually 4, 6 or 8 bp in length. Such areas are often termed palindromes. In general, the larger the recognition sequence the fewer such sequences present in a given DNA molecule and, hence, the smaller the number of DNA fragments that will be generated. Depending upon the specific RE utilized, DNA cleavage may yield blunt ends (e.g. BsaAI and EcoRV) or staggered ends – the latter are often referred to as sticky ends.

An essential feature of the cloning vector used is that it must be capable of self-replication in the cell into which it is introduced, which is usually *E. coli*. Two of the most commonly used types of vector in conjunction with *E. coli* are plasmids and bacteriophage λ. Plasmids are circular extrachromosomal DNA molecules, generally between 5000 and 350,0000 bp in length, that are found naturally in a wide range of bacteria. They generally house several genes, often including one or more genes whose product renders the plasmid-containing cell resistant to specific antibiotic(s). One plasmid often used in cloning experiments with *E. coli* is pUC18. Bacteriophage ('phage') are viruses capable of infecting and replicating inside bacteria. Bacteriophage λ DNA is approximately 48,500 bp in length. Another vector type sometimes used are the bacterial artificial chromosomes (BACs), which are effectively very large plasmids used to clone very large stretches of DNA (usually DNA fragments above 100,000 bp).

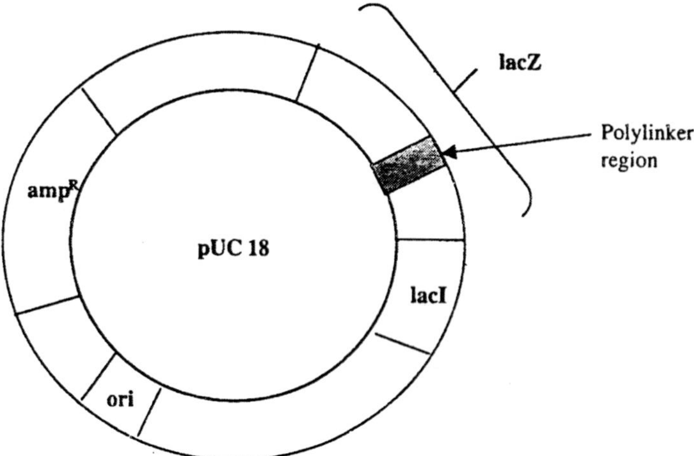

Fig. 21.11. The plasmid pUC18 is often used for cloning purposes.

Table 21.2 Some commercially available REs, their sources, DNA recognition sites and cleavage points

Restriction enzyme	*Source*	*DNA recognition sequence and cleavage site*
BclI	*Bacillus caldolyticus*	5'-T↓GATCA-3' 3'-ACTAG↑T-5'
BglII	Recombinant *E. coli* carrying *BglII* gene from *Bacillus globigii*	5'-A↓GATCT-3' 3'-TCTAG↑A-5'
BsaAI	Recombinant *E. coli* carrying *BsaAI* gene from *Bacillus stearothermophilus* A	5'-PyAC↓GTPu-3' 3'-PuTG↑CAPy-5'
BsaJI	*B. stearothermophilus* J	5'-C↓CNNGG-3' 3'-GGNNC↑C-5'
BsiEI	*B. stearothermophilus*	5'-CGPuPy↓CG-3' 3'-GC↑PyPuGC-5'
EcoRV	Recombinant *E. coli* carrying *EcoRV* gene from the plasmid J62 pIg 74	5'-GAT↓ATC-3' 3'-CTA↑TAG-5'
MwoI	Recombinant *E. coli* carrying cloned *MwoI* gene from *Methanobacterium wolfeii*	5'-GCNNNNN↓NNGC-3' 3'-CGNN↑NNNNNCG-5'
Tsp509I	*Thermus* sp.	5'-↓AATT-3' 3'-TTAA↑-5'
XbaI	Recombinant *E. coli* carrying *XbaI* gene from *Xanthomonas badvii*	5'-T↓CTAGA-3' 3'-AGATC↑T-5'
XhoI	Recombinant *E. coli* carrying *XhoI* gene from *X. holcicola*	5'-C↓TCGAG-3' 3'-GAGCT↑C-5'

Integration of the DNA fragments into the chosen vector is undertaken by 'opening up' the circular vector via treatment with the same RE as used to generate the DNA fragments for cloning, followed by co-incubation of the cleaved vector and the fragments under conditions that promote the annealing of complementary sticky ends. Some vectors may simply recircularize to reform their original structure, but pretreatment of the vector in various ways can prevent this from happening. Most of the recircularized plasmids will have incorporated a fragment of DNA to be cloned. The plasmids are then incubated with another enzyme, a DNA ligase, which catalyses the formation of phosphodiester bonds in the DNA backbone and thus will seal or 'ligate' the plasmid. The next stage of the cloning process entails the introduction of the engineered vector into *E. coli* cells. This can be achieved by a number of different means. One approach (called *transformation*) involves co-incubation of the plasmids and cells in a solution of calcium chloride, initially at 0°C, with subsequent increase in temperature to 42°C. This temperature shock facilitates entry of plasmids into some cells.

The *E. coli* cells are next spread out on the surface of an agar plate and incubated under appropriate conditions in order to kill cells that have not taken up plasmid. Each individual cell will thus form a colony (clone of cells). Three main types of cell will be initially transferred onto these agar plates: (a) some cells will have failed to take up any plasmid; (b) some transformed cells may have a plasmid in which no foreign DNA had been inserted; (c) some cells will house a plasmid that does carry a fragment of the target DNA. These latter cells are the only ones of interest, and various strategies may be adopted to identify them. Once the various *E. coli* clones (colonies) containing vector into which DNA fragments have been successfully integrated (i.e. clones containing rDNA) have been identified, all that remains to be achieved is to pinpoint which colony harbours the rDNA fragment containing the gene of interest.

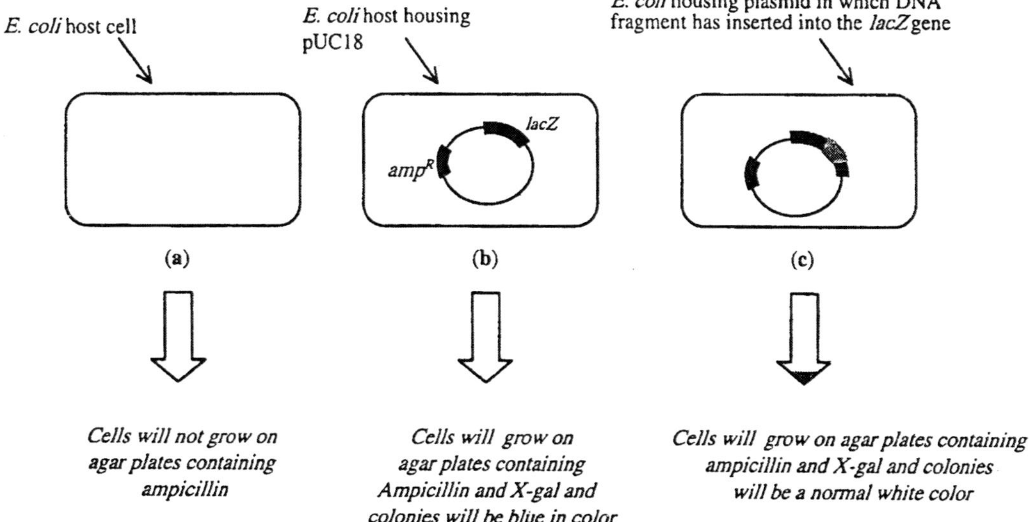

Fig. 21.12. Identification of E. coli host cell clones containing rDNA using pUC18 vectors.

Assuming you started off with whole genomic DNA, the procedure thus far has effectively generated a library of clones containing different genomic DNA fragments. The final task remaining, therefore, is to identify which specific clone/clones harbour the actual DNA fragment of interest (in our context this would be the fragment containing the gene coding for the desired therapeutic protein). This can be a major task, as libraries often consist of 10^9 or more clones. The most common means of achieving this is via sequence-based hybridization studies. The basic approach taken entails the use of a labelled (e.g. radioactive) probe that is a single-strand DNA fragment or an RNA fragment synthesized to have a base sequence complementary to a sequence within the gene of interest. Genome projects now mean that such sequence information is known for many proteins. Alternatively, likely base sequences can be deduced if a partial amino acid sequence of the protein is known. Hybridization studies are usually initiated by physically pressing a nitrocellulose paper onto the agar plates containing the recombinant colonies. A replica of the plate is thus created on the paper, as some cells from each colony adhere to it. Subsequent treatment of the paper with alkali lyses the cells, releasing and denaturing the DNA within. The DNA adsorbs tightly to the paper.

The paper is then exposed to a solution containing the labelled DNA probe under conditions that allow it to anneal to the target DNA, if it is present. After washing (to remove unbound probe), any probe retained on the paper surface can de detected by an appropriate visualization technique (e.g. autoradiography if the probe is radiolabelled), and the positioning of the label on the paper surface pinpoints which colony on the agar surface houses the desired DNA fragment. Cells from the appropriate colony can then be grown up in larger amounts by submerged fermentation in order to produce larger amounts of the desired (now cloned) gene. The cells can be collected, lysed and the vector therein recovered by standard microbiological techniques. The cloned gene can then be excised from the vector via treatment with an appropriate RE and purified by standard molecular techniques.

cDNA Cloning

An alternative to cloning genomic DNA, as outlined in the sections above, entails beginning the process not with chromosomal fragments but with mRNA. This is often an approach taken when cloning eukaryotic genes in particular. Total eukaryotic cellular mRNA can be purified from the cell via an affinity-based mechanism. The mRNAs recovered in this way reflect only the polypeptide-encoding genes that are expressed in the cells at the time of their extraction. Incubation of the mRNA with the enzyme reverse transcriptase results in the conversion of the single-stranded mRNA into double-stranded DNA known as cDNA. These cDNA fragments can then be cloned to generate a cDNA library, and the desired cDNA clone can be identified by means similar to those already described in the context of cloning genomic DNA. cDNA libraries are smaller than genomic libraries as they are derived only from expressed genes. Non-coding regions in the genome (as well as quiescent genes and genes coding for rRNA and tRNA) are not represented in the library. Therefore, cDNA libraries are more manageable to work with, assuming that the gene of interest is being expressed.

Cloning via Polymerase Chain Reaction

An enormous number of individual genes have been sequenced over the last two decades or more. Of latter years in particular, genome projects have also begun to make available the sequence of the entire complement of genes present in many species. The bulk of this sequence information has been made publicly available by its deposition in sequence databases. As a result, scientists who now wish to clone a particular gene will usually have prior access to partial/entire sequence information from the relevant organism or a closely related species. This sequence information allows them to obtain large amounts of the gene of interest by using the PCR technique. This approach to cloning has now come to the fore, as it is faster and more convenient than the more classical methods described above. The process begins by extraction of total genomic DNA from the source of interest (e.g. human cells if you wish to clone a specific human gene).

Oligonucleotide primers whose sequences flank the target gene/DNA segment are synthesized and used to amplify that portion of DNA selectively. Recognition sites for REs can be incorporated into the oligonucleotides to allow cloning of the amplified gene, as outlined earlier. Because the target gene sequence is the only segment of the extracted DNA to be amplified by the prior PCR step, the vast majority of clones in the library now generated should contain the desired gene. This can be confirmed by direct sequencing of the inserted DNA fragment from several of the colonies. Sequencing is important not only to prove definitively that the cloned DNA is the target gene, but also that its sequence perfectly matches the published sequence. The PCR process is prone to the introduction of sequence errors.

Expression Vectors

The vectors described thus far have been designed to facilitate the cloning of genomic DNA/ cDNA sequences, ultimately in order to identify and isolate a gene/cDNA coding for a particular polypeptide. The genetic construction of these vectors normally does not support the actual expression (i.e. transcription and translation) of the gene. Once the gene/cDNA coding for a potential target protein has been isolated, the goal usually becomes one of achieving high levels of expression of this target gene. This process entails ligation of the gene into a vector that will support high-level transcription and translation. In addition to the basic vector elements (e.g. an origin of replication and a selectable marker, such as an antibiotic resistance gene), expression vectors also contain all the genetic elements required to support transcription and translation, as described earlier in this chapter (e.g. promoters, translational start and stop signals, etc.). A wide range of such expression vectors is now commercially available and, obviously, each is tailored to work best in a specific host cell type (e.g. bacterial, yeast, mammalian, etc.).

Protein Engineering

The advent of rDNA technology renders straightforward the manipulation of a protein's amino acid sequence. This process, termed site-directed mutagenesis or protein engineering, entails the controlled alteration of the nucleotide sequence coding for the polypeptide of interest such that specific, predetermined changes in amino acid sequence are introduced. Such changes can include insertions, deletions or substitutions. Site-directed mutagenesis is now most often undertaken by using a variant of the basic PCR method already described, known as '*overlap PCR*', in which primers of altered nucleotide sequences are used for the PCR reactions.

Protein engineering facilitates a greater understanding of the link between a polypeptide's amino acid sequence and its structure. It also provides a powerful method of studying the relationship between structure and its function. As such, this technique will help greatly in achieving the much pursued, but still distant, objective of *de novo* protein design. Protein engineering is also used to tailor structural or functional attributes of therapeutic and other commercially important proteins. An increasing proportion of therapeutic proteins gaining approval for general medical use display an engineered amino acid sequence, altered in order to fulfil a predefined therapeutic goal better. An alternative approach to protein engineering entails the covalent attachment or the alteration of specific molecules/groups to or on the polypeptide's backbone.

Plasmid DNA

Extracted from the nucleus of human cells in the kitchen of Tubingen's castle (Germany), Nuclein is an heterogeneous product that was introduced in 1868 by further fractionated Nuclein and isolated in 1889 the substance that he named "*nucleic acids.*" These molecules were characterized by Albrecht Kossel (1853–1927, winner of the Nobel Prize for Medicine in 1910). Kossel used chemical hydrolysis of nucleic acids to identify their basic components: the nucleotides. Five nucleotides are found in the Nuclein: two purines [adenylic acid (A) and guanylic acid (G)] and three pyrimidines [cytidylic acid (C), uridylic acid (U), and thymidylic acid (T)]. In 1910, Kossel could also distinguish between two families of nucleic acids present in Nuclein: one is degraded at high pH and contains A, C, G, and U; one is resistant and contains A, C, G, and T. The precise chemical structure of the nucleotides was deciphered by a student of Kossel: Phoebus Levene (1869–1940) together with Walter Abraham Jacob (1883–1967) in 1929.

These researchers found that nucleotides consist of a nitrogen base (Adenine, Guanine, Cytosine, Thymine, or Uracile), a sugar (pentose), and a phosphate group. They also found that nucleotides are linked linearly in the order of phosphate-sugar thanks to phosphodiester bonds. This way, they generate a polymer with a phosphodiester backbone. The pentose in the high-pH-sensitive nucleic acid is a ribose, whereas in the high-pH-resistant nucleic acid, it is a 2′-deoxyribose. Based on this chemical difference are the names of the two nucleic acids: RNA for the ribonucleic acid and DNA for the deoxyribonucleic acid. Although the Nuclein contains RNA and DNA, the cytosole of cells was shown by Tornbjorn Caspersson (1911-1998) and Jean Brachet (1909-1988) to contain only RNA.

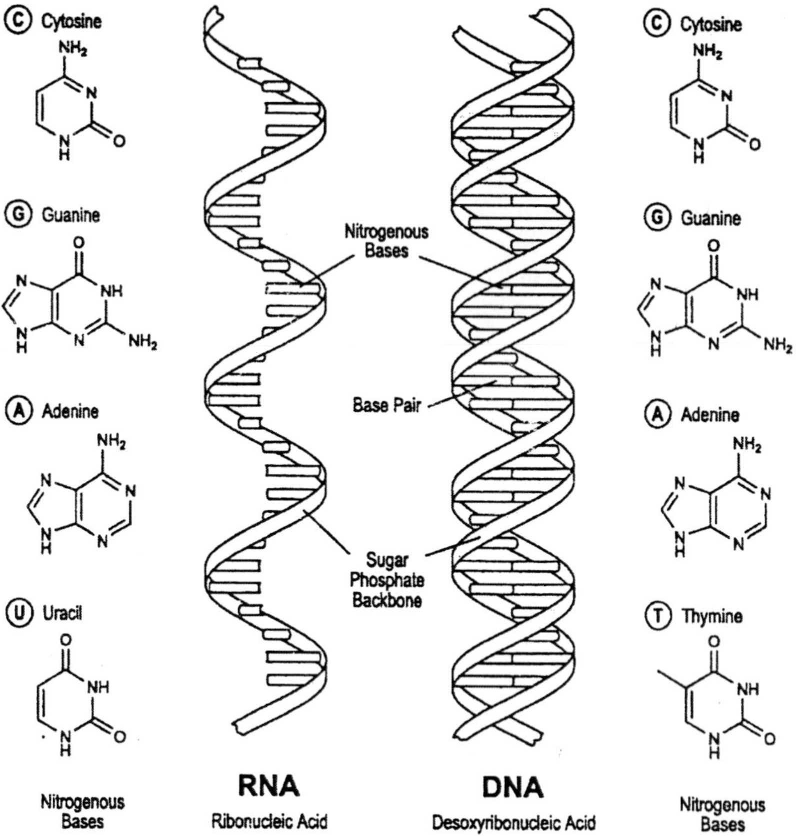

Fig. 21.13. Structure of DNA and RNA molecules.

In 1953, Jim Watson (1928), Francis Crick (1916-2004), and Maurice Wilkins (1917), who received the Nobel Prize in 1962 for their resolution of the structure of DNA, demonstrated that, thanks to specific hydrogen bonds between their base moieties, nucleotides are complementary: A pairs with T or U using two hydrogen bonds and G pairs with C using three hydrogen bonds. Helped by the x-ray photograph of DNA obtained by Rosalind Franklin (1920–1958), they proposed that DNA is a molecule with two antiparallel strands shaped in a regular helix of a 2 nm diameter and 3.4 nm step (10 nucleotides for one turn) with its phosphodiester backbone on the outside and the bases on the inside of the helix. One year earlier, in 1952, Alfred Hershey (1908–1997, Nobel Prize winner in 1969) and Martha Chase (1 927–2003) demonstrated using T2 phages that DNA is the genetic material in bacteria. There results confirmed the conclusions of Oswald Theodore Avery (1877–1955) who showed in 1943 that the "*transforming principle*" that can modify *Pneumococcus*'s phenotype from "smooth" to "rough" is DNA. By deduction and because of the location and behavior of DNA in eukaryotic cells, it was admitted, before being experimentally demonstrated, that DNA is the genetic material in higher organisms as well.

Meanwhile, the characterization of the cytosolic RNA-rich granules called ribosomes and identified by Albert Claude (1898–1983, Nobel Prize in 1974) indicated that RNA is involved in protein synthesis. Such a function of RNA was first hypothesized by Torbjoern Caspersson (1910–1997) and Jean Brachet (1909–1998) at the end of the 1930s and was then based on the relation between the RNA content of cells and their activity (proliferation). Ribosomes contain ribosomic RNA (rRNA) and are the site of protein production. The key intermediate between nucleic acids and proteins is the hybrid aminoacyl-RNA molecule called transfer RNA (tRNA) identified in 1958. It consists in a family of at least 20 members in any organism. A tRNA is a short (between 75 and 85 nucleotides) RNA molecule linked at its 3′ end to one amino-acid. Finally, the identification of an unstable RNA called messenger (mRNA) which is a copy of genes to be translated into proteins completed the basic description of the fundamental protein machinery. It is summarized in Crick's central dogma of molecular biology: DNA contained in the nucleus is transcribed into (messenger) RNA, which is translated into proteins. Since the formulation of this central dogma, the molecular mechanisms involved in these processes have been characterized in detail.

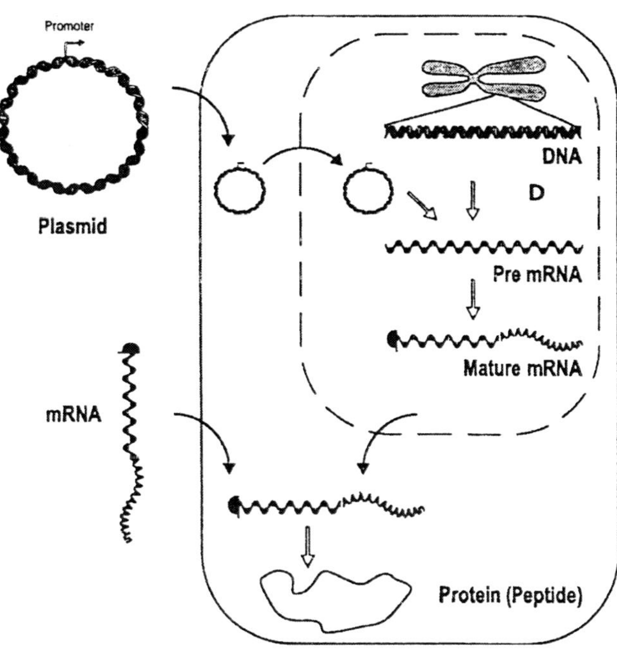

Fig. 21.14. *Central dogma.*

Of interest, we now know that the transient nature of all RNA molecules compared with DNA is not due to the chemical structure difference (in cells, pH are neutral or acidic: DNA and RNA are practically equally stable at the chemical level) but due to the abundance inside and outside the cells of potent and stable ribonucleases (RNases). We have also learned that RNA has more functions than initially postulated: It can replace DNA as genome in viruses and eventually (i.e., in retroviruses) be reverse transcribed into DNA. Moreover, several types of RNA molecules with various biological activities (structure, enzyme activities, containment of gene information) are involved in each step of gene expression. Nowadays, thanks to the molecular biology methods, we can also introduce designed foreign DNA and RNA molecules into cells. As proposed by Crick et al. in 1961, through a genetic code based on three letters (three consecutive bases: a codon), the nucleic acid information copied from the DNA genome into mRNA is translated in proteins. Each possible codon ($4^3 = 64$ possibilities) corresponds to one precise amino acid. This genetic code is universal: It is conserved between all living organisms. As there are only 20 amino acids, most of them are encoded by more than one codon.

Some codons are favored (more frequently found in highly expressed genes) in a species-specific manner. For example, alanine, which is encoded by four codons would be preferably encoded by GCA in *Bacillus subtilis*, by GCC in *Homo sapiens*, by GCG in *Escherichia coli*, and GCT in *Saccharomyces cerevisiae*. The correspondence between codons and amino acids, i.e., the fundamental translation process, is performed by specialized enzymes called aminoacyl tRNA synthetases. There are at least 20 different aminoacyl tRNA synthetases in any organism. Each is responsible for loading one amino acid on the adequate tRNA(s). By transferring a specific amino acid on a specific tRNA, which has the adequate anticodon (complementary to the codon in the mRNA), aminoacyl tRNA synthetase convert genetic information (nucleotides) into protein information (amino acids).

DNA: Stable Genetic Information Store

In eukaryotic cells, DNA molecules are located in the nucleus. During the interphase (between two cell divisions) of the cell cycle, DNA molecules are packed by histones into an heterogenic structure called the chromatin. Through intense condensation of the chromatin, each DNA molecule can be visualised as a chromosome during mitosis or meiosis. A human cell contains 23 pairs of DNA molecules that consist altogether ca. 3.15×10^9 bases. These molecules stretched would represent altogether a ca. 2-m-long chain. They have a stable nucleotide sequence that is eventually modified only at the ends (the telomeres). At this location, an inducible ribonucleo–protein complex that contains a reverse transcriptase (telome rase) uses a matrix RNA molecule to elongate the DNA molecules with a repetitive sequence motif. In proliferating cells not expressing the telomerase, the telomeres shorten at each division due to incomplete replication of DNA molecules at their extremities.

Below a certain size of the telomeres (the Hayflick limit), the cell undergoes senescence and starts a self-destruction program (apoptosis). Thus the shortening of telomeres at each replication cycle is a method to "date" a cell: to know how many times it divided. For cells that need to proliferate (germ and stem cells, for example), the telomerase complex is induced and maintains or extends the telomeres' length, keeping the cell "young." Aside from the telomeres, the sequence of the chromosomic DNA molecules is unmodified in healthy cells. However, genomic DNA molecules have a dynamic structure in constant reorganization and modification: Methylations of residues, condensation into a closed chromatin configuration, opening into an accessible chromatin configuration, or changes of the double-helix structure (A, B or Z) can affect the availability of the DNA sequences for gene expression. Several important conserved sequences define a functional DNA stretch. Many of them have a role that is not yet characterized. Only ca. 2% of the human genome is functionally identified as being genes. These entities are characterized by a promoter that is the starting point of mRNA transcription. Promoters are recognized by the RNA polymerase II (the RNA polymerase responsible for the production of mRNA in eukaryotes). They have a minimal core sequence of a few nucleotides [usually a "TATA(A/T)A (A/T)" sequence called a TATA box or Hogness box], 19 to 27 bases upstream of the initiation site of the mRNA. The TATA box is usually surrounded by G- and C-rich sequences. Its efficacy largely depends on upstream proximal control sequences.

The so-called "CAAT Box" (consensus GG(C/T)CAATCT) and "GC box" (consensus GGGCGG) enhance the activity of the promoter, i.e., its utilization by the RNA polymerase II. Distal upstream and downstream sequences called "Enhancers" also impact the activity of the promoter. An efficacious promoter in eukaryotic cells requires ca. 100 bases upstream from the TATA box. Highly specialized promoters such as "Locus Control Regions" that also affect the local chromatin structure and keep it in an opened configuration can increase the efficacy of transcription. Downstream of the promoter is the transcribed sequence that is segmented between exons (sequences that will be present in the cytosolic mRNA) and introns (sequences that will be spliced-out from the neotranscribed mRNA in the nucleus). Transcription of mRNA stops at a transcription stop signal, which is usually a U-repeat. Before it leaves the nucleus, the immature mRNA is further processed as described bellow.

RNA: Multi-Function Molecule

RNA molecules can have all functions of leaving: storage of genetic information, enzymatic activity, and construction of defined three-dimensional structures. RNA is the only biomolecule that has all of these activities. Thus, it was proposed as the primordial macromolecule that, on its own, started the concept of life 4.2 billion years ago.

Structure-related functions (rRNA, tRNA, aptamers)

Because of its single- stranded nature, RNA refolds according to the most thermodynamically favored base-pairing. This way, it generates stem loops which position each other into complex three-dimensional structures. It is still hard to predict the dominant structures that will adopt a precise RNA sequence, but several algorithms can help in predicting them.

The sequence-dictated three-dimensional conformation of an RNA molecule is essential in the functionality of several RNA types: The ribosomic RNAs fold into structures that scaffold the ribosomes, and the tRNAs fold into defined structures that allow their recognition by both amino-acyl tRNA synthetase and ribosomes. In both cases, some nucleotide sequences that remain single stranded are involved in the enzymatic processes performed by the molecules. Thus, the sequence of an RNA dictates its structure and allows it to perform its function. Both are strictly connected. One single mutation in a rRNA or a tRNA may completely change the favored three-dimensional structure of the molecule and totally impair the RNA's function(s).

The scaffolding characteristic of RNA molecules is used in drugs under the generic name of aptamers. Selected for their capacity to interact precisely with a target structure similarly to the antibody–antigen interaction, aptamers can specifically bind to any molecule or complex of interest. The first pharmaceutical aptamer is Macugen. It recognizes and neutralizes specifically the vascular endothelial growth factor, thus inhibiting pathologic blood vessel growth. It is used as treatment against age-related acute macular degeneration.

Regulation of protein expression-related functions (antisense, siRNA, miRNA)

Small RNA molecules of ca. 20 nucleotides in length can remain linear with all their bases available to pair with a complementary sequence present on another RNA molecule. Such "antisense" RNA oligonucleotides can this way impair the function (block translation) of mRNA. Another type of short RNA molecules of ca. 20 nucleotides in length is double stranded and has two bases overhangs. It is called small inhibitory RNA (siRNA) when naturally produced in the cytosole out of foreign double-stranded RNA molecules or micro-RNA (miRNA) when encoded in the DNA genome. Through its recognition by a proteic complex called RISK, one strand is discarded (the sense strand) and the other strand (the antisense) is used as a guide to direct RISK to a complementary sequence in a mRNA and induce a cleavage on this target molecule. Thus, siRNA or miRNA are a catalytic version of antisense RNA: one molecule can inhibit (induce the degradation of) many mRNA. Some miRNAs can also modify the DNA sequence in the promoter region by inducing methylations. This way, they dictate the level of packaging into the chromatin and the expression of a gene.

Enzymatic functions (ribozymes)

Through a fixed three-dimensional structure and the availability of certain nonpaired residues, RNA molecules can fold into enzymes called ribozymes. The evidence of such an enzymatic capacity of RNA was discovered by Altmann and Cech. It was acknowledged with a Nobel Prize. Initially, this enzymatic activity was restricted to the capacity of ribozymes to recognize and cleave or religate in an autonomous way a target RNA (mRNA) sequence. Later, other enzymatic capacities of ribozymes were evidenced: Selected ribozymes can catalyse the synthesis of nucleotides or the creation of amide bonds.

Coding functions (mRNA)

The pre-messenger RNA produced by transcription of the genomic DNA is processed before leaving the nucleus: Splicing of introns is made by spliceosomes that are ribo–proteic complexes. Within these structures, the RNA provides the sequence specificity of the spliceosome's activity. An exon does not have any sequence recognized by the spliceosome. It is the intron, and its borders that are recognized and excised. Evolutionarily, introns may derive from movable genetic elements called transposons. Thus, theoretically, introns can be introduced naturally (through evolution) or experimentally (thanks to molecular biology methods) within any coding sequence. They present the advantage that they enhance the efficacy of gene expression, probably through the facilitation of mRNA export to the cytosole. Moreover, thanks to regulated alternative splicing mechanisms, some specific exons may be spliced out with flanking introns. Such alternatively spliced mRNAs encode proteins with missing domain(s) and thus with different function(s). Meanwhile, the deregulation of the splicing mechanisms in dysfunctional cells, such as tumor cells, may allow introns to remain in the mature mRNA. Then, a protein with an extra domain and eventually truncated (if the intron contains a stop codon in the frame of translation) is generated. Aside from being spliced, the immature mRNA is also capped at its 5′ end (the addition of a methylated guanine followed by three phosphates bonds) and poly-adenylated at its 3′ end (the addition of several hundreds of adenine residues).

The spliced, capped, poly-adenylated mRNA is exported to the cytoplasm through nuclear pores. In the cytosole, several elongation initiation factors recognize the Cap structure, whereas the poly-A binding protein binds to the 3′ poly A tail. These proteins allow the ribosomes to bind to the mRNA and start to scan from the 5′ end the nucleotide sequence until it finds a start codon (ATG) in a "Kozak" surrounding (A/GNNNAUGG). At this location, the first amino acid, always a Methionine, is brought by a tRNA that has the 5′ CAU 3′ anticodon. Then, the ribosome translocates toward the 3′ end to the next codon where an adequate tRNA will bring the second amino acid encoded by the gene. The process continues toward the 3′ end of the mRNA and stops when the ribosome meets a UGA, UAA, or UAG "termination" codon. The neosynthesized protein and the ribosomes are then released. Several ribosomes are sitting on one mRNA. According to its stability and efficacy of translation, one mRNA can produce many proteins.

Ultimately, the mRNA is degraded by intracellular RNases. This catabolic process is highly regulated: Several sequences in the mRNA, and especially at its ends, before and after the coding sequence, have primary and secondary structures that are recognized by specific proteins in the cytosole. Those proteins may induce or, on the contrary, prevent the detection and degradation of the mRNA by the intracellular RNases, which are in general exonucleases.

This means that they degrade the mRNA starting by the 5′ or 3′ ends. Both ends are protected in the mature mRNA: the Cap on the 5′ and the poly-A tail covered by the poly-A binding proteins on the 3′. Specific and regulated mechanisms of decapping and deadenylation will render the mRNA accessible to the exonucleases. Accelerated degradation (shortening mRNA half-life) can be induced by the presence of AU-rich sequences called AUREs in the 3′ UTR, or by the presence of a specific restriction site. This latter possibility is illustrated by the regulation of iron metabolism: An iron-induced endoribonuclease recognizes a sequence present in the mRNA coding for the transferrin receptor (TfR) that is responsible for iron-loaded transferin uptake.

The presence of high iron stocks in the cell induces the endonuclease, which cleaves the TfR-encoding mRNA. Thus, it prevents TfR expression and further iron uptake. Inhibition of mRNA degradation (increasing mRNA half-life) involves other untranslated sequences as illustrated with the very stable globin mRNAs: They contain in their 3′ UTR, pyrimidine-rich sequences that are recognized by a ubiquitous protein complex called the alpha-complex. It stabilizes the poly-A binding proteins associated with the poly-A tail and secures the integrity of the 3′ end of the mRNA, thus increasing the half-life of the whole RNA molecule. Depending on the presence of stabilization and destabilization sequences in its UTRs, its length, structure, and efficacy of translation, the intracellular mRNA can have a half-life varying from minutes to weeks. Outside the cells, naked mRNA are degraded within seconds because of the abundant, ubiquitous, stable, and processive extracellular RNases. The presence of such an efficacious machinery to degrade extracellular RNA may have been developed as a protection against viruses, especially those with RNA genomes. It may also control the secretion and recapture of RNA by neighboring cells, which is hypothesized to represent a way for cells to communicate.

Recognition of Nucleic Acids by Immune Cells

In eukaryotic cells, DNA is strictly in the nucleus and in energy-producing sub-compartments (mitochondria and chloroplast), whereas RNA is strictly in those same compartments plus the cytosole. In healthy situations there is no nucleic acid in the endoplasmic reticulum, golgi apparatus, endosomes or lysosomes, and associated vesicles. The immune system developed the tools to scrutinize for the presence of nucleic acids in those compartments because it would be associated with a pathogenic situation such as the presence of an infectious agent. A family of receptors similar to immunity-related receptors from flies called Tolls receptors is dedicated to the detection of such "*danger signals.*" This family of Toll-like receptors (TLRs) contains 11 known members. Four of them were shown to recognize nucleic acids: TLR3 is specific for double-stranded RNA (dsRNA), TLR7 and TLR8 recognize single-stranded RNA (ssRNA), and TLR9 recognizes an unmethylated DNA pattern ("*CpG motif*") that is found specifically in the genome of microorganisms such as bacteria. These four receptors are located in the lumen of cytoplasmic vesicles (mainly endosomes) in immune cells like B cells, NK cells, granulocytes, macrophages, or dendritic cells (DCs). TLR3, 7, and 8 detect the infection by viruses such as influenza (dsRNA genome) or HIV (ssRNA genome), whereas TLR9 signals the presence of bacteria in the endosomes. Upon engagement of TLRs, immune cells are activated. They trigger an adaptive (involving T and B lymhocytes) immune response specific for the antigens associated with or encoded by the foreign nucleic acid(s). This natural immune detection of exogenous nucleic acids is an advantage for the utilization of these molecules in vaccines but a dis advantage for the utilization of nucleic acids in gene therapy.

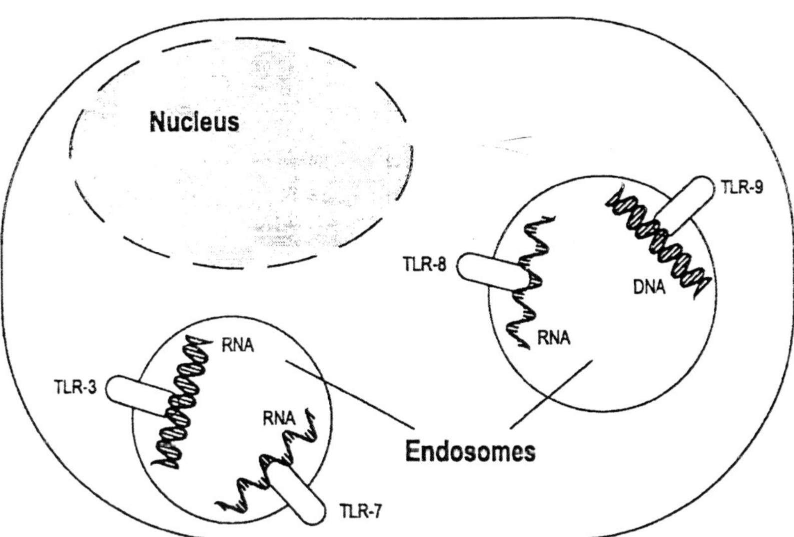

Fig. 21.15. Recognition of nucleic acids by TLR.

Production of Plasmid DNA and Messenger RNA

Plasmid DNA

Plasmid DNA (pDNA) are small (from 2 to 15 kb) circular DNA molecules that contain a bacterial origin of replication. They can proliferate within a bacteria and represent up to 1% of the microorganims's mass. They are manipulated to code for a protein that neutralizes an antibiotic. Moreover, they can contain any desired sequence, such as for example a promoter, a gene from bacterial or non-bacterial origin, and a poly-adenylation signal. Plasmids are purified from bacteria grown in the presence of the antibiotic that they can neutralize. This guarantees that the bacteria will conserve and amplify their plasmids during fermentation. Frequently, the antibiotic is ampicillin, which is deactivated by the protein β-lactamase encoded by many standard plasmid vectors. The bacteria are pelleted, usually by centrifugation, and cells are lysed, usually thanks to sodium dodecyl sulfate (SDS) and sodium hydroxide. After neutralization with potassium acetate, most proteins and the genomic DNA precipitate while the plasmids remain in the aqueous phase. Several methods exist to purify pDNA from these solutions, but the most commonly used is anionic exchange chromatography. Protocols are available to eliminate most lipopolysaccharides coming from the bacteria and that may affect the functionality of the pDNA for therapeutic utilizations. However, standard purification methods will provide the pDNA with three topologies: Most is supercoiled circular DNA, but some is in the form of a relaxed circle (one strand has at least one nick) or linear (both strands were broken at the same place). The supercoiled plasmid is the form that should be used for research and therapy because, based on *in vivo* transcription studies, it is the most active form. Although the nicked pDNA molecules are most often not strongly affecting the functionality of the plasmid *in vitro* or *in vivo*, it is custom to use pDNA with a low amount of these topologies for preclinical and clinical utilizations. At laboratory scale, the purification of the supercoiled pDNA can be obtained using caesium chloride gradients. For larger scale and clinical trials, specialized companies offer the production of high-quality pDNA for research and therapy. One liter of bacteria culture can yield up to 30 mg of pDNA.

Messenger RNA

Messenger RNA are produced from purified pDNA using bacterial RNA polymerases in a reaction called "*in vitro* transcription." The pDNA used for *in vitro* transcription must contain a specific promoter recognized by the bacteriophage RNA polymerases T3, T7, or SP6 in front of the coding sequence of interest. It is linearized using a unique restriction site that must be at the end of the sequence to be transcribed. Then, the linearized plasmid is mixed with the RNA polymerase and the four nucleotides plus, in standard reactions, an excess of Cap analog (m7G(5′)ppp(5′)G) compared with GTP. Usually the Cap analog is at ca. 6 mM in the reaction; ATP, UTP, and CTP are at 4 mM; and GTP is at 1.5 mM in the final reaction. The RNA polymerase synthesizes more than 100 mRNA molecules from one pDNA template. After the synthesis of the mRNA, 1 hour at 37°C, the DNA is destroyed by a DNase and the mRNA is recovered by precipitation, usually with lithium chloride. Afterward, the mRNA is resuspended in the adequate solution.

Packaging of Nucleic Acids for Therapy

Although some cells in skin, muscle, brain, and so on can spontaneously take up exogenous injected naked pDNA or mRNA, this process is relatively inefficient and can consequently be used only when a local expression of a protein is desired, i.e., for vaccination. Even if physical methods exist to enhance the uptake of naked nuclei acids, increasing the efficacy of transfection *in vivo* is best reached using encapsulation of the nucleic acids. Two methods are used: cationic polymers or liposomes.

Polymeric particles

Cationic polymers can spontaneously associate with the anionic nucleic acids. Such complexes can keep a positively charged surface that allows an interaction with the negatively charged cell surfaces. Commonly used cationic polymers for the production of micro- or nanoparticles include chitosan, protamine, poly-L-lysine (PLL), poly-ethylenimine (PEI), and polyamidoamine dendrimers. Usually, a simple mixing of the cationic polymers and the nucleic acid, eventually with high-speed homogenization, is enough to obtain particles. Thus, production is very easy and upscalable. However, some of these cationic polymers, such as PEI or PLL, are toxic or have secondary effects (for example, chitosan induces hypocholesterolemia). Moreover, particles generated by simple mixing of nucleic acids and cationic polymers may be very heterogenous in size and physical properties, making them hard to qualify for pharmaceutical use.

A more controlled method to produce particles is based on poly(lactide co-glycolide) (PLG). It is a biodegradable and biocompatible molecule used for several biomedical products including sutures. As it is a negatively charged molecule, it needs to be mixed with cationic polymers such as those listed above or chemical products [cetyltrimethylammonium bromide (CTAB), dimethyl dioctadecyl ammonium bromide (DDA), or 1,2-dioleoyl-1,3-trimethylammoniopropane (DOTAP), for example]. Optimally, a mixture of several reagents allows the production of homogenous particles with a defined size (from ca. 100 nm up to μm) and surface charge (zeta potential). When using PLG, protocols based on the solvent evaporation process are used. Cationic particles can be manufactured and then coated with the nucleic acid or produced in the presence of the nucleic acid. In the first case, the genetic material is on the outside of the particles, and in the second in case, it is inside. Because the production of the PLG particles involves high shear, organic/aqueous interface, high temperature, and freeze-drying, the nucleic acid may be denatured or degraded during the process. Thus, for a production that is reliable, reproducible, and easy to upscale in GMP conditions, the coating of nucleic acids on the surface of premade cationic PLG particles is preferred. In both cases, the nucleic acid associated to the particles is protected from the activity of nucleases and can be applied by injection (the particles are phagocytosed by cells) or, for vaccination, by gene-gun.

The release of the nucleic acid is largely determined by the nature of the polymers used for the preparation of the particles. *In vitro*, the particles may readily release quickly a significant amount of nucleic acid in the injection solution. For example, PLG/CTAB microparticles released ca. 35% of their loaded pDNA within 1 day. For this reason, particles should be stored lyophilized and injected quickly after reconstitution in the injection's buffer. *In vivo*, the biodegradability of the polymers and the site/method of delivery will dictate the release of the genetic information. For some particles, the release may be performed slowly, over several days. Polymers with specific degradation patterns (for example, in endosomes: at low pH) can be engineered to increase the efficacy of delivery and regulate the time frame in which nucleic acids are available for expression within the cell. Some layer-per-layer production processes allow the production of particles with several layers of nucleic acids separated by layers of polymers. The choice of the polymer(s) will dictate the degradation profile of the particles and thus the release of the several layers of nucleic acids. Theoretically, such a strategy allows the slow release of nucleic acids within cells over a long time.

Liposomes

Liposomes are vesicles that consist of an aqueous compartment enclosed in a phospholipids bilayer. As they lack proteinaceous components, liposomes are not immunogenic. A broad variety of cationic liposomes containing eventually modified lipids have been used to deliver pDNA and mRNA for therapeutic utilizations. These formulations are usually based on a cationic lipid such as 1,2-dioleol-3-trimethylammonium propane (DOTAP) and a fusogenic lipid such as 1,2-dioleoyl-sn-glycero-3-phosphoethanolamine (DOPE). Despite their ease of production and efficacy *in vitro* for transfecting cultured cells, cationic liposomes face toxicity issues *in vivo*. Meanwhile, their heterogeneous size and instability are drawbacks for a pharmaceutical production and qualification. Moreover, cationic liposomes are often inactivated in the presence of serum. As possible improvements of cationic liposomes, immunoliposomes, which are liposomes coated with an antibody, are developed. Thanks to their targeting, they are more efficacious than classic liposomes and can consequently be administered at a lower dosage. This way, the immunoliposomes are less toxic. Another variation of liposomes are called stealth liposomes. They consist in poly(ethylene glycol) (PEG)-coated liposomes. PEG prevents adsorption of the liposomes by endothelial cells after intravenous delivery. Thus, stealth liposomes are remaining in the circulation and are distributed more homogenously through the body than classic liposomes.

Plasmid DNA and Messenger RNA for Therapy

Plasmid DNA (pDNA) and messenger RNA (mRNA) are attractive tools for therapy because they are simple molecules that are easy to produce, store, detect, and manipulate using molecular biology techniques. They can be used to quickly turn into a drug any genetic information. Alternatives to pDNA and mRNA are virus- or bacteria-derived vehicles that can contain the genetic information to be expressed as a drug. The drawbacks of these methods are as follows:

1. *Safety issues*: The modified infectious agents may revert to a wild-type phenotype or may recombine with wild-type viruses to produce new sorts of pathogens.

2. *Specificity*: Not only the gene of interest is injected into a patient but also the proteins and eventually parts of the genetic information of the pathogen. The function of these proteins may interfere with the function of the transgene (in vaccination, for example, some pathogen-specific mechanisms may interfere with the priming of the immune response against the transgene), and moreover, an immune response against the vehicle (virus or bacteria) may be dominant. Not only could this hide the response against the relevant antigen for vaccination, but it could also prevent the repeated or chronic delivery of the drug for gene therapy.

Plasmid DNA and mRNA, which are both nonviral coding nucleic acid vehicles, are minimal genetic vectors: in their human host, they express only the therapeutic protein of interest. The two main utilizations of pDNA and mRNA for therapy are as follows:

1. Vaccination using simply the gene sequences of pathogens (viruses, bacteria, parasites, or tumors).
2. Genetic complementation after the gene responsible for a genetic disease is characterized.

Vaccination is by far the most exploited feature of nonviral coding nucleic acids. This is due to

1. The fact that a local, transient expression of a foreign protein is enough to trigger an immune response.
2. The natural capacity of pDNA and mRNA to stimulate the immune system through TLR.

As the production of nucleic acids is barely affected by their sequence, generic production facilities and methods were developed to produce GMP-certified pDNA or mRNA. Several specialized bioindustries throughout the world can supply within a few weeks any nucleic acid to be used in therapy. This feature is unique because all other polymeric biomolecules used in therapy (synthetic peptides, recombinant proteins, or viruses) face more or less severe production and storage issues that are changing depending on their sequence. Thus, pDNA and mRNA seem to be the most versatile and simplest biomolecules to be used as active pharmaceutical ingredients in new drugs. Both nucleic acids were used in clinical trials and are known to be safe. Efficacy was reported, but pDNA- and mRNA-based drugs should be optimized before such treatments are available on the market.

Design and Optimization of pDNA and mRNA Vectors

Coding sequence

As mentioned above, most amino acids are encoded by several codons, some of them being more favorable because they correspond to more abundant tRNA. Unfavorable codons or "rare" codons (as opposed to frequent, i.e., favorable codons) force the ribosome to pause during translation, and this may result in the premature ending of translation that generates abortive proteins. In any case, unfavorable codons decrease the efficacy of translation of full-length proteins. This phenomenon is particularly pronounced when the vaccine nucleic acid is a copy of a gene from a non-mammalian organism: Genes from bacteria or parasites have a codon usage very different from mammals. Moreover, some human virus genes and some endogenous human genes have an unfavorable codon usage that may be part of the mechanisms of regulation of their specific expression. For example, the HIV GAG gene has a "bad" codon usage that will limit the efficacy of gag production. This is actually important in the regulation of the virus replication's cycle. Thus, for human genes and more importantly for nonhuman genes, a codon optimization should preferably be performed in the coding part of therapeutic nucleic acids. The design of the gene is performed starting from the protein sequence to be expressed. Through algorithms that are based on the precise human codon usage a coding sequence will be proposed that should be ideally translated by the human cell machinery. The corresponding gene is synthesized by assembly of synthetic oligonucleotides. This process has another advantage, which is to generate a totally synthetic gene that can be very well documented and consequently easily introduced in a GMP manufacturing process.

Noncoding sequences

The nucleic acid vector can be optimized in the noncoding (untranslated) parts of the mRNA. Mainly, the AURES destabilizing sequences should be deleted because they would destabilize the mRNA and limit the expression of the antigen. In general, only the coding sequence of the gene of interest should be used for constructing the therapeutic vector; any sequence upstream of the ATG and downstream of the stop codon should be avoided. Meanwhile, stabilization thanks to 3′ UTR in the form, for example, of the ca. 180 bases or ca. 80 bases UTR from the β- or α-globin genes, respectively, can be added after the coding sequence of interest (after the stop codon). Both of these sequences are recognized by the ubiquitous α-complex, which stabilizes the mRNA and enhances its translation rate. They are routinely used in the pDNA and mRNA vectors used for therapy.

Specific optimization of pDNA vectors

The promoter used for the expression (transcription) of the transgene offers the possibility to control the level, site, and eventually time of expression of the transgenic protein. Concerning the level of expression, strong ubiquitous promoters helped by enhancers will be adequate when a high and broad expression of the transgene is needed. However, if an expression of the transgene is expected in specific cell types, investigators can use the large panel of restricted promoters that are active thanks to cell-type-specific transcription factors. This way, the expression of the transgene can be restricted to the liver (albumin promoter, for example), lymphocytes (immunoglobulin promoter or CD2 locus control region, for example), antigen presenting cells (fascin promoter for example), and so on. The drawback of these promoters is that they may lead to a relatively weak transcription activity compared with ubiquitous promoters. The control of time of expression is a critical parameter for all pDNA-based approaches because a long-term expression may have serious negative effects on the efficacy of the treatment (immune tolerance instead of immune activation, for example) or unacceptable side effects (overexpression of growth factors or other proteins with physiological activity that are used in gene therapy). A way to finely tune the expression of a transgene is to use an inducible promoter such as the Tet-On or Tet-Off promoters. Their activity depends on the Tet-On or Tet-Off transcription factors that must be constitutively encoded by the therapeutic pDNA construct. The Tet-On and Tet-Off proteins should be expressed thanks to ubiquitous promoters. The presence of tetracyclin or its analog Doxicyclin, which can just be added in the drinking water, will activate (Tet-On) or deactivate (Tet-Off) the transcription capacity of the Tet protein. Accordingly, it will turn on (Tet-On) or off (Tet-Off) the transcription of the transgene of interest. The drawback of these systems is that they are "leaky," thus always giving a basal expression of the transgene even in conditions where it should be silenced (in the presence of Doxicyclin for Tet-off and in its absence for Tet-On).

The other functional parts of the plasmid such as the transcription termination signal, the bacterial origin of replication, and the antibiotic used for production of the plasmid do not impact the efficacy of the pDNA as a therapeutic vector. However, the antibiotic-resistance gene expressed by the plasmid when it is in a bacteria (the gene is expressed thanks to bacteria-specific controlling sequences) is relevant for the regulatory aspects. Moreover, the overall sequence of the plasmid is active at the level of immune stimulation: The more the plasmid contains unmethylated CpG immnostimulating motifs, the more it may induce signaling through TLR9 in human immune cells, and consequently, the stronger may be the priming of the immune response. Thus, for vaccination approaches, pDNA vectors should be enriched in CpG motifs, whereas for gene therapy approaches, pDNA should be depleted of such sequences.

Specific optimization of mRNA vectors

As mentioned, a 3′ globin (α or β) UTR at the end of the mRNA provides higher intracellular stability to the mRNA, which is of advantage whether the mRNA is the vaccine vector or a product of the vaccine vector (with pDNA vaccines as mentioned in the above paragraph). Aside from this, specific modifications of the mRNA vector are the poly-A tail and the 5′ Cap structure. Concerning the poly A tail, it should be of a minimum of 30 residues and preferably exceed 100 residues. To generate the poly-A tail, there are two methods: Either it is encoded in the plasmid DNA that is used as a matrix for *in vitro* transcription or it is added by a specific polymerase (Poly(A) polymerase) at the end of the mRNA transcripts. In the first case, a A-tail can be of a maximum of ca. 120 As because more residues would titrate the adenosine triphosphate in the transcription reaction and limit its output. The other method is ·to submit the *in vitro* transcribed mRNA to the activity of the Poly(A) polymerase, which is a commercially available enzyme that polymerizes A residues at the 3′ end of a ribonucleic acid, in a matrix-independent manner. The enzyme can add several hundred A residues at the 3′ end of the mRNA molecules. This method is preferred to produce efficacious and stable mRNA for research purposes. However, the production of such poly-adenylated mRNA in GMP conditions is limited by the fact that the poly-adenylation process is not totally controlled and may generate heterogeneous molecules with more or less long A tails. This could make endproduct controlling, characterization of a batch, and batch-to-batch reproducibility more difficult than when the poly-A tail is encoded in the plasmid and is consequently clearly defined in length.

As mentioned above, at the 5′ end of mRNA molecules to be translated by eukaryotic cells, there is the characteristic Cap structure. It consists of a 7-methylated guanine residue linked through three phosphates to the first residue of the mRNA. A noncapped mRNA is not translated in eukaryotic cells. Not only is this structure essential for recognition of the mRNA by the translation machinery (the cap is recognized by the initiation factor 4: eIF4), but it also protects the 5′ end of the mRNA against exonucleases. Similarly to what was described for the poly-A tail, either the Cap structure is incorporated during the transcription process or it is added afterward on the *in vitro* transcribed mRNA.

In the first case, a fourfold excess of synthetic Cap analog (m7G(5′)ppp(5′)G) versus GTP in the transcription mixture guarantees that ca. 80% of the produced molecules will start with a Cap instead of a canonical G residue (the T7, T3, or SP6 promoters are made in a way that they will start transcription with a G residue). The drawback of this method is that the GTP content in the transcription reaction must be lowered compared with the other residues and thus becomes the limiting factor for the transcription. It significantly reduces the amount of recovered mRNA compared with an *in vitro* transcription reaction without Cap and with an identical concentration of all four residues. However, this method to produce capped mRNA is efficacious, fast, and reliable. Some modifications of the Cap analog can improve the efficacy of the mRNA vector: The standard synthetic Cap is a di-guanine molecule with one of its G methylated and three phosphates in-between the nucleotides. It can be incorporated at the start of the mRNA in two orientations: the methylated G being at the 5′ end or the non-methylted G at the 5′ end. Only the former situation will give a functional mRNA. Thus, statistically half of the capped mRNA molecules are nonfunctional. Strategies to avoid this phenomenon include the anti-reverse Cap structure (ARCA). It consists in a Cap analog in which the sugar carrying the methylated guanine is modified in its 3′ position (OCH_3). Thus, the dinucleotide can be used as the start nucleotide by the RNA polymerase only in the functional orientation where the 3′ OH of the non-methylated based is used to extend the mRNA. ARCA Cap enhances the functionality of *in vitro* transcribed mRNA vectors. However, ARCA Cap is relatively difficult to synthesize and consequently more costly than the standard Cap analog.

The second method for capping mRNA takes advantage of the activity of the vaccinia virus capping enzyme, also known as guanylyltransferase. This enzyme is commercially available. In the presence of GTP and S-adenosyl methionine (SAM), it can add a natural Cap structure (7-methylguanosine) to the 5′ triphosphate of a RNA molecule. As it is an enzymatic reaction, it can bring a correct Cap to all mRNA molecules, and thus, it is optimal compared with *in vitro* transcription in the presence of standard Cap but similar theoretically to *in vitro* transcription in the presence of ARCA Cap.

Because of the lack of a reliable quantitative assay to control for the presence of the Cap structure, aside from a functional assay of the mRNA expression (transfection of the mRNA in cells and detection of the translated protein). the enzymatic capping of mRNA is rarely used to produce mRNA for research or therapy. The utilization of the synthetic Cap (nonmodified analog or ARCA) in the *in vitro* transcription reaction is the standard method to produce capped mRNA.

Aside from the 5′ and 3′ ends, some internal modifications of the mRNA such as a phosphorothiate backbone or 2′ modifications of residues can be brought into the mRNA as long as the modified residues are substrate for the RNA polymerases routinely used for *in vitro* transcription (T7, T3, or SP6 RNA polymerases) and do not interfere with the translation process. It seems that only a few modifications such as phosphorothioate nucleotides and 2′ amino residues can be used. However, they lower the efficacy of transcription and translation while they do not noticeably increase the stability of the mRNA toward RNases. Some more work may allow the identifications of modifications that may allow the efficacious production of mRNA, which resists extracellular RNases and remains well translatable by the ribosome. Such mRNA would be optimized compared with native mRNA for therapeutic uses.

Vaccination

Upon entry of a pathogen (virus, bacteria, or parasite) or upon pathologic genetic modifications of a cell of the body (tumors), pathogen associated molecular patterns (PAMPs) or "*danger signals*" such as dsRNA or stabilized ssRNA (virus), CpG DNA or flagelin (bacteria), uric acid, or heat shock proteins (tumors), for example, are recognized by immune receptors such as TLR receptors or scavenger receptors. These activating receptors are expressed by cells of the innate immunity such as macrophages and DCs that are professional antigen presenting cells (APCs). Some PAMPs also stimulate B cells, NK cells, or NKT cells. Professional APCs loaded with a pathogen's derived material and stimulated by the associated PAMP migrate from the site of detection of the danger signal to the draining secondary lymphoid organs such as lymph nodes and activate antigen-specific T and B lymphocytes through their clonotypic receptors: T-cell receptor (TCR) for the former and surface immunoglobulin for the latter. There are approximately 5×10^9 T cells (ca. 70% are CD4 positive helper cells and ca. 30% are CD8 positive cytotoxic cells called CTLs) and 2×10^9 B cells in an adult human body. Generally, only a few hundred naïve lymphocytes specific for a precise antigen are available (frequency ca. 10^{-7}). Upon an encounter with the antigen-loaded activated APC, specific lymphocytes are triggered and proliferate. A lymphocyte clone may expand so much that it reaches a frequency of 10^{-2}.

Activated lymphocytes become armed effector cells. Armed B lymphocytes secrete the clonotypic immunoglobulin that sprays through the body, recognize its antigen, and inactivate it or target it to destruction by effector mechanisms of the innate immunity. Armed CD4-positive T lymphocytes secrete cytokines (mainly interferon-γ for Th1 cells and Il-4 for Th2 cells) that are necessary for immune cells' activity and they stimulate APCs. Armed CD8-positive T lymphocytes migrate to the site of antigen expression and kill cells expressing it. Upon disappearance of the antigen (complete elimination of the pathogen), armed effector cells disappear (contraction of the immune response) and some memory cells remain for the individual's whole life. Not only does this memory cell allow a higher number of specific lymphocytes to be present in the body at an eventual second appearance of the antigen than at the time of the primary encounter, but also memory lymphocytes have the peculiarity to react very quickly and efficiently (higher affinity of the antibodies for example). Thus, in the case of reappearance of the antigen, the neutralization of the pathogen (infectious agent or tumor cells) will be much faster than at the time of first priming. Prophylactic vaccination mimics a first contact between the immune system and a pathogen. It guaranties that, should the pathogen be present in the body, its recognition and elimination will be efficient and fast, preventing acute or chronic (persistent) disease. Therapeutic vaccination or immunotherapy aims at boosting the more or less preexisting immune response (triggered naturally by the already present pathogen), sustaining its strength (stimulating the proliferation of specific lymphocytes) and broadness (stimulating a larger spectrum of lymphocytes specific for the pathogen) to enhance its efficacy. As shown for several pathogens such as for example, Hepatitis B Virus (HBV), Human Immunodeficiency Virus (HIV), or tumor, a strong immune response against the pathogen is associated with a better control of the disease. High morbidity and mortality is often due to a weak immune response against those pathogens. Thus, immunotherapy aims at enhancing the natural capacity of the immune system to help control the pathogens. Another type of vaccination is used to shift or tolerize a preexisting pathologic immune response: in allergies or autoimmune diseases. Those immunotherapeutic regimen allow the manipulation of a preexisting immune response to render it armless.

Nucleic acids for vaccination

In all cases where the antigen of interest is a protein, nucleic acids can be used as a method to vaccinate. An adequate pDNA or mRNA vector can be produced *in vitro*, formulated for the delivery and eventually co-injected with an adjuvant in the form of a danger signal or cytokine. The local expression of the foreign nucleic acid-encoded protein associated with the local activation of innate immunity will trigger a T- and B-lymphocyte-mediated antigen-specific immune response that can protect against a challenge with the pathogen (infectious agent or tumor cell) that expresses this protein. It can also modify an existing pathologic immune response (autoimmunity, allergy) to render it armless. Both pDNA- and mRNA-based vaccines were reported to be capable of inducing humoral and cellular immunity. The particularly advantageous feature of this vaccination technique is that because antigens are made by the cells of the body, their epitopes are presented on major histocompatibility complex (MHC) I molecules and a CTL response is generated. Other vaccine methods based on proteins or inactivated infectious agents do not usually efficiently induce CTL. These cells are particularly relevant for antivirus, anti-intracellular pathogen and antitumor immunity. Thus, nucleic-acid based vaccines are theoretically very attractive modalities in the context of these pathogens.

It is usually accepted, although not firmly demonstrated, that the stronger is the transgene's expression (the highest is the amount of produced antigen), the better is the triggering of the immune response. Thus, enhancing the injected nucleic acid's translation is a common method for improving the efficacy of nucleic acid-based vaccination. Improving the efficacy of the processing and presentation of the coded antigen was also reported to strongly impact the vaccine's potential. However, of foremost importance is probably the site of delivery, the formulation, and the used adjuvant, which have a very strong and documented impact on the efficacy of the pDNA- or mRNA-based vaccines.

Optimization of the antigen processing and T-cell priming

When the antigen encoded by the nucleic acid is to be recognized by T lymphocytes, its derived peptide epitopes must be efficaciously presented by MHC class I or class II molecules. Although any cytosolic, membrane or secreted protein can be used to produce MHC I and MHC II associated epitopes, several methods to enhance this presentation were described.

For augmenting the presentation by MHC I molecules, a sequence coding for ubiquitin can be inserted at the beginning of the gene. The produced protein will be cleaved after the ubiquitin, thus exposing a non-methionine N-terminal residue. Should this residue be a "destabilizing" one, the protein is quickly degraded by the proteasome and its derived epitope efficiently presented on MHC I proteins. Another method to enhance MHC I epitope presentation is to insert a sequence coding for Herpes Simplex Virus (HSV) VP22 protein or heat schock protein 60 or calreticulin at the beginning of the gene. HSV VP22, HSP60, and calreticulin moieties have the particularity to enhance MHCI-antigen presentation of the conjugated protein. For augmenting the presentation by MHC II molecules, the engineering of genes encoding Invariant chain (Ii) or lysosome-associated membrane protein-1 (LAMP-1) fused to the antigen is recommended. Both Ii and LAMP-1 can direct the foreign nucleic acid-encoded protein to the cellular compartments where the degradation of antigens and the loading of MHC II molecules take place.

Shipping the antigen to the extracelullar compartment and at the same time targeting it to APC is another method to enhance T-cell priming: Whatever cell expresses the foreign nucleic acid, the antigen will be released and captured by APCs. To this end, the antigen can be fused for example to CD40L, Flt-3L, or CTLA4 because these molecules bind to APC-specific surface proteins. These strategies enhanced the efficacy of pDNA-based vaccines but may have the theoretical drawback of triggering an immune response against the self-protein used as fusion. Such an immune response would lead to autoimmune disorders targeting the immune system.

Finally, for enhancing the priming of the T cell, especially when the immune system may be tolerant (self-proteins used in anticancer vaccination), the addition of a "foreign" sequence to the antigen such as for example the Pan DR Epitope (PADRE: AKFVAAWTLKAAA) or the utilization of a xenogenic antigen (the sequence of the antigen in species other than human) that has a ca. 90% homology to the nominal antigen are shown to increase the vaccine potential of nucleic acids.

Specific functional optimization of pDNA vectors for vaccination

For a good expression of the vaccine transgene, a strong promoter must be used. Investigators can chose between (1) ubiquitous promoters such as the commonly used promoter of the early genes of CMV, eventually enhanced using additional regulatory elements; and (2) cell-type specific promoters such as those that can promote transcription only in APCs (promoter exclusively used by dermal dendritic cells such as the fascin gene, for example) or locus control regions. In the first case, independently of the site of injection and of the cell type that take up the pDNA, there will be a local expression of the protein, and through direct presentation (when the plasmid was taken by APC) or cross-presentation (when the plasmid was taken up by a somatic cell and the produced protein phagocytosed by neighboring APCs), specific lymphocytes are activated.

In the latter case, expression of the antigen is limited to APCs. This has several advantages: As APCs are terminally differentiated cells, they cannot persist or proliferate; thus, longterm uncontrolled expression of the transgene and risks of transformation (when the transgene is an oncogene to be used in antitumor vaccination) are excluded. The induction of immune tolerance due to long-term expression of the antigen by somatic cells is also excluded. Moreover, the delivery of vaccine plasmids that have an expression restricted to APCs was reported to enhance the efficacy of vaccination compared with ubiquitously expressed plasmids.

Should the plasmid contain no CpG motifs, the introduction of some of these sequences outside of the functional sequences (i.e., origin of replication, antibiotic resistance, and relevant gene expression cassette) would be needed to render the plasmid functional for vaccination purposes.

Delivery of nonviral coding nucleic acids for vaccination

Injection of naked nucleic acids

Although *in vitro* cultured cells do not usually take up naked nucleic acids (pDNA or mRNA) spontaneously, skin cells and muscle cells do in vivo. The direct injection of pDNA or mRNA resuspended in an isotonic buffer results in the local uptake of the nucleic acid that can be visualized by the expression of the encoded protein (luciferase, EGFP, CAT, or β-galactosidase are easily detectable markers) or by the induction of an immune response directed against the encoded protein. This is true whether the injection is made intramuscular, intradermal, or subcutaneous. To get an immune response, standard injections in mice consist of 50 to 200 μg of nucleic acids. A great optimization is obtained by direct intra-lymph-node injections, which proved in preclinical models to be much more efficacious than other routes, i.e., giving similar immunity than a 100-fold higher dose injected intramuscularly or intradermally. Such a method was evaluated in clinical trials and found to be a feasible and safe approach.

The mechanisms and molecules necessary for the spontaneous uptake of exogenous nucleic acids are not fully characterized. However, it is probable that both pDNA and mRNA are phagocytosed, eventually in a receptor-mediated way (the reporter gene expression, after pDNA or mRNA injection, is a saturating process that can be competed with irrelevant nucleic acids), and travel through endosomes before they can reach, in an unknown way, the cytosole and, for pDNA, subsquently the nucleus. As pDNA and mRNA vectors contain intrinsic danger signals (non-methylated CpG sequences recognized by TLR9 for the former and any nonmodified ribonucleic acids recognized by TLR7 and TLR8 for the latter) that are detected in the endosomes of cells that have phagocytosed the exogenous nucleic acid, the expression of the encoded protein parallels a local activation of the immune system. This results in the development of a B-cell- and T-cell-mediated immune response specific for the protein encoded by the injected nucleic acid. After the antigen is not expressed any longer, the triggered immune response becomes a memory response that provides an advantage to the treated individual, should he be re-exposed to the nominal antigen expressed by a pathogen.

An *in vivo* electroporation method was developed and tested in order to enhance the penetration of injected naked nuclei acids in cells at the site of delivery. After the injection of the nucleic acid, a short electric pulse is given through the injected tissue thanks to electrodes connected to a programmed generator. This method allows a strong enhancement of the uptake of the injected pDNA. So far, however, it has not been successful in enhancing the uptake of injected mRNA. For pDNA vaccination, *in vivo* electroporation is becoming a standard method to enhance the efficacy of vaccination in mice and it is being tested in a phase I trial in humans.

Delivery of vaccine nucleic acids using particles or cells

One problem when using injections of naked nucleic acids for vaccination is that a big amount of vector is needed to vaccinate mice and *a fortiori* humans. This is partly due to the quick degradation of the extracellular vector (half-life within seconds for the mRNA and eventually minutes for pDNA) and its relatively poor uptake by cells. Only a few thousand plasmids are expressed at the site of injection. For vaccination, three strategies were developed that can protect the nucleic acid and/or deliver it efficiently to its functional site (cytosol for mRNA and nucleus for pDNA): Gene Gun, *in vitro* transfection of professional APCs before adoptive transfer, and finally encapsulation in particles or liposomes.

Gene-gun. The gene-gun technology is based on a ballistic delivery. The nucleic acid is precipitated on micrometric gold particles that are resuspended in a buffer and quickly injected into an horizontal tubing of 4 mm in diameter and 75 cm in length. The particles are left there to sediment. Thereafter, the buffer is slowly discarded and the tube is turned 180° along its axis in a way that the initial bead's bed is on the "roof" and disperses slowly through gravity on the inside of the tubing, covering it homogeneously. After it is dried in the inside, the tube is chopped into the size of cartridge. The cartridges are placed in the cartridge holder of a gun that is connected to pressured helium. Upon firing, the gas goes through the cartridge and propels the beads with high speed. Should the gun be a few centimeters from the skin, the beads penetrate the *stratum corneum* and stop in the dermis. They release the nucleic acid in the hit cells or cells' nuclei. Within these cells are dermis DCs and Langerhans cells. They are activated probably through signaling by TLR9 (pDNA vaccines) or TLR7 and TLR8 (mRNA vaccines) and migrate to the draining lymph node where they can activate antigen-specific lymphocytes.

Adoptive transfer of in vitro transfected APCs. As the key event in vaccination is the presentation of the antigen and its derived epitopes by professional APCs, researchers investigated the possibility of generating a pure APC population out of blood cells and of modifying these cells with exogenous nucleic acids before reimplanting them in the body. Because the transfection of pDNA in APCs such as DCs is inefficient and, when successful, induces apoptosis, the methods of genetic modification of APCs were principally developed using mRNA vectors. As APC, the monocyte-derived dendritic cells are most often used. They are easily produced, even in GMP conditions, starting from blood monocytes that are extracted from total blood either using their characteristic to stick quickly on plastic surfaces or by sorting (magnetic beads or FACS) with monoclonal antibodies specific for monocytes such as CD14. The monocytes are cultivated 1 week with GM-CSF and interleukine-4 to generate immature DCs. These cells can be easily transfected with mRNA using simple co-incubation or, for a more efficient, more controlled uptake, electroporation.

Eventually, the cells are rendered mature by the addition of one or several danger signals and further cultivated 1 or 2 days. Then the cells are re-injected into the patient. Although the method was shown to work in animals and in humans, the optimal danger signal(s) and site of injection are still to be precisely defined. For the maturation, a cocktail containing IL-1β, IL-6, TNF-α, and PGE2 may be optimal to generate mature DCs that can migrate to the lymph nodes draining the site of adoptive transfer without dying too early from over-stimulation. Using this type of cocktail, DCs injected subcutaneous or intradermally are expected to go to the secondary lymphoid organs and prime antigen-specific lymphocytes. Alternatively, the direct intra-lymph-node injection of mature transfected DCs may be the best method to guarantee that most *in vitro* generated APCs are at their site of activity after adoptive re-implantation. The utilization of this method in many human clinical trials is ongoing throughout the world, and optimized protocols will soon be deducted from these studies.

Particles. Both pDNA and mRNA vectors entrapped in particles or coated on particles were shown to be potent vaccines. In all cases, the particle strategy allowed a drastic reduction of the amount of the nucleic acid needed to get a significant immunity. For mRNA vectors, Martinon et al. were the first to report that influenza nucleoprotein coding mRNA entrapped in liposomes can induce an immune response against influenza virus in mice. It was then shown that minimal amounts of mRNA (down to 1 μg of encapsulated mRNA injected intradermal or intravenous) are enough to prime an antigen-specific immune response. This technology has not yet been transferred to human clinical trial. Encapsulated pDNA, however, were shown earlier to be potent vaccine formulations. Plasmid DNA entrapped or coated on cationic microparticles or enclosed in liposomes are more potent than naked pDNA as vaccines. Using either intramuscular or intravenous routes of delivery, doses as low as 1 μg of encapsulated pDNA were shown to prime humoral and cellular immune responses in mice. Using these formulations, oral, intranasal, or other mucosal delivery routes (intrarectal, for example) can be used to stimulate mucosal and systemic immunity in animals (mice or macaques).

Adjuvants

Although nucleic acids have the intrinsic capacity to signal "danger" through TLR7, 8, or 9, extra-immunostimulation can enhance or polarize the immune response. It can be achieved by injection of cytokines or nucleic-acid-coding cytokines together with the vaccine. The cytokine GM-CSF is one of the most studied adjuvants in the context of nucleic acid vaccinations. It was shown to enhance and to polarize toward Th1 immune responses after pDNA or mRNA applications. The optimal timing of application of such an adjuvant is not clearly established. Theoretically, the local delivery of GM-CSF should attract immature DCs that would render the site more reactive to a consecutive nucleic acid injection. However, practically, in mice it looks like the injection of GM–CSF should at best follow the injection of pDNA or mRNA. The optimal timing of GM–CSF injections in humans would need to be deducted from clinical trials especially designed to decipher this matter. Inflammatory cytokines such as IL-12 are also foreseen as promising adjuvants to be used in combination with nucleic acid vaccines.

Preclinical results and clinical applications

Both pDNA- and mRNA-based vaccinations were demonstrated to be efficacious in animal models as prophylactic or therapeutic immunotherapies against tumors, infectious diseases, and allergy. Two pDNA-based vaccines are commercialized for veterinary use: an anti-equine fever and an anti-infectious hematopoietic necrosis virus (IHNV) for farm-raised salmons. In humans, several formulations of nucleic acid vaccines are tested in clinical trials. Although pDNA-based vaccine trials were reported in the context of antitumor, antivirus (HIV, influenza virus, HBV) and antiparasite (*Plasmodium falciparum*) approaches, mRNA-based vaccines were up to now tested only as immunotherapies against cancer.

Anti-infectious diseases vaccines (HIV, Plasmodium falciparum, influenza virus, HBV, Mycobacterium tuberculosis)

Theoretically, any infectious agent can be recognized by the immune system, and thus, vaccination is of interest to prevent acute infection or reduce chronic replication. Preclinical results have shown at least in mice that for all economically or socially relevant pathogens, pDNA-based vaccination is a robust method to prevent or treat the infections. Several trials in the human population are ongoing and address the safety of pDNA vaccines designed to trigger immunity against HIV, *Plasmodium falciparum*, influenza virus, HBV, *Mycobacterium tuberculosis*, severe acute respiratory syndrome (SARS) virus, West Nile Virus, or Ebola virus. Most are phase I trials and thus address only the safety and dose.

Aids. The Acquired Immunodeficiency Syndrome (AIDS) is the fourth cause of death in the world (an estimated 3.5 million people die from AIDS every year). An estimated 40.3 million persons are living with HIV, and 5 million people per year become infected. An affordable and efficacious anti-AIDS vaccine is urgently needed. Due to the potency of pDNA vaccines to induce CTL in mice and the known efficacy of these cells to control HIV replication in humans, the first trials using direct injection of nucleic acids were performed in HIV-infected individuals in the mid-1990s. Follow-up trials were performed in uninfected volunteers. These studies showed that anti-HIV pDNA vaccines are feasible and safe. The induced immune responses were less strong than expected based on preclinical studies. However, CTL responses could be recorded after injection of naked pDNA. Interestingly, in infected patients, the pDNA vaccines could induce new anti-HIV immune specificities, not triggered by the infection itself. Thus, in the context of immunotherapy, pDNA vaccination has indeed the potential to boost the preexisting immunity but also to broaden it by inducing new virus-specific CTL and antibodies. Up to now, no clinical efficacy of pDNA vaccines against HIV could be demonstrated. However, strategies using pDNA as a prime followed by recombinant viruses or proteins as boost are being evaluated as vaccine protocols in high-risk populations.

Malaria. Plasmodium falciparum (*P. falciparum*) is the most pathogenic parasite causative of malaria. Yearly, 300–400 millions clinical cases of *P. falciparum* infections are reported, among which 2–3 million are deadly. Moreover, an increase of the incidence of the disease has been observed due to the emergence of drug-resistant parasites and of insecticide-resistant mosquitos. For these reasons, a protective and cost-effective vaccine against *P. falciparum* is needed. *P. falciparum*, being an intracellular parasite, its control requests the recognition by CTL. Thus again, nucleic acid-based immunotherapies are theoretically adapted for the development of a preventive or therapeutic vaccine against malaria. The same year as the report of anti-HIV pDNA-based vaccines was published so was the result of the first anti-malaria pDNA-based vaccine. In this and follow-up studies, the induction by the pDNA vaccine of CTL against *P. falciparum* epitopes was documented. However, no antibody response was induced. The codon usage of *P. falciparum* is very inadequate. for mammal cells. Thus, the pDNA vaccines based on native *P. falciparum* genes may have been relatively inefficiently translated *in vivo*. This may account for the generation of CTL, which are recognizing fragments of the protein but fail to generate antibodies that require the production of the full-length foreign protein. To conclude, although the documented induction of anti-malaria T cells by pDNA applications is an encouraging progress toward the development of an antimalaria vaccine, a randomized placebo-controlled phase III trial is required to see whether pDNA-induced anti-*P. falciparum* immunity results in the reduction of the burden of infection, morbidity, and mortality within populations living in endemic areas.

Hepatitis B. The hepatitis B virus (HBV), which may have infected more than one third of the population, is responsible for approximately 1 to 2 million deaths every year. After infection, most people clear the virus through an efficient immune response. However, the virus persists in ca. 10% of the people and eventually leads to liver diseases such as hepatocellular cancer. Although the anti-HBV vaccine based on the recombinant surface antigen is efficient and safe, 5% to 10% of healthy immunocompetent subjects do not respond to it. For those people and the ca. 350 million carriers, an alternative vaccine that would trigger a B-cell but also a T-cell response is of great interest. Indeed, a potent T-cell response of the Th1 type is believed to lead to the control of HBV. Several prophylactic and therapeutic trials are ongoing.

One of the most successful methods to trigger immunity against HBV using pDNA is based on the utilization of the gene-gun: A trial showed that ballistic delivery of pDNA coding HBS could induce CD4 and CD8 T cells as well as protective levels of antibodies in all treated hepatitis-naïve volunteers. Moreover, no or low responders to the standard vaccine were found to respond to the pDNA applied with the gene-gun (12 out of 16 patients responded). Each dose of the vaccine contained no more than 4 μg of plasmid. Subjects received between one and three doses, with a two-month interval in-between applications. Thus pDNA-based vaccination is a safe, feasible, cost-effective, and promising prophylactic and therapeutic approach against HBV. The results of phase II and III trials are needed to prove clinical efficacy and allow commercialization of this vaccine.

Tuberculosis. Mycobacterium tuberculosis is the etiologic agent of tuberculosis. The disease is due to the immune response against the pathogen more than to the pathogen itself. Immunotherapy using the whole inactivated pathogen or BCG may enhance rather than decrease the disease. Nucleic acid vaccination offers the possibility to perform immunotherapy with the immunogenic parts of the pathogen that are associated with a protective immune response rather than with a pathologic immune response. Heat Shock Protein (HSP) 65 is a dominant mycobacterial antigen. Vaccination with HSP65-encoding pDNA in mice was superior to infection in priming protective T cells. In this model, the same method was found to be efficacious in a therapeutic setting. However, these results were not confirmed by another laboratory, where vaccination of mice with pDNA encoding mycobacterium HSP65 enhanced the pathology. These contradictive results may be due to the ratio of Th1 versus Th2 cells primed by the vaccine, which may be linked with the purity of the nucleic acid (the presence of endotoxin, which orientate the response toward Th2), the site of injection (intradermal delivery orientates the response toward Th2), or the level of immunological naivety of mice that depends on the clean conditions in which they are kept. As an improvement of the approach, a combination between efficacious anti-mycobacterium chemotherapy and pDNA vaccination may allow a sustained immune control of the pathogen. This regimen may be used in infected patients suffering from tuberculosis. However, the risk of increasing rather than decreasing the pathologies associated with *Mycobacterium tuberculosis* using pDNA vaccination is a drawback that limits the testing of this immunotherapy.

Antitumor vaccines. Many, if not all, tumor cells express characterized specific antigens (self-proteins or virus-encoded proteins) that make them recognizable and controllable by the immune system, especially by T cells. The capacity of immune- stimulation approaches, among them, nucleic acid-based vaccines, to control tumors was clearly proven in many animal models. For this reason, nucleic acid vaccines coding tumor antigens such as virus-encoded oncogenes (for example, HPV 16 E7), self-proteins (prostate antigens for prostate cancer, clonotypic antibodies for B-cell leukemia, melanocyte-specific proteins for melanoma, or shared tumor antigens such as testis-antigens for many tumor types, for example) or mutated oncogenes (p53 or cRas, for example) were tested as immunotherapy in cancer patients. Prophylactic vaccination against cancer is validated in mice but not yet transferred to healthy, tumor-prone individuals identified thanks to family history and detection through genotyping using known tumor-predisposition markers.

Plasmid DNA-based anti-tumor vaccines. One of the first reports of an antitumor pDNA-vaccine phase I trial used a dual expression plasmid coding HBS and carcino embryonic antigen (CEA), a protein overexpressed on many epithelial cancers. The plasmid was repetitively injected intramuscularly. Per injection, up to 2 mg was applied. Some patients developed a good immune response toward HBS, but there was only a very limited response toward CEA. No objective clinical response was recorded. Similar results were obtained in another phase I trial using a pDNA coding gp100 (an enzyme involved in melanine synthesis and expressed in most melanoma) whether the DNA was injected intramuscularly or intradermally. As a superior vaccination strategy that may allow breaking tolerance, the intranodal delivery of pDNA coding tyrosinase (like gp100, it is a protein expressed in melanocytes and melanoma) was tested in melanoma patients. Patients received up to 800 μg of pDNA every 2 weeks for four cycles.

The treatment was feasible and safe. Nearly half of the patients (11 of 26) showed the triggering of an immune response against tyrosinase. Overall survival in this small cohort was found to be higher than expected. Meanwhile the utilization of an adjuvant in the form of recombinant cytokines (IL-2 and GM-CSF) applied subctaneously was tested in a phase I trial involving prostate tumor patients. The pDNA (up to 900 μg per injection, five cycles) was given intramuscularly and intradermally. Cellular and humoral immune responses targeted to PSA could be detected in two of three patients injected with the highest dose. Biochemical regression was recorded in these two immunologically responding patients. Finally, as an immunotherapy strategy targeting the idiotype of B-cell lymphoma, pDNA expressing patient-specific clonotype were delivered with a needleless device. Patients received monthly injections of up to 1800 μg of pDNA. Here again, an immune response (B or T cell) could be triggered against the tumor-specific antigen (the antibody's idiotype) in most patients (7 out of 12).

Viral oncogenes are a privileged target for antitumor immunotherapies: Being foreign molecules, they are usually efficaciously recognized by the immune system and can be used as prophylactic antitumor vaccination targets. Human Papilloma Virus-16 (HPV-16) encodes two oncogens: E6 and E7. PLG-encapsulated pDNA coding for a few HLA-A2 epitopes of HPV-16 E7 administered intramuscularly could induce an immune response against HPV-16 in most treated patients suffering from HPV-16 associated anal dysplasia or cervical intraepithelial neoplasia. Clinical responses (histological responses) were observed in some patients. Thus, pDNA-based vaccinations against HPV can be envisioned as a possible prophylactic and therapeutic antitumor immunotherapy regimen. This technology may become a standard anti-HPV therapy in the relatively near future.

Messenger RNA-based antitumor vaccines. The only published results where mRNA vectors were used to vaccinate cancer patients are based on the utilization of mRNA-transfected DCs as described above. This popular method first described in 1996 was validated in several preclinical mouse models and used to vaccinate prostate or renal cancer patients with different mRNA preparations. In most patients. an increased T-cell immune response against the antigen(s) encoded by the mRNA(s) could be observed. Thus, mRNA-based vaccines using *in vitro* transfection of autologous DCs is a feasible and efficacious approach to stimulate a T-cell immune response against tumor antigen. Phase II and III trials are needed to show the clinical efficacy of mRNA-transfected DCs as anticancer immunotherapy. However, the need for a large amount of blood to prepare a few vaccine doses, the costly and variegating production of DC in GMP-conditions, as well as the logistic issues restrict the utilization of this technology. As an alternative, direct injections of naked or protamine-encapsulated mRNA was shown to be efficacious for priming cellular and humoral immune responses in mice. It is being evaluated in human as anticancer immunotherapy (ongoing phase I/II studies).

Conclusion on antitumor vaccines based on pDNA or mRNA. Most published results show limited efficacy of nucleic acid-based vaccines as anticancer immuno-therapies, highlighting the need for improving these strategies. However, the possibility of triggering an immune response against self-tumor antigens with pDNA or mRNA vaccines sustains the hope that once the correct antigens and optimized immunization methods will be identified, antitumor vaccinations would be a way to get regression or at least stabilization of tumor diseases in many patients.

The fundamental knowledge of immune-tolerance and control of autoimmunity will help to find the protocols that will allow nucleic-acid based vaccines to become potent antitumor therapies. Of particular and new interest is the role of regulatory T cells (Treg) that can suppress immunity and are usually increased in number in the blood of tumor patients. Antitumor vaccination may enhance the activity of suppressive cells rather than the one of effector antitumor cells, thus leading to a failure of the therapeutic approach. Controlling, i.e., reducing, the activity of Treg and of other immunomodulatory cells or molecules may be crucial for the success of anticancer immunotherapies. Methods such as chemotherapies, which are lymphoablative or specific inhibition of gene expression using siRNA (anti-TGF-β or IL-10, for example), may allow a transient reduction of natural immunosuppression that could be used for intensive vaccination protocols. Such combinations are being evaluated in clinical trials.

Anti-allergy vaccines

Allergic diseases affect approximately one third of the population, and for unclear reasons, prevalence of these diseases is increasing. Through the triggering of Th2 type of T helper cells, environmental antigens induce the release of Il-4, Il-5, and Il-13 activate basophil, eosinophil, mast cells, and IgE, which eventually induce the development of inflammatory allergic diseases such as asthma, eczema, hay fever, and rhinitis. The desensitization of a patient can be obtained through repeated injections of increasing doses (starting at very low doses) of the nominal allergen over the course of several years. However, this protocol has been reported to have inconsistent efficacy and in rare cases very strong toxicity. As vaccination with pDNA was reported to induce a Th1 response and inhibit the Th2 response, it was anticipated that pDNA vaccines could have a potential for the prevention and cure of allergic diseases. Indeed, it was demonstrated in animal models that the injection of pDNA coding for an allergen (β-galactsidase in experimental models or relevant allergen such as house dust mite Derp5, latex Hevb5, peanut Arah2, honeybee venom phospholipase A2, pollen allergen Cryj1, or Betv) can be a prophylactic or therapeutic treatment against allergies. However, a clear control of the Th2 response, eventually using the co-injection of the vaccine with nucleic acids coding Il-12 or IL-15 as enhancers of the Th1 response, is needed before pDNA desensitization protocols can be planned for testing in the human population.

Conclusion on vaccination using nonviral coding nucleic acids

Both pDNA and mRNA vectors can induce a antigen-specific humoral and cellular immunity of the Th1 and/or Th2 types. When using direct intramuscular injections of naked plasmid, a minimum of 800 μg of pDNA seems to be necessary to get a detectable immune response. Optimization of the vectors is a standard way to increase the efficacy of the nucleic acid-based vaccines and should be used for any clinical trials. The choice of the relevant pathogen-derived antigen, especially in the case of antitumor immunotherapies, is critical: This antigen should be well immunogenic and recognized by T and/or antibodies on pathogenic cells (infected and malignant) or by antibodies on infectious agents. The delivery method should be cost-efficient, praticable, and result in the induction of a strong immune response. Although the efficient intra-lymph-node delivery method may be adequate for therapy of a limited number of patients with advanced nontreatable diseases (tumor patients, for example), the gene-gun delivery sounds like the most favorable delivery method for easy, painless, efficacious, and cost-effective nucleic-acid-based vaccination of large populations.

The utilization of a nontoxic adjuvant is always relevant, and at the moment, GM–CSF, which is the most frequently used cytokine in the context of nucleic acid vaccination trials, looks like a fairly good candidate. Meanwhile the control of Tregs is fundamental to trigger efficient immunity, especially in anticancer immunotherapies. The choice of the vehicle (pDNA or mRNA) needs to be addressed in clinical trials where both vectors are compared. Although mRNA looks safer due to its transient nature, pDNA may be more efficacious and require less injections for reaching protective immunity (high antibody titers and high T-cell frequencies).

On another hand, long-term persistence of antigen expression when using pDNA may interfere with the development of memory T cells and thus render a prophylactic vaccine inefficient. The induction of memory cells by mRNA- and pDNA-based vaccines needs to be evaluated and compared in human populations, especially when prophylactic vaccination is envisioned. Thus, it could be stated that the prevention of diseases or the treatment of chronic non-life-threatening diseases (i.e, allergy) may be most adequately addressed by mRNA vectors, whereas the treatment of late-stage patients (AIDS or tumor patients, for example) may be at the moment best addressed with pDNA vectors.

Gene Therapy

Known mutated genes that are the cause of recessive genetic diseases are, for example, adenosine deaminase in severe combined immunodeficiency disease (SCID), cystic fibrosis transmembrane conductance regulator gene (CFTR) in cystic fibrosis, hypoxanthine-guanine phosphoribosyl transferase in Lesch-Nyhan disease, glucocerebrosidase enzyme in Gacher disease, dystrophin in Duchenne muscular dystrophy, and factors XIII and XI for some hemophilia. In these cases, using foreign recombinant nucleic acids, it is possible to bring the protein that is missing or deficient. This technology is called gene complementation.

The challenge of nucleic-acid-based gene therapies is to bring in all defined target cells an amount of nucleic acid that would provide a functional quantity of the encoded protein without over- or under-expression by some cells and without stimulating immunity or inducing apoptosis. General optimizations of gene expression as described for vaccination with pDNA and mRNA vectors should be performed to obtain the highest possible expression, thus efficacy, from the nuclei-acid-based drugs. At the same time, the vectors should be designed to have low immunogenicity, for example, by eliminating CpG sequences in pDNA vehicles. Using pDNA vectors, the utilization of promoters that specifically drive gene expression in the adequate tissue or cell type is a method to lower side effects such as expression of the exogenous vector in irrelevant organs or cells.

Although delivery of naked nucleic acid is evidenced *in vivo* and can be used for some approaches, the efficacious systemic delivery of nucleic acids needed for gene therapy is best obtained thanks to encapsulation. Both methods are presented below. None of them has been used in human clinical trials. Up to now, gene therapy approaches tested in humans are based on virus-derived constructs that can efficiently penetrate cells and integrate in the nucleus. However, because of safety issues, pDNA and eventually mRNA (not used in preclinical models up to now) may appear again as favorable vehicles for gene complementation.

Naked pDNA for gene therapy

As published by Wolff et al. in 1990, the injection of naked pDNA in the mouse skeletal muscle results in local transgene expression. Since then, other species such as rats, cats, or monkeys and other sites such as skin, liver, brain, urological organs (assisted by *in vivo* electroporation), thyroid, and tumors were shown to be permissive to the local uptake of injected naked pDNA. However, the local transgene expression obtained by direct injection of naked pDNA into an organ is usually too low to be used in the context of genetic disease, even when the missing function is contained in a soluble protein secreted in the bloodstream (for example, coagulation factors in hemophilia). It was estimated that after injection of naked pDNA, only a few thousand plasmids are functionally retained within cells of the injected tissue.

To treat a genetic disease, a physiological expression of the therapeutic molecule by all cells that need the missing function or a functional level of the protein in the body fluids is required. For this reason, gene therapy approaches based on naked pDNA use a systemic delivery method such as intravenous or, at best when organs other than lungs are targeted, intra-arterial injections. Indeed, the intravascular injection of naked pDNA surprisingly results in the expression of the encoded protein, especially in the liver. As it is the case for intramuscular and intraskin injections, the intravascular injection of naked pDNA was initially a (negative) control of experiments designed to test the potency of transfection reagents.

To reach a good expression level in mouse hepatocytes, the pDNA should be injected in a relatively large volume and short delivery time ("*hydrodynamic*" delivery) through the tail vein, the portal vein, the hepatic vein, or the bile duct. One injection can transfect about 1% of the hepatocytes throughout the entire mouse liver. This method can be used to produce *in situ* liver-specific proteins and soluble proteins such as coagulation factors XIII and XI that are missing in hemophilic patients. The production of critical proteins such as growth hormones with this technology is theoretically possible but would be hazardous because the amount of protein produced and the duration of the expression are not controlled. Although naked siRNA can be delivered using the same procedure, naked mRNA would not be suitable because it is degraded within seconds in the serum.

Using hydrodynamic injection in a muscle's artery or vein, the expression of naked pDNA can also be obtained in the muscle. However, for a high expression, the blood flow through the targeted vessel must be stopped surgically during the injection. Expression of the naked pDNA can also be obtained in the cardiac myocytes after injection in the left ventricular wall.

These preclinical observations made in mice, rats, and monkeys allow us to foresee the utilization of naked pDNA as a treatment of muscle diseases such as Duchenne muscular dystrophy, peripheral limb ischemia, and cardiac ischemia. However, the methods described above for animals (hydrodynamic injection, transient stop of blood flow through a muscle) are difficult to transpose to the human situation. Instead of an hydrodynamic delivery, human may benefit from the utilization of a vasodilator before pDNA injection. This treatment could increase the permeability of discontinuous endothelium such as those in liver, spleen, and bone marrow and induce permeability through continuous endothelium such as those in the brain. This way, plasmid DNA may go through the vascular wall and reach the target cells of the organs. As mentioned, the utilization of pDNA for gene therapy in humans has not yet been evaluated in clinical trials. Virus-based gene complementation is still observed as the most feasible method although safety issues are raised. Encapsulated pDNA is possibly an improved version of naked pDNA for gene therapy and has better safety features than virus-based delivery systems.

Encapsulated pDNA for gene therapy

Both cationic liposomes and polymeric particles were used to deliver efficiently pDNA in animal models for gene therapy approaches. Although in these preclinical assays the expression of the transgene vanished after few days, the uncontrolled long-term expression as well as a possible overexpression after repeated delivery of encapsulated pDNA are safety issues that must be addressed before these methods are evaluated in clinical trials. However, thanks to the recent knowledge on gene regulation (utilization of inducible promoters such as Tet On and Tet Off promoters), immune activation (CpG motifs), immune modulation (Tregs for immunosuppression, for example), we can anticipate new generations of safe (controllable and non-immunogenic) encapsulated plasmid constructs that will be the basis of future drugs designed to treat genetic diseases.

Preclinical results obtained with liposome formulations

One of the most frequent genetic diseases with high morbidity and mortality for which the deficient gene has been identified is cystic fibrosis. It is due to mutations in the CFTR, which is a transporter of chloride anions. This deficiency is recessive: Bringing the correct gene in the cells can correct it. As cystic fibrosis affects the lung, local gene therapy approaches where the genetic vehicle is delivered through airways is foreseen as an efficacious and safe method. As early as 1992, liposomes encapsulating pDNA coding for CFTR were found to be capable of bringing this protein function to airway epithelium of the lung after intratrachea instillation in mice. Optimization of the delivery can be obtained by modifying the liposome formulation. This promising method was not evaluated in patients.

Meanwhile, the intravenous delivery of lipid-entrapped pDNA was shown to efficaciously lead to gene expression, especially in liver, lung, and kidneys. The addition of targeting molecules can efficiently target the vesicles to specific cells. For example, the utilization of galactosyl-cholesterol or mannosylated-cholesterol in the liposome formulation allows efficient delivery of the pDNA to the liver in mice.

To conclude, cationic liposome formulations were shown in animal models to be efficient, safe, and versatile delivery vehicles for pDNA molecules. The engineering of liposomes coated with targeting molecules is one method to enhance the efficacy and specificity of these vehicles. Clinical trials in humans are needed to demonstrate the feasibility, safety, and efficacy of these approaches.

Preclinical results obtained with particles

Poly-L-lysine and poly-L-Ornithine were used to generate particles that can entrap pDNA. The cationic polymers can be coupled to a targeting molecule such as galactose or mannose for enhanced delivery to the liver after intravenous or intraportal injections in mice. Expression in other organs than the liver (for example, kidneys) is observed; however, expression in the liver using these particles is dominant. Such particles are found to be more efficient and to persist for a longer time in the circulation than liposomes. Hepatic expression of the pDNA delivered by poly-L-Lysine particles can be found several months after delivery. These promising formulations were not evaluated in humans.

Conclusion on gene therapy using nonviral coding nucleic acids

As opposed to vaccination strategies, the local delivery of naked pDNA in an organ is not foreseen as a possible gene therapy approach because the protein expression is too low. However, the systemic delivery through the blood circulation of naked or entrapped pDNA was found to result in strong expression of the transgene, mainly in the liver. The utilization of hepatocyte-specific promoters in the pDNA would allow us to turn these methods into liver-specific expression systems. They may be used to produce soluble proteins such as coagulation factors XIII and XI or erythropoietin in patients suffering from genetic deficiencies for these molecules. Encapsulated pDNA expressed by hepatocytes could also theoretically be used for the sustained production of therapeutic monoclonal antibodies (the anti-Her-2/neu antibody: Herceptin, for example) by the body's own cells in tumor patients. Aside from that, some methods (hydrodynamic delivery, occlusion of veins, particles) can allow delivery of pDNA in the muscle as a possible treatment for myopathies. Finally, inoculation through the airways can result in gene expression in the lung and could be used as a treatment against cystic fibrosis. Thus. although they are not yet tested in humans, the gene therapy approaches based on simple pDNA coding for a therapeutic protein are very exciting and promising approaches that offer a broad range of applications. However, several issues have to be addressed:

1. *The natural immunogenicity of the pDNA*. Even without any known CpG sequence in the plasmid, repeated applications may still induce the activation of the immune system. This immune response could neutralize the produced transgenic protein and result in the specific killing of cells expressing it. As a remedy, the utilization of immunosuppressive drugs concomitantly with the application of pDNA-based gene therapies should probably be envisioned.
2. The uncontrolled persistence and expression of the transgene prevents its utilization for the production of active molecules such as growth factors. Repeated applications may result in some patients in the accumulation of pDNA and overexpression of the transgene. This would have negative effects on the producing organs (necrosis) and pathogenic systemic effect due to the protein's own activity. The utilization of inducible promoters and a careful monitoring of the patients before each application of the pDNA would be needed to perform safe clinical trials.

Cationic liposomes that were frequently used and validated in several laboratories and animal models may be the first approaches used for gene therapy using pDNA in humans. Meanwhile, the utilization of encapsulated mRNA appears theoretically as a method to circumvent all limitations of pDNA-based approaches for gene therapy. Encapsulated mRNA were not yet reported as gene therapy tools but because they are transient molecules, readily expressed in the cytosole, and if nonstabilized, barely activate immunity (TLR7 and TLR8), they can be foreseen as safe (transient), efficient (expressed in the cytosole), and nonimmunogenic (not stabilized) genetic information vehicles to be used in gene therapy.

Pharmaceutical Production and Regulations

Plasmid DNA

Several companies in the United States and Europe offer the contract manufacture of documented pDNA for preclinical use and of GMP-certified pDNA for clinical utilisations. It is regulatory practice that ampicilin is not used in GMP productionin order to avoid cross-contaminations and concerns with penicillin-allergies. Instead, plasmids containing a kanamycin-resistance gene are frequently used. At best, the starting material is a pDNA containing a synthetic gene constructed by assembly of oligonucleotides. This way, the history of the pDNA can be clearly reported in the production's file. The whole manufacturing process is free of bovine- derived products. The plasmid of interest is tested in different *E. coli* strains and several culture media to find out the best conditions for producing the highest amount and best quality plasmid. It should appear as a clear and colorless solution by visual inspection. The final controls must meet the following criteria:

1. *Identity*: Sequencing should show 100% identity with the expected sequence. Electrophoresis or chromatography studies should be used to show that the pDNA is predominantly supercoiled. The restriction enzyme digest pattern analyzed by gel electrophoresis can be included. Susceptibility to DNase can also be used as a proof of molecular identity.
2. *Content*: Quantification should be performed by absorbance at 260 nm. Osmolarity and pH should also be measured using standard methods.
3. *Purity*: Residual proteins, chromosomal bacteria DNA, RNA, and endotoxin must be below specified limits. Sterility must be controlled by standard microbiological assays.

Moreover, some tests can be performed to check counter-ions (should be NaCl, thanks to precipitation of the pDNA with alcohol plus NaCl), residual solvents (if they are used during the production), and potency (functional assay using, for example, transfection of cells and verification of the expression of the protein of interest or testing of the immune response after injection in an animal model).

Production of pDNA using up to 100-m^3 scale fermentation is performed by specialized industries. Batches of more than 1 kg of pDNA can be produced. As functional doses for vaccination in humans were of ca. 800 μg (intra-muscular injection) or 4 μg (gene-gun), 1 kg of pDNA is enough for 1,250,000 or 250,000,000 doses, respectively. This is largely enough for pDNA-based therapies to be commercialized worldwide as treatments against infectious diseases, cancer, or genetic diseases.

Preclinical toxicology studies should address the standard systemic and local reactogenicity, histopathology, and toxicity (acute and chronic dosage) in rodent and nonrodent animals. Also, as pDNA-based therapies are classified as gene therapy approaches, additional strict safety issues must be addressed before starting a clinical trial. The potency of the pDNA to integrate in the genome of the injected animal must be tested using assays that can detect one integrated pDNA in more than 150,000 nuclei. The potential of the pDNA preparation to induce anti-DNA antibodies (the etiologic agents of systemic lupus erythematosus) must be evaluated. The biodistribution and persistence of the pDNA must also be measured: Tissues and body fluids are analyzed at different time points for the presence of the pDNA using PCR methods. Of particular relevance is the study of pDNA in germ cells because such an event could theoretically generate transgenic descendants.

These toxicology studies were performed many times using many different pDNA batches. Close to no integration of pDNA in genomes, no induction of pathogenic anti-DNA antibodies, and a clearance of injected pDNA within days were reported. However, long-term (months) antigen expression in mice using intramuscular injections of a pDNA that may replicate in mammalian cells was found. In this case, the cellular response triggered by the vaccine was weak and may in part account for the persistence of the foreign nucleic acid. The antigen coded by the vaccine in this preclinical study (Hepatitis Surface Antigen) associated with specific antibodies formed circulating immune complexes that caused pathologic lesions in liver and kidney. Thus, special care should be devoted to the design of the plasmid to guarantee that it cannot replicate in mammalian cells. Meanwhile, the regulatory authorities acknowledged the fact that since the first report of trials in humans using injections of up to 800 μg of nonviral coding pDNA (1998), no adverse events have ever been registered. Thus, especially for phase I trials, the toxicology studies can now be facilitated in agreement with the relevant authorities. For vaccination, gene-gun offers the extra-safety advantages that very low doses are used and that the pDNA is delivered exclusively in the dermis, avoiding systemic distribution and potential side effects while guaranteeing the elimination of most of the injected product through natural skin regeneration.

Messenger RNA

Two companies offer contract manufacture of mRNA at laboratory and clinical grade (GMP-certified): Asuragen, a spin-off of Ambion, in the United States and CureVac in Europe. Here again, the whole manufacturing process is free of bovine-derived products. There are no official guidelines for the production of mRNA; however, it can be proposed that the final product should be checked by the standard quality controls. It should appear as a clear and colorless solution by visual inspection. The following criteria would have to be met by the results of the final controls:

1. *Identity*: Sequencing of the plasmid used for *in vitro* transcription should show 100% identity with the expected sequence. At best, reverse transcription and sequencing of the final mRNA could be performed. It should also show 100% identity with the expected sequence. Susceptibility to RNase could additionally be used as a proof of molecular identity.

2. *Content*: Quantification should be performed by absorbance at 260 nm. Osmolarity and pH should also be measured using standard methods.
3. *Purity*: Residual proteins, chromosomal bacteria DNA, plasmid DNA, bacteria RNA, aberrant mRNA transcripts (smaller or larger by-products of the transcription) and endotoxin shoud be below specified limits. Sterility must be controlled by standard microbiological assays.

As is the case for pDNA, some physical tests can be performed to check counter-ions, residual solvents (if they are used during the production), and potency (functional assay using, for example, transfection of cells and verification of the expression of the protein of interest or testing of the immune response after injection in an animal model).

Preclinical toxicology studies should address the standard systemic and local reactogenicity, histopathology, and toxicity (acute and chronic dosage) in rodent and nonrodent animals. Since the FDA and some European authorities decided to classify mRNA-based therapies as no-gene therapy, the implementation of clinical trials does not require additional specific toxicology testing.

Future Perspectives

Since the initial publication by Wolff et al. showing that the injection of pDNA or mRNA simply coding for a protein can result in gene expression *in vivo*, many studies have been performed in animal models and humans showing that this method is safe and can elicit the expected results, which is the expression of the protein. Because pDNA and stabilized mRNA have the natural capacity to activate the immune system through the triggering of TLR, pDNA- and mRNA-based therapeutic utilizations are mostly tested in the field of vaccination. However, since gene therapies based on viruses have shown severe toxicity features in recent human trials, some pDNA or mRNA formulations may now be intensely developed as safer alternatives. Of special interest is the yet unexplored use of (encapsulated) mRNA for gene therapy. As this transient nucleic acid cannot persist or accumulate and would not generate unwanted long-term side effects even after repeated injections, it may seem as the optimal active pharmaceutical ingredient for gene therapies. Meanwhile, vaccination strategies based on nonviral coding nucleic acids are very advanced in terms of time to commercialization. The injection of naked pDNA and the adoptive transfert of APCs transfected with mRNA were demonstrated in many human clinical trials to be feasible and safe and to result in the development of the expected antigen-specific immunity. Optimal formulation, dosage, frequency of application, and adjuvant still need to be clearly defined.

Improvements of the methods include the optimization of the gene sequence, the optimization of the antigen processing, the enhancement of uptake using for example electrical methods, or the use of particles for formulating the vaccines. Concerning the last point, three types of particles were evaluated: liposomes, cationic degradable polymers, and coated gold particles delivered by gene-gun. This latter technology seems to be at the moment the most efficacious, versatile, cost-efficient method for vaccination with nucleic acids. Moreover, it is painless for the patient and very reproducible because the operator cannot influence the delivery (as opposed to injections, especially intradermal injections). The company Powdermed is developing and implementing the utilization of gene-gun-based therapies to deliver pDNA as vaccines against infectious diseases and cancer.

Meanwhile, for autologuous vaccination, which may be needed for example with the mutating and patient-specific HIV virus, vaccination with adoptively transferred mRNA-transfected DCs as developed by Argos pharmaceuticals may be of high potency. The choice between pDNA and mRNA for clinical utilizations is a matter of cost and efficacy. Although there was an intense development and optimization of pDNA-based vaccines, accompanied by the implementation of industrial production facilities, mRNA was until recently, relatively unexplored. However, mRNA offers many advantages over pDNA in the context of therapeutic utilizations. Being active in the cytosole, mRNA does not need to cross the very selective nuclear envelope to be expressed. Being transient, mRNA can allow the controlled production in terms of quantity and time frame of the protein of interest. Moreover, as it is a single-stranded molecule, mRNA does not have the discrete topologies that have pDNA and that could affect its clinical efficacy. This feature allows mRNA to have theoretically a higher functional batch-to-batch reproducibility. At the level of efficacy for vaccination, pDNA is assumed currently to be superior to mRNA; however, the direct comparison of optimal formulations of pDNA and mRNA using gene-gun delivery, for example, as a consistent and reliable method, still needs to be performed. Meanwhile the unique possibility that offers mRNA to transfect, without inducing death, DCs *in vitro*, is a guarantee of vaccine efficacy using a minimum amount of nucleic acid. Thus, although pDNA-based vaccination approaches are very advanced and may soon be commercialized, it can be envisioned that due to their safety features, mRNA-based approaches will be the second generation of nucleic-acid-based vaccination strategies.

Several companies active in the field of nucleic-acid-based vaccines will probably manage to get their product(s) and methods brought to the market for disease-specific utilizations. Prevention and treatments of hepatitis B, AIDS, influenza, and some cancer are the most advanced. Thus, in the near future, drugs containing pDNA or mRNA as an active pharmaceutical ingredient should be available in pharmacies and help in treating or preventing pandemic infections (HIV, influenza virus, *plasmodium falciparum*, etc.) as well diseases with unmet medical needs such as certain types of cancers. The continuous optimization of these methods ensures that the future pDNA- or mRNA-based drugs will get more and more efficacious and will be used for a large area of therapeutic applications.

22

PROTEOMICS

As the sequences of the genomes of several species are completed, interest is growing in the functional component of biological systems, the "*proteome*." Proteome refers to the complete protein expression profile of a biological system. Examination of the proteome will allow one to determine important proteins, enzymes, and pathways involved in disease states by comparing the proteome of normal and diseased tissues. One may determine alteration in protein expression of tissues or cells in response to stresses such as exposure to drugs or toxins. Thus the proteome is a rich source for identification of protein targets or therapeutics for drug development. Another important aspect of studying the proteome is the discovery of novel proteins.

One of the most useful techniques for visualization of the proteome is two- dimensional sodium dodecyl sulfate-polyacrylamide gel electrophoresis (2-D SDS-PAGE). This technique possesses unmatched resolving power for separation of proteins and has been used extensively to analyze proteins, their regulation, and posttranslational modifications. Several techniques have been used to identify proteins from various organisms following separation by 2-D PAGE. These techniques include amino acid analysis, Edman sequencing, immunological methods, and mass spectrometry. Mass spectrometric technologies are particularly attractive because of their high sensitivity and adaptability to high-throughput analysis.

However, protein extracts from cells or biological fluids such as serum contain thousands of proteins in varying abundance, and only the most abundant protein species are visible in the 2-D gels of these samples. The minor protein components are either below detection levels or are obscured by the abundant species.

For example, of the possible 1700 gene products in *Haemophilus influenzae*, only about 400 are visible on a Coomassie-stained 2-D gel of an extract of this organism. In the case of *Saccharomyces cerevisiae*, even a 2-D gel image generated by [^{35}S]methionine-labeled polypeptides contains about 1200 spots, corresponding to roughly 20% of the gene products. Wilkins et al. have pointed out that this discrepancy arises due to two factors, poor electrophoretic behavior and low copy number. Using a graphical model, these authors predict that proteins present at less than 1000 copies per cell cannot be visualized on 2-D gels considering the current maximum 2-D gel loading capacity. Similar observations are made with many biological systems, where only a fraction of the proteins are visualized on a 2-D gel. Therefore the challenge is to enhance the sensitivity of detection of the low-abundance proteins. This chapter describes approaches that accomplish this enhancement in sensitivity and help to identify novel low-abundance proteins.

PROTEOMICS

Two-Dimensional SDS-PAGE

High-resolution 2-D gel electrophoresis involves separation of proteins based on their isoelectric point (pI) in the first dimension and size in the second. Originally, the first dimension consisted of isoelectric focusing (IEF) tube gels with carrier ampholytes. These gels were irreproducible, difficult to transfer to the PAGE gel, and were limited in the amount of protein that could be loaded. Recently, immobilized pH gradients (IPGs) have gained popularity. These IEF strips are produced by copolymerization of ampholytes within the fibers of a polyacrylamide matrix on GelBond film. The IPGs are compatible with various additives used in 2-D gel electrophoresis, such as urea (8 M), and nonionic and zwitterionic detergents which improve the solubility and resolution of proteins. The high degree of reproducibility in spot position, ease of handling, and improved protein capacity have made this technique an improvement over tube gels and has increased the sensitivity of the 2-D gel technique. After isoelectric focusing on the IPG, the proteins are further resolved by applying the IPG strip to the top of an SDS-PAGE gel and transferring the proteins electrophoretically into the second-dimension gel. Following electrophoresis the proteins are visualized by a variety of staining techniques. The most common stain used is Coomassie blue, which can detect as little as 50 ng of an individual protein. More sensitive stains such as silver may detect as little as 1 ng of an individual protein.

Identification of Protein Spots on 2-D Gels Using Mass Spectrometry

The method of choice for identification of proteins separated by 2-D PAGE is mass spectrometry (MS). Recent developments in mass spectrometry have enabled the rapid identification of proteins separated by 2-D PAGE with sensitivities routinely in the femtomole range and, in some cases, the attomole range. Two mass spectrometric methods utilized in the analysis of proteins and peptides are matrix-assisted laser desorption ionization–time-of-flight mass spectrometry (MALDI-Tof MS) and electrospray ionization. The identification by these mass spectrometric techniques is done after proteolytic digestion of the protein in the gel, typically using the enzyme trypsin, and extraction of the resulting peptides.

The most widely used mass spectrometric identification procedure is MALDI-Tof analysis of the entire peptide mixture. Gas-phase matrix interaction with peptide ions in MALDI-Tof results in singly charged ions, giving a mass profile that is highly characteristic of the protein from which the peptides are derived. These peptide masses (actually protonated peptide molecular ions, MH^+) can be used to search databases (either protein or nucleic acid databases) to identify the proteins. The two most important factors in successfully identifying proteins by this approach are the number of matching peptide masses and the accuracy of the peptide mass determination.

In some cases the identification of proteins based on peptide masses is ambiguous or a suitable match cannot be found. Further information may be obtained by performing a collision-induced dissociation tandem mass spectrometry (CID MS/MS) experiment, in which the peptide molecular ions are fragmented in a collision cell and the resulting product ions are analyzed. These product ions often reveal sequence information that can then be used to identify the protein.

The sensitivity of these techniques is excellent when applied to the levels of protein present in spots from a 2-D gel. The most sensitive staining technique visualizes a nanogram of protein, a level well within the detection limits of mass spectrometric techniques. However, many proteins, such as cytokines, nuclear factors, transcription factors, etc., are present at levels far below these limits of detection and are not visible on gels using any of the available staining methods. Therefore, enrichment methods are critical for successfully applying the techniques of 2-D PAGE and mass spectrometry to interesting biological questions.

Prefractionation as an Approach to Enhancement of Sensitivity

One approach to detection of low-abundance proteins is to increase the amount of sample loaded on the IPG strips. While this increases the amount of low- abundance proteins on the gels, it also increases the high-abundance proteins. This causes problems with the running of the IPG strips and excessive streaking in the second dimension. Higher protein loads lead to spot overlapping and decreased resolution. In biological samples such as serum, where one or two species (albumin and immunoglobulins) predominate, isoelectric focusing encounters severe problems due to protein precipitation and gel expansion in those regions. Simply increasing total protein loads is not a solution to visualization of low- abundance proteins. Fractionating the protein complex prior to running the 2-D gel can be used to accomplish two purposes, removal of the abundant species and enrichment of low-abundance species. A variety of high-resolution chromatographic modes for fractionation of proteins exists, and many of these are readily adaptable to 2-D gel electrophoresis. We have utilized ion-exchange chromatography as a method for separation of proteins in complex mixtures. By careful selection of buffer and pH, subsets of proteins in a mixture may be bound to ion-exchange resins. The bound proteins may be further fractionated by elution with salt gradients. Protein not bound in the first round of chromatography may be bound and fractionated by altering conditions and rechromatographing or by chromatography in a different mode. We have used a chromatographic prefractionation approach in the analysis of serum proteins. Serum contains two major protein fractions, albumin and immunoglobulins. In addition, serum contains thousands of proteins in very low abundance. The presence of huge quantities of a single protein, albumin, negates high loads of serum on IPG strips for isoelectric focusing. Serum loads above 100 μl on a 17- to 18-cm IPG strip cause severe problems in the isoelectric focusing and hence improper running of the strip. In addition, the presence of relatively high amounts of certain other proteins, such as transferrin, alpha 1-antitrypsin, etc., causes extensive spot overlapping. We have used anion- exchange and cation-exchange chromatographic procedures to enrich lower- abundance acidic and basic proteins from rat serum.

PROTEOMICS: GENERAL METHODS

Chromatography

Anion-exchange chromatography was performed at pH 4.5 in 50 mM sodium acetate buffer on a DEAE column (0.75 × 7.5 cm, Tosohaas). Rat serum (5 ml), dialyzed in the same buffer, was loaded at 1 ml/min and the column was washed with 20 ml of buffer followed by 10 ml of 0.1 M NaCl. Proteins were eluted with a linear gradient of NaCl (0.1–1.0 M) over the next 30 min and a final isocratic elution at 1.0 M NaCl for an additional 20 min. The elution was monitored at 280 nm, and 1-ml fractions were collected.

Cation-exchange chromatography was performed at pH 7.5 in 50 mM sodium phosphate buffer on a sulfopropyl column (0.75 × 7.5 cm). The run conditions were maintained as above except in the present case the rat serum was dialyzed in 50 mM sodium phosphate buffer, pH 7.5.

Two-Dimensional Gel Electrophoresis

Chromatographic fractions were pooled, dialyzed extensively against water, and lyophilized. Prior to electrophoresis, samples were dissolved in approximately 0.4 ml of rehydration solution (0.3% dithiothreitol, 2% 3-[(3-cholamidopropyl)-dimethylammonio]-1-propanesulfonate (CHAPS), 8 M urea, 2% immobilines, pH 4–7, and bromophenol blue) and applied to immobilized pH gradient strips (Pharmacia, linear gradient, pH 4–7, 18 cm). The rehydration of the IPG strips was performed overnight in a rehydration tray (Pharmacia) with 400 μl of sample applied to each strip. The rehydrated IPG strips were focused for 50,000 V-hr with a slow voltage ramp for the first 4 hr reaching a maximum of 2500 V. Following focusing, the proteins on the strips were reduced by immersing the strips in a buffer (0.1 M Tris-HCl, pH 6.8, 6 M urea, 2 M thiourea, 1% SDS, 6.4 mM dithiothreitol (DTT), 30% glycerol, and a few grains of bromophenol blue) for 15 min at room temperature. Alkylation was achieved by incubating for 15 min at room temperature in a second solution containing 24 mM iodoacetamide instead of DTT. The IPG strips were then overlayed on SDS PAGE gels (11–18% acrylamide) using 1% agarose to hold them in place. The gels were subjected to electrophoresis at an initial low voltage (50 V) until the dye front had entered the gels and then at a higher voltage (200 V) overnight. The tank buffer (24 mM Tris, 200 mM glycine, and 0.1% SDS) was maintained at 5°C throughout the electrophoresis run. The gels were fixed by soaking in 50% ethanol, 2% phosphoric acid, and 48% water for 14 hr. Proteins were visualized by staining with colloidal Coomassie blue in Neuhoff concentrate (17% w/v ammonium sulfate, 34% methanol, and 3% phosphoric acid in water) for 2 days.

Protein Spot Digestion

Protein spots of interest were excised from the gels, suspended in 50% acetonitrile in 50 mM ammonium bicarbonate, and crushed using a plastic pestle. The Coomassie blue was extracted from the gel pieces by repeated washing with the same buffer. The pieces were finally suspended in a small volume of acetonitrile and dried completely using a concentrator (Savant). Protein in the gel pieces was proteolyzed by swelling the gel in a solution of trypsin (Promega, sequencing grade, 50 μg/ml) in 50 mM ammonium bicarbonate and incubating overnight at 37°C. Peptides were extracted from the gel three times using trifluoroacetic acid/ acetonitrile/50 mM ammonium bicarbonate. The combined extracts for each digest were dried completely and washed with 200 ìl water four times. Each extract was finally dissolved in 10 μl of 50% acetonitrile/1% acetic acid in water and used for further mass spectrometric analyses.

Mass Spectrometry of Digests

Peptide extracts prepared as described above were analyzed on a MALDI-Tof mass spectrometer. A small portion of the extract was mixed with an equal volume of α-cyano-4-hydroxycinnamic acid (alpha CHC) matrix in methanol and loaded onto a MALDI plate. Calibration of the flight tube was performed with the internal standards angiotensin I and adrenocorticotrophic hormone.

When identification of the protein could not be achieved using MALDI data alone, peptides were fragmented and the product ions analyzed. Peptide fragmentation was performed on a Micromass quadrupole time-of-flight (Q-Tof) mass spectrometer. The peptide extracts were desalted on a 0.5-ml C18 reverse-phase column and dried in a Speed Vac concentrator, then suspended in 10 μl of 50% acetonitrile/1% acetic acid in water. An infusion pump was used to introduce the sample into the Q-Tof and the peptide ions fragmented by varying the collision gas (nitrogen) energy. Information from the fragmentation pattern was used for protein identification.

Protein Identification

Proteins from the gels were identified by searching protein sequence databases with data derived from the mass spectrometric analyses described above. In most cases, positive identifications could be made by searching tryptic peptide masses derived from the MALDI-Tof experiments. Programs used to perform this type of search include PeptideSearch and MS Fit from Protein Prospector. When a positive identification could not be made by searching the peptide masses, searches were carried out using peptide fragmentation data from the Q-Tof experiments. The programs used for these searches were PeptideSearch and MS-Tag from Protein Prospector.

Enrichment and Identification of Low-Abundance Serum Proteins

It is readily apparent from the pattern that even though serum contains thousands of proteins, the 2-D gel pattern is dominated by a relatively small number of proteins. Our first step in enrichment of

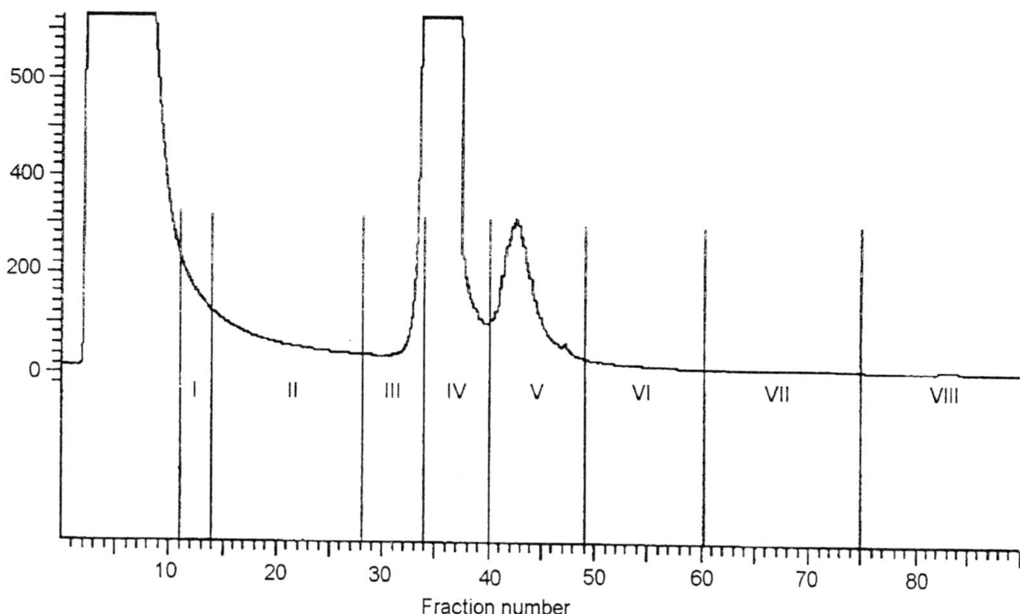

Fig. 22.1. Chromatographic profile of separation of proteins in rat serum on a DEAE anion-exchange column at pH 4.5.

low-abundance proteins was anion-exchange chromatography. Retention of a small percentage of the total serum proteins was observed and almost all of the retained proteins eluted at salt concentrations lower than 0.4 M. Several chromatographic runs were made, indicating the high degree of reproducibility of this process. The chromatographic fractions were pooled as shown and were run on 2-D gels after extensive dialysis against water and lyophilization to dryness.

The 2-D gels of three chromatographic portions from anion-exchange column separation of 10 ml of rat serum are shown. We observed from the gel patterns that almost 90% of the albumin was removed from the fractions shown. In addition, almost all of the immunoglobulins were removed and the amount of alpha 1-antitrypsin was greatly reduced. The reduction in these major protein species has helped overcome the issues related to improper running of the gels, spot overlapping, and resolution. A comparison of the whole-rat serum gel and the chromatographic fractions highlights this point.

Several spots that were not visible on the stained gel of whole serum were now predominant. Although several protein spots not seen in the unfractionated rat serum gel were visible, many of these proved to be fragments of abundant proteins such as alpha 1-macroglobulin, albumin, alpha 1-antitrypsin, etc. The low-abundance proteins that were enriched are indicated by arrowheads. Many of these protein spots are at the acidic end of the gel, indicating that the anionic chromatographic fractionation not only accomplished removal of major protein species but also enriched several low-abundance acidic proteins. We next enriched basic proteins by cation exchange. From the chromatographic profile of 10 ml of whole serum separated on a strong cation-exchange resin at relatively high pH, it can be seen that only a small portion of the proteins bound to this column. These proteins were also eluted with salt concentrations below 0.4 M. A striking feature seen in these gels is the complete removal of the abundant protein species in serum—albumin, immunoglobulins, and trypsin inhibitors—indicating the usefulness of this approach. The protein pattern is concentrated more toward the basic end of the gel. As in the case of the anion-exchange fraction gels, these gels reveal several proteins not represented in the whole-rat serum gel. While enrichment of protein spots on 2-D gels is qualitatively interesting, the full power of proteomics may not be realized without identification of these proteins. Following digestion

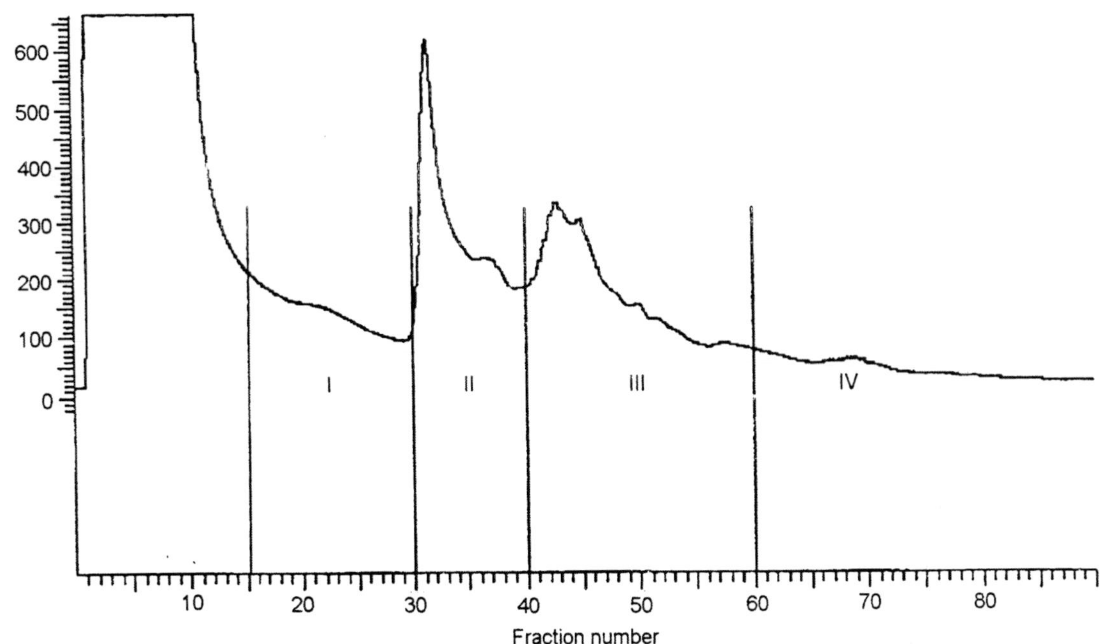

Fig. 22.2. Chromatographic profile of separation of proteins in rat serum on a SP cation-exchange column at pH 7.5.

of the proteins in the gel spots with trypsin, the tryptic peptides were analyzed by two mass spectrometric techniques, MALDI-Tof and Q-Tof. A MALDI-Tof mass spectrum obtained from the tryptic digest of a spot from a 2-D gel of rat serum fractionated by cation-exchange chromatography. Three ions in the spectrum, 842.50, 2211.14, and 2261.24, represent auto-catalytic fragments of trypsin. These ions, as well as the ions at 1296.69 (angiotensin D) and 2465.20 (ACTH), have been used to calibrate the mass analyzer. With careful calibration, accuracies better than 100 ppm are routinely achieved.

Thirteen ions were selected from the spectrum and used to search the SwissProt protein sequence database. The program MS-Fit, which is part of the Protein Prospector package of programs, was used to conduct the search. Eight of the m/z values searched matched within 0.1 dalton of the theoretical MH^+ of ions from the protein "mouse pigment epithelium-derived factor precursor (PEDF)," also known as stromal cell-derived factor 3 (SDF-3). Interestingly, the protein identified in the SwissProt database was a mouse protein, whereas the sample being analyzed was obtained from rat serum. A more careful examination of the databases revealed no entry for a rat homolog of this protein. This represents the first report that pigment epithelium-derived factor is found in the rat.

Occasionally, a protein was not identified by MALDI-MS methods. This may occur when more than one protein is present in a spot. Protein identification may still be accomplished by fragmentation of peptide ions by an MS/MS technique. This requires the use of mass spectrometers equipped with collision chamber or an ion-trap type of instrument. We have used the Q-Tof using the general procedure as follows. The ions in the protein digest were first identified by an initial ion scan in the quadrupole of the instrument. The ionization potential was set such that doubly charged ions predominate in the spectra. An individual ion (known as the precursor ion) was selected and diverted into a collision chamber, where it was fragmented into a series of product ions. The most scissile bonds are the peptide bonds, fragmentation of which yields a series of product ions differing in mass by the mass of successive amino acid residues in the peptide sequence. A fragmentation obtained on a Q-Tof will generate b-ions (N-terminal fragments) and y-ions (C-terminal fragments) which are passed into the

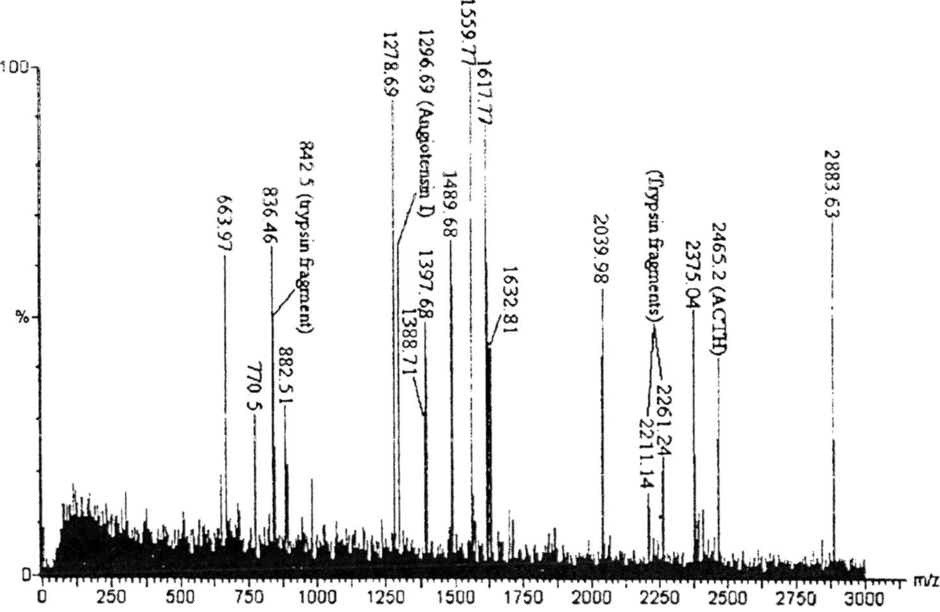

Fig. 22.3. MALDI-Tof mass spectrum.

flight tube for mass analysis. Charge tends to be retained on the most basic residues (which are the C-terminal amino acids in tryptic peptides) and so y ions tend to be the most intense in MS/MS spectra. Interpretation of the MS/MS spectra may be accomplished using sequence tags generated by manual interpretation of the MS/MS spectrum. More automated programs such as Protein Prospector, PeptideSearch, or Sequest are capable of searching databases with MS/MS data in tabular format. One such fragmentation pattern for the parent ion 537.83 (+2 charge state) of a peptide obtained from the tryptic digest of the spot. Calculation of the differences in the y-ion series in the spectra between masses 414.32 and 860.55 yielded the sequence I/LVSF (read in C-terminal to N-terminal order). This partial sequence information along with the masses of the product ions encompassing the sequence (414.32 and 860.55 in this case) is termed a "*sequence tag*," which was used to search a database. Such a search using the PeptideSearch program identified the peptide, K<TLFSVLPGLK>M, which is present in two isoforms of the inter-alpha-inhibitor 4 protein. Many of the theoretical MS/MS ions of this peptide can be identified in the actual MS/MS spectrum. The sequence FSVL (read from N-terminal to C-terminal) matches the sequence determined from the y series in the MS/MS spectrum.

Using approaches described above, the low-molecular-weight spots that were enriched in the acidic region have been characterized to be different peptides of rat kininogens from which bradykinin peptides originate. The higher-molecular-weight enriched proteins were identified to be several different forms of serpins. In addition a novel rat form of the thrombospondin 1 protein was discovered in one of the 2-D gels. In the case of unfractionated serum this protein would not have been identified, due to the highly abundant immunoglobulins appearing in the same region and the relatively lower abundance of this protein in serum.

Cation exchange-enriched spots that were identified include several forms of the APO-E protein. The most striking feature was the enrichment of a low-abundance novel rat homolog of stromal cell derived factor 3 represented as a series of protein spots on the 2-D gel differing by charge (due to variations in the glycosylation state). The location of this protein spot on the gel indicates that this charge series would have overlapped with the alpha 1-antitrypsins and other serpins had the entire 10

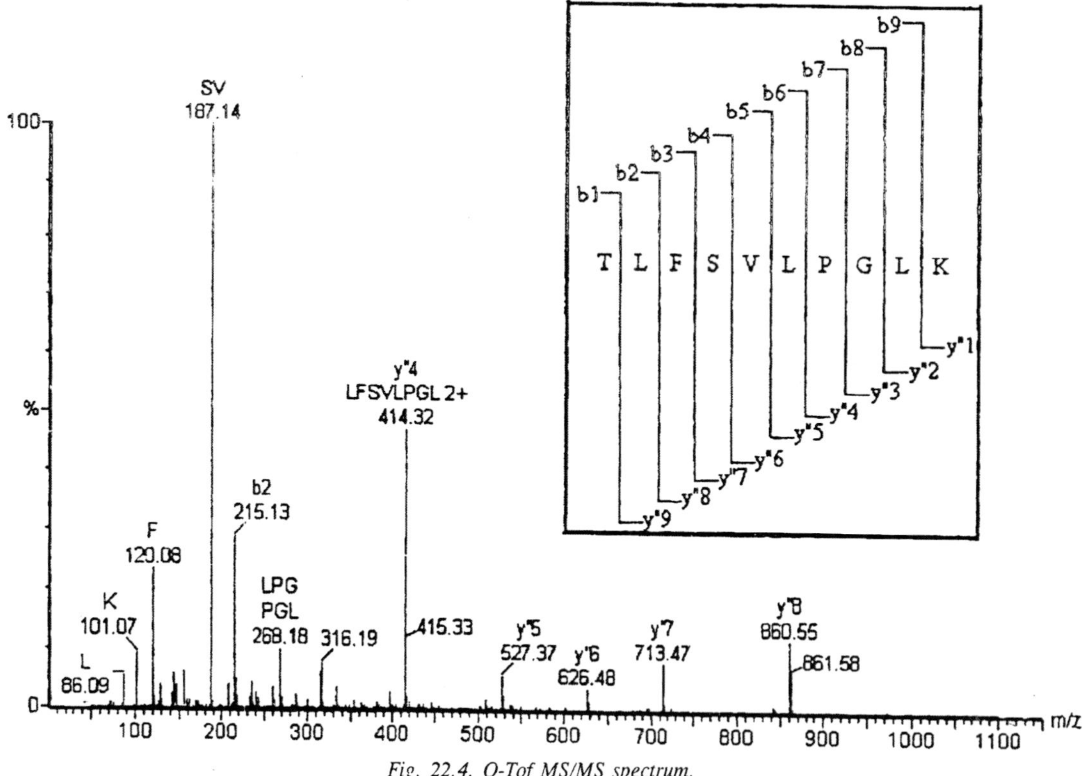

Fig. 22.4. Q-Tof MS/MS spectrum.

ml of serum been run. We also found fragments of a stem-cell factor receptor precursor, indicating that this fractionation approach has enabled us to enhance the sensitivity of the 2-D gel approach.

Use of Other Prefractionation Methods

Examples have been reported in the literature in which other forms of chromatography have been used for prefractionation of sample prior to the use of 2-D gel. Fountoulakis et al. have used hydroxyapatite chromatography to enrich low-abundance proteins in *Escherichia coli*. In this study, about 130 proteins not detected in the 2-D gel of the total extract were identified. The same group has reported the use of a heparin-affinity approach in the identification of low-abundance proteins in *Haemophilus influenzae*. The availability of other affinity approaches to enrich protein classes of interest, such as metal-affinity chromatography used to enrich phospho-proteins, lectin chromatography to enrich glycoproteins, and antibody columns targeted to phosphorylated amino acids or certain protein domains, makes this technique a very versatile one. Enrichment and identification of low-abundance proteins in *H. influenzae* by hydrophobic interaction chromatography has been reported.

Different physical techniques can also be used for prefractionation of samples to be analyzed by 2-D gels. Corthals et al. have fractionated human serum by an electrokinetic technique. Fountoulakis et al. have used chromatofocusing as a prefractionation step in the analysis of low-abundance proteins in *H. influenzae*. Ultrafiltration in conjunction with other chromatographic methods offers an attractive approach to enrich proteins of the desired size and characteristic, although nonspecific binding of proteins to the membrane limits the use of this method. Several reports have appeared in the literature recently using multidimensional chromatographic approaches in tandem with ESI mass spectrometry in the identification of proteins.

Future Directions in Proteomics

Currently, efforts are being made by a number of companies in the automation of 2-D gel technology and protein identification by mass spectrometry. These advances will be critical to the success of characterizing complete proteomes of organisms. Automation will address the problems of separating and identifying large numbers of proteins, but issues in identification of low-abundance proteins will remain. We believe that prefractionation of proteins either by multidimensional chromatography or other techniques prior to 2D-gel electrophoresis will be needed in order to obtain complete characterization of the proteome. Already, some genomics companies have begun to address the proteome and consider the problems associated with protein analysis. Fractionation of proteins and protein classes will play an important role in the ultimate success of proteome characterization.

Index